A History of the Medicines We Take

From Ancient Times to Present Day

A History of the Medicines We Take

From Ancient Times to Present Day

Anthony C. Cartwright and
N. Anthony Armstrong

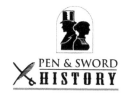

PEN & SWORD
HISTORY

First published in Great Britain in 2020 by
Pen & Sword History
An imprint of
Pen & Sword Books Ltd
Yorkshire – Philadelphia

ISBN 978 1 52672 403 8

Printed and bound by CPI Group (UK) Ltd, Croydon, CR0 4YY

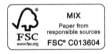

Pen & Sword Books Limited incorporates the imprints of Atlas,
Archaeology, Aviation, Discovery, Family History, Fiction, History,
Maritime, Military, Military Classics, Politics, Select, Transport,
True Crime, Air World, Frontline Publishing, Leo Cooper, Remember
When, Seaforth Publishing, The Praetorian Press, Wharncliffe
Local History, Wharncliffe Transport, Wharncliffe True Crime
and White Owl.

For a complete list of Pen & Sword titles please contact

PEN & SWORD BOOKS LIMITED
47 Church Street, Barnsley, South Yorkshire, S70 2AS, England
E-mail: enquiries@pen-and-sword.co.uk
Website: www.pen-and-sword.co.uk

Or

PEN AND SWORD BOOKS
1950 Lawrence Rd, Havertown, PA 19083, USA
E-mail: Uspen-and-sword@casematepublishers.com
Website: www.penandswordbooks.com

Contents

List of Picture Illustrations

Front cover: Cartoon etching of an apothecary using a pestle and mortar to make up a prescription (Wellcome Images).

Back page: An apothecary, John Simmonds, and his boy apprentice, William, working in the laboratory of John Bell's pharmacy. Engraving by J.G. Murray, 1842, after W. Hunt (Wellcome Images).

1. Cuneiform medical clay tablet BCE. (Wellcome Images)
2. Section of the Ebers Papyrus from National Library of Medicine in Egypt from 1550 BCE, with an asthma remedy to be prepared as a mixture of herbs heated on a brick so that the sufferer could inhale the fumes. (Wellcome Images)
3. Roman mosaic from the third to fourth century CE Villa Romana del Casale in the province of Enna in Sicily, showing animals being loaded onto a ship in North Africa to go to Rome. (© Author photograph)
4. Facsimile page from the Anglo-Saxon Leechbook of Bald, written about 950 CE in Winchester, which is a copy of a text written about fifty years earlier in the reign of Alfred the Great. (Wellcome Images)
5. English tin-glazed earthenware drug jar dated 1700–1720 labelled E. MITHRIDATUM – Electuarium Mithridatium. White glaze with bluish tinge and design in blue. (Royal Pharmaceutical Society Museum image reference LDRPS:KCY1)
6. English ceramic, tin-glazed earthenware drug jar dated 1700–1725 labelled THER. LOND – Theriaca Londinensis or London Treacle. (Royal Pharmaceutical Society Museum image reference LDRPS:KCY1)
7. Two distillation alembic stills from the laboratory in the Hospices de Beaune Museum, Beaune, France, founded in 1443. (© Author photograph)
8. Late eighteenth-century pill tile made by Mander Weaver, Wolverhampton. Used for rolling the pill mass into a long 'pipe'

before dividing it into individual pills. (Royal Pharmaceutical Society Museum image reference ATB2)

9. Hand pill-making equipment, twentieth century. For dividing the pill mass into individual pills, and rolling them into round pills. (© Author photograph)

10. Punch and die set as patented by William Brockedon in 1843 to produce single tablets. Set shown was manufactured by S. Maw, Son and Thompson 1870–1900. (Royal Pharmaceutical Society Museum image reference ATA3)

11. Hand-operated single punch tablet-making machine made by J.W. Pindar and Company 1901–1920 for use by a community pharmacist. (Wellcome Images)

12. Rubber tablet triturate mould. Manufactured by Whitall Tatum Company, late 1800s or early 1900s. (Royal Pharmaceutical Society image reference ATA1)

13. Empty gelatin capsules, as patented by James Murdoch in Britain in 1847. Capsules were filled by the pharmacist or by a pharmaceutical manufacturer. (© Author photograph)

14. Wet-seal cachet machine from early 1900s. Used to fill the lower halves of the cachet with powder fill, then moistening the rims of the upper and lower halves and bringing the two halves together to seal. (© Author photograph)

15. Anel ophthalmic syringe from the seventeenth century. Dominique Anel (1679–1730). (Wellcome Images)

16. Dr Alexander Wood's hypodermic syringe of 1853, the first used in Great Britain. (Wellcome Images)

17. Becton Dickinson insulin syringe introduced in 1924. (Image courtesy of Becton Dickinson)

18. Omnipod® Insulin Management System Product. (Image used with permission. © Insulet Corporation. All Rights Reserved)

19. Smiths Medical Graseby® 2000 syringe infusion pump. (Image used with permission of Smiths Medical)

20. Becton Dickinson Alaris CC Plus syringe pump. (Image courtesy of Becton Dickinson)

21. Syrian glass ointment jar, 400–550 CE. (Wellcome Images)

22. Plaster irons, 1800s or early 1900s. These were used to spread plaster mass onto sheepskin, calico, linen or silk. One shown was gas-heated,

the other was heated over a flame. (Royal Pharmaceutical Society Museum image references APC1/D and APC1/L)

23. S. Maw and Sons ceramic double-valved vapour inhaler devised by Dr Nelson in 1861. (Royal Pharmaceutical Society Museum image reference GIA12)

24. Oxford ceramic creamware vapour inhaler, c.1880. (Royal Pharmaceutical Society Museum image reference GIA22)

25. French Salès-Giron Pulvisateur vapour spray inhaler device of 1858. (With permission from www.inhalatorium)

26. Alfred Newton's dry powder inhalation device of 1864. (With permission from www.inhalatorium)

27. Dr John Adams' spray nebuliser inhalation device of 1868. (With permission from www.inhalatorium)

28. Parke Davis Glaseptic Nebuliser, 1907. (With permission from www.inhalatorium)

29. Abbott Laboratories powder Aerohaler, 1948. (With permission from www.inhalatorium)

30. Roman collyrium stamp inscribed with names of four remedies prepared with saffron by Junius Taurus from a prescription of Pacius. Dated between 1 and 299 CE. Used for marking sticks of eye ointment before they harden. From Lorraine, France. (Wellcome Images)

31. Single dose Levofloxacin antibiotic eye drops. (Wellcome Images)

32. Diagram of Iluvien fluocinolone acetonide intravitreal implant. This is an implant injected into the eye and used for the treatment of diabetic macular oedema. It releases the drug over three years. (© Alimera Sciences Limited)

33. Photograph of Iluvien implant to show its size compared to a pencil tip. (© Alimera Sciences Limited)

34. Roman bronze pessary ring in two halves used to treat uterine prolapse. Dated 200 BCE–400 CE. (Wellcome Images)

35. Nickel-plated brass pessary mould to produce six pessaries. Marked 120 grain (7.2 grams) which is the pessary size. (Royal Pharmaceutical Society Museum image reference APA2)

36. French ivory enema syringe, dated 1701-1800. (Wellcome Images)

37. Black and white etching, entitled 'Apotekeren / l'Apothicaire', designed by Jacques Antoine Arlaud, dated around 1730. It depicts

a young, thin and bespectacled apothecary, kneeling in profile to the right, his eyes staring and lips pursed as he prepares to administer a huge clyster (enema) to an unseen lady – only her discarded shoe is visible next to a steaming jug. (Royal Pharmaceutical Society Museum)

38. Metal suppository mould to produce twelve suppositories. Marked 15 grain (900 mg), which is the suppository size. (Royal Pharmaceutical Society Museum image reference ASE3/I)

Preface

This book is about the history of medicines and the preparations made for patients to take, which are the dosage forms. Despite what many writers on pharmaceutical medicine imply, patients do not usually take active drugs alone; they take a preparation such as an injection, tablet, ointment, or inhalation which delivers the drug to them.

From early products to today's high technology products, this book tells the story of both medicinal substances and the medicinal dosage forms which we take. It follows the development of medicines from traces of herbs found with the remains of Neanderthal man from 50,000 years ago, to prescriptions written on clay tablets from Mesopotamia in the third millennium BCE, through the active drugs extracted from plants in the nineteenth century to the latest biotechnology monoclonal antibody products. The history of dosage forms and their inventors from powders and liquid extracts used by early man through pills and tablets to needle-free injections is also covered.

The simplest dosage form was the powder made by grinding down the drug in a pestle and mortar, then weighing it out and wrapping it up in individual sheets of paper. Other early products given by mouth were extracts made with water, wine or beer. Sweetened medicines were popular in the seventeenth and eighteenth centuries, where the herbal extract was dissolved in syrup or honey. This idea persists in modern cough mixtures.

Pills were made by mixing the powdered ingredients together with a liquid binding agent to make a pill mass, rolling it out into a cylinder and cutting it and rolling the individual sections. Five thousand could be made by hand in a day, but machines were developed to manufacture them. In 1844, the artist, travel writer and inventor William Brockedon devised a means of making compressed tablets using a simple die and punch (shown in Picture 10). Other manufacturers took up the idea, and automated it so that large quantities could be made in a day. In the early nineteenth century, manufacturing laboratories, such as John Bell in London and Squibb in the United States (US), were established to make bulk drugs and preparations. They were followed by others such as Burroughs Wellcome and John Wyeth and Brother to create the companies that became the basis of the modern multinational pharmaceutical industry. These came to dominate the production of medicines, so that fewer and fewer medicines were made in individual pharmacies.

During the seventeenth and eighteenth centuries, medicines were prepared by apothecaries from scratch using drugs and other ingredients. This was time-consuming. By the middle of the nineteenth century, pharmacies had taken over much of the work of dispensing medicines, but the number of prescriptions remained small. In Britain, the 1911 National Insurance Act brought in by Lloyd George as Chancellor of the Exchequer in the Liberal Government enabled access to a contributory system of insurance against illness and unemployment for workers, but not their families. This improved access to medical care and increased the number of prescriptions which were written and dispensed in pharmacies. Following the Second World War, the National Health Service (NHS) was established in 1948 and this provided universal health care provision. The wider access meant another leap in the number of prescriptions.

Changes in the numbers of prescriptions dispensed from 1880 to 2017

Before the establishment of the NHS there were no central records of prescriptions, but we can get an idea of the numbers by looking at the records in the prescription books of dispensing chemists held in the archives of the Wellcome Library in London. For the purposes of this book, two chemists were chosen: a provincial chemist, R. Woollatt and Boyd Chemists in Taunton,[1,2] and a metropolitan one, Armitage Dispensing Chemist in Blackheath.[3,4] During the period 1880 to 1900, they dispensed 300–700 prescriptions per year. By 1938–9, the Armitage Dispensing Chemist was dispensing just over 2,500 prescriptions per year.[4]

By 1994–5, the average number of prescriptions dispensed by each pharmacy in England had risen to over 43,000, sixty times more than the levels before the First World War and seventeen times higher than levels just before the Second World War. The numbers have continued to escalate, and as can be seen from the graph in Figure P1, in 2016–7 the average pharmacy in England was dispensing about 95,000 prescriptions per year. This equates to over 300 prescriptions each day that they were open for business, which is almost as many as they dealt with in a whole year before 1900.

Changes in patterns of prescribing from 1880 to 2017

The first medicines taken by our remote ancestors were herbs such as yarrow and camomile, which they chewed. As the practice of medicine progressed, the herbs and other materials were processed to make them easier to take. By the time of the ancient Egyptians, a wide range of dosage forms were available. The Egyptian Ebers papyrus dating from 1550 BCE mentioned draughts (single dose liquid medicines), liquid mixtures and pills; creams, ointments, lotions, liniments, poultices and pastes; powders to be applied to wounds or infections; inhalations; eye drops and eye ointments; and enemas, pessaries and suppositories. The most frequently mentioned products were those taken by mouth.

The majority of the products dispensed by R. Woollatt and Boyd in Taunton and Armitage Dispensing Chemist in Blackheath before 1900 were liquid medicines – mainly mixtures. About 6–13 per cent of the prescriptions were for pills which would have been made by hand using a pill machine such as the one shown in Picture 8. Less than 1 per cent were tablets. Looking at the Drug Ledger of the Royal London Hospital, they purchased twenty-three different tablets in the period 1899–1902.[5] But in 1910–14 the hospital purchased forty-eight different tablets, and twenty-two different capsules.[6]

The hospitals were providing patients with a wider range of products than they received from their general practitioners (GPs). Later in the century, hospitals started to make their own tablets. The Royal Brompton Hospital, which specialised in respiratory medicine, manufactured sixty-two different tablets in 1944–5.[7]

By 1938–9, at Armitage Dispensing Chemist 17.7 per cent of the prescriptions were for tablets and 1.7 per cent for capsules, all of which they would have purchased from manufacturers. But they were still making up 2.3 per cent of prescriptions for pills. Shortly after 1970, nearly all prescriptions were dispensed using commercial products which they purchased, and most pharmacies did not even have a set of weighing scales to make up products from scratch.

A special analysis has been carried out by the NHS Business Services Authority for this book on the type of product dosage form dispensed in 2015 from GP NHS prescriptions. These are summarised in the Table P1.

The numbers in the table are expressed as a percentage of the 1,083,663,000 items dispensed in this year. Items not included in this list are dressings, appliances, stoma care products, diagnostics and some nutritional products. Nearly three-quarters of the items dispensed were tablets and capsules, and because of the extent of their use, Chapter 12 of this book, on products taken by mouth, is the longest and most detailed chapter.

The range of different products also increased dramatically during this period as new medicines were developed. The list of products that GPs are allowed to prescribe for patients is set out in the *Drug Tariff*. In 1925, the *Drug Tariff* included forty-seven different tablets (including different strengths of the same tablet), and eleven capsules. By 2010, the *Drug Tariff* included 884 tablets and 220 capsules.

Table P1: Summary of items dispensed by pharmacies in England in 2015 by type of dosage form.

Type of product	Number of items dispensed	Percentage of total items dispensed
Tablets	638,930,422	58.9
Capsules	162,595,167	15.0
Creams	22,282,359	2.1
Drops	19,253,087	1.8
Injections	16,028,959	1.5
Inhaler	10,333,381	1.0
Lotions	6,966,097	0.7
Ointments	6,924,771	0.6
Patches	4,668,619	0.4
Inhalant	1,018,972	0.09
Suppositories	878,772	0.08

Base Data, NHSBSA Copyright 2017.

Trends in the costs of GP primary care prescribing, hospital prescribing and total prescribing

In 2003, nearly 22 per cent of the total cost of NHS prescribing in England was due to pharmaceutical products provided by hospitals. From 2003 to 2017, the cost of primary care prescribing by GPs for patients in England rose about 22 per cent; in the same period the cost of hospital issues of pharmaceutical preparations rose over 400 per cent (see Figure P1). The cost of hospital issues of drugs now exceeds GP prescribing.

Figure P1: Cost of GP and Hospital Prescribing in English NHS 2003–2017.

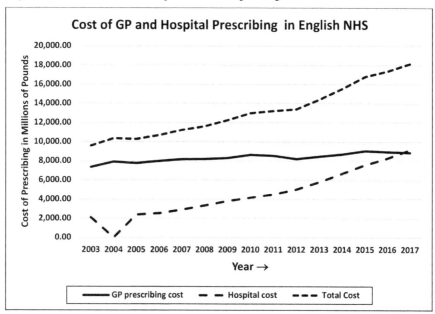

NHS Digital data under terms of Open Government Licence v3.0.

Which are the most prescribed drugs?

The top twenty drugs in terms of cost prescribed on the NHS in 2016–7 include only four drugs mainly prescribed by GPs. The top drug in cost was adalimumab; this was issued in hospital and it cost the NHS 2.6 per cent of its drug bill. See the list in Table P2:

Table P2: Top 20 most prescribed drugs in 2016/2017 in England in the NHS.

Name of drug	Condition treated	Where prescribed	Cost in £ millions
Adalimumab	Rheumatoid arthritis, Crohn's disease, ulcerative colitis	Hospital	461.9
Aflibercept	Age-related macular degeneration	Hospital	292.1
Etanercept	Rheumatoid arthritis	Hospital	202.9
Infliximab	Rheumatoid arthritis, Crohn's diseases, ulcerative colitis	Hospital	185.8
Ranibizumab	Age-related macular degeneration	Hospital	185.2
Rituximab	Autoimmune diseases and some cancers	Hospital	157.5
Trastuzumab	HER-2 positive breast cancer	Hospital	151.8
Rivaroxaban	Prevention or treatment of deep vein thrombosis	GP	145.2
Lenalidomide	Multiple myeloma and myelodysplastic syndromes	Hospital	144.2
Ombitsavir-parataprevir-ritonavir combination	Hepatitis C	Hospital	114.0
Enzalutamide	Prostate cancer	Hospital	112.7
Apixaban	Deep vein thrombosis	GP	107.7
Imatinib	Anti-cancer	Hospital	96.2
Dimethyl fumarate	Multiple sclerosis	Hospital	89.1
Insulin glargine	Type 1 diabetes	GP	83.6
Alemtuzumab	Multiple sclerosis	Hospital	81.1
Ledipasvir-sofosbuvir combination	Hepatitis C	Hospital	80.5
Buprenorphine	Opioid addiction	GP	72.4
Doxacetal	Breast cancer	Hospital	70.5
Ibrutinib	Anti-cancer	Hospital	67.5

NHS Digital data under terms of Open Government Licence v3.0.

Of the top twenty products in terms of cost, half were injectable products and the remainder were capsules and tablets.

Many of the top twenty products were biotechnology products, which are further described in Chapter 10 of this book. The cost of many of them will come down appreciably as they are replaced with 'biosimilar' products once the original patents expire and additional manufacturers can produce copy products.

Natural products in medicine

The picture painted by most of the conventional medical historians is that of a gradual evolution away from the herbal remedies used since the time of the ancient Egyptians and continued through to the eighteenth century, to the modern synthetic chemical and biotechnology drugs. The reality is more complex and interesting. Throughout the Middle Ages, physicians mainly used herbal products to treat their patients, but information on their use was also available to a wider public through popular books on domestic remedies. The use of herbal remedies has continued in parallel to the developments in modern medicine. In Victorian times many of the over-the-counter products used herbal ingredients. The global herbal medicine market size was valued at US $71.19 billion in 2016.[8] In 2017, German consumers spent €1.95 billion (retail prices) on herbal medicinal products. In the UK the market for herbal products is now over £500 million, and about a third of the population consumed herbal products in the first decade the twenty-first century.[9] The European Medicines Agency established a Herbal Medicinal Products Committee to review information and set standards for products. A scheme was set up in 2004 for European Union countries to register herbal remedies using a Traditional Herbal Medicinal Product procedure. In the UK there are 355 Traditional Herbal Registration medicines which have been approved. Most of these products use herbs such as valerian, St John's wort, milk thistle, senna, hops and dandelion. These were included in the *London Pharmacopoeia* of December 1618, so that they have had centuries of continuing tradition of use.

Historical dates in the book

We have used the BCE/CE method of identifying historical dates in the book, as we deal with medicines used over millennia by different religions and cultures. CE means **Common Era** and is used in place of AD. The dates are the same i.e., AD 2019 is 2019 CE. BCE means **Before Common Era**. For example, 400 BC is 400 BCE.

Acknowledgements

The authors gratefully acknowledge the help of librarians and archivists at a number of institutions, including the British Library, the Wellcome Library, the Royal Pharmaceutical Society Library, the Worshipful Society of Apothecaries Archives, the National Archives, the Royal London Hospital Archive, Boots UK Corporate Records and Archives, and the Hertfordshire Archive and Library Service. The assistance of John Betts and Matthew Johnston from the Royal Pharmaceutical Society Museum is acknowledged in accessing some pictures in their archives and in allowing Anthony C. Cartwright to take photographs of some of the society's artefacts in the museum for this book. Dr Alan Hunter kindly agreed to host a visit to see his personal collection of pharmaceutical antiques and allowed Anthony C. Cartwright to photograph several of them. The help of the Science Museum staff in organising a research visit to Blythe House to look at an early Pindar hand tablet-making machine is also acknowledged. The NHS England dosage form prescribing information included is 'Base Data, NHSBSA Copyright 2017'. This information is licenced under the terms of the Open Government Licence. The analysis of information on UK Traditional Herbal Remedy registrations is reproduced with permission of the MHRA under the terms of the Open Government Licence (OGL) v3.0. Lastly, our thanks are due to Dr Brian Matthews, an old friend and colleague, who kindly reviewed and commented on the draft manuscript.

Part One

A History of Medicines

Chapter 1

Early Medicines: From Prehistory to Mesopotamian and Egyptian Medicine

T he earliest written recorded accounts of the use of medicines in man are on the Mesopotamian clay tablets which are about 5,000 years old and then in Egyptian papyri from about 2000 BCE. However, earlier prehistorical use of medicines by Neanderthals and man can be inferred from the behaviour of animals voluntarily consuming medicinal plants for a variety of reasons, then being copied by the local indigenous population. There is also archaeological evidence from Neolithic and ancient human sites of the use of herbal medicines to treat illness and the use of what are now called 'herbal highs' – psychoactive drugs for recreational purposes or used as part of religious rituals.

Animals and psychoactive plants

The perennial plant *Nepeta cataria*, catmint or catnip, is known to many for its attractive properties to cats, who delight to roll in the plant, bruising the stem and leaves to release nepetalactone, which causes an intoxicating effect. Other species of animals also seek out psychoactive drugs.[1] Siberian reindeer feed on a variety of fungi during the summer, but they prefer the hallucinogenic fungus *Amanita muscaria*, fly agaric, with its distinctive bright red cap with white spots. This fungus contains muscimol and ibotenic acid which are hallucinogenic compounds. Canadian caribou during their migrations will also seek out this fungus, leaving individual animals drugged and vulnerable to prey.

In North America, horses and cows can become addicted to various species of wild grasses such as *Astralagus lambertii* in Nebraska, and *Astralagus mollissimus* in Mexico, Montana and Arizona. The animals will desert their normal pasture in favour of these grasses, known as locoweed, then eat them until they become intoxicated. The toxic chemical in the weed is the alkaloid swainsonine.

In the Canadian Rocky Mountains, wild bighorn sheep scramble over rocky ledges and into deep ravines in search of the vividly coloured yellow and green lichen, which has narcotic properties.

In Africa and Asia, various animals seek out fallen fruit which has begun to ferment to use as a source of alcohol so that they can become drunk. African elephants find marula, mgongo and palmyra fruits, while Asian elephants in Bengal and Indonesia are attracted to the fruits of the durian, *Durio zibethinus,* as are many other animals – monkeys, orangutans, squirrels and flying foxes.

The *Tabernanthe iboga* shrub grows in Gabon and the Congo.[2] Boars have been seen to dig up and eat the roots of the plant and then go into a wild frenzy. Porcupines and gorillas occasionally do something similar. The roots contain a number of alkaloids with ibogaine the most abundant. Ibogaine is a central nervous stimulant and can cause hallucinations.

Gorillas are known to eat many species of cola plants, particularly for their seeds. The seeds of *Cola pachycarpa* contain caffeine and theobromine, which are stimulants.

Animals and medicinal plants

Animals have the ability to exploit ingredients in plants, or use physical characteristics of plants. Many species are known to self-select items as part of their diet that can cure ailments such as parasitic infections, or to minimise the symptoms of disease.[3] The study of how animals self-medicate with medicinal compounds from plants and other materials is called 'zoopharmacognosy' – from the Greek words 'zoo' meaning animal, 'pharmaco' remedy and 'gnosy' knowing. Plants contain secondary ingredients, which can reduce palatability or be toxic to the predator, to protect themselves against the effects of animals which eat them. However, these same plant-defence compounds can also be useful to some animals as part of their diet. Parasites play a key role in the lives of wild animals since their welfare and survival is linked to their ability to deal with parasites and pathogenic organisms. If a species can defend itself against a life-threatening or debilitating infection, this enables it to thrive and is an adaptive advantage.

The work of Michael A. Huffman and his colleagues at the Primate Research Institute at Kyoto University has provided much of the evidence on animal self-medication.[4] African chimpanzees in the rainy season are liable to become infected with nodular worms, which can cause secondary bacterial infections, diarrhoea, pain, weakness and weight loss. They are also liable to infection with a primate tapeworm. Infected chimpanzees have been observed to chew the bitter pith of Bitter Leaf herb *Vernonia amygdalina* and recover from their symptoms within a day.[5] The chimpanzees remove the outer bark and leaves to chew on the pith to extract the bitter juice. The pith contains a steroid glucoside vernonioside B1 and a lactone vernodaline, which are both active against adult worm parasites and inhibit the female worms' ability to lay eggs.

Swallowing of leaves of *Aspilia* species of plants was first reported in African chimpanzees at Gombe by Jane Goodall in the early 1960s, and again in 1983 by Wrangham and Nishida.[6] The leaves are folded in the mouth and individually swallowed. The leaves control parasites by increasing the motility of the animal's gut. The mechanism is that stiff silicate hairs on the surface of the leaf are abrasive and difficult to digest. The leaves are defecated, usually undigested, together with adult worms. Since then, this behaviour has also been seen in bonobos and lowland gorillas in Africa, and reported by Barelli and Huffman in 2016 in white-handed gibbons in the Khao Yai National Park in Thailand.[7] Over forty different plant species have been involved in leaf-swallowing by animals. The same behaviour has also been seen in wolves, dogs, the North American brown bear, Canadian geese and the Chinese lesser civet.

Pith and fruit of the *Afromum* species, the wild ginger family of plants, are eaten by gorillas, bonobos and chimpanzees. These plants are known to have bactericidal activity against a number of pathogenic bacteria – including *Escherichia coli*, *Pseudomonas aeruginosa*, and *Proteus vulgaris*, and they are also active against a range of fungi.

Many species of primates eat figs, which contain the proteolytic enzyme ficin, effective against nematode worms *Ascaris* and *Trichuris*.

Geophagy, or eating soil or clays, has been seen in a wide range of animals.[8] Bird species which show geophagy include pigeons, grouse, hornbills, cassowaries and crows, and it is particularly well known in some parrot species. The exact function of geophagy probably varies – in some cases as a source of sodium, as an aid to digestion, and as a buffer. Gilardi *et al* in 1999, suggested from their studies of parrots in Peru that they select specific clay soils to reduce the toxicity of a diet rich in alkaloids and other bitter compounds from unripe fruit.[9]

Copying animal self-medicating behaviour by indigenous local human populations

The indigenous inhabitants of Gabon and the Congo were found to be using the root bark of *Tabernanthe iboga* plant as a stimulant and aphrodisiac. Some tribes found that larger doses caused hallucinatory visions. The discovery of the properties of the iboga plant has been related to their seeing wild boars dig up the roots and going into a frenzy. The plant is used in an initiation rite by the Bwiti cult secret society in Gabon, when young men are fed shavings of iboga root for several hours and then involved with a sorcerer in a torchlit dance ceremony. The roots contain the alkaloid ibogaine, which has stimulant and aphrodisiac properties.

Humans have probably copied self-administering plant medication by observing the behaviour of animals from the earliest times, and there are folklore stories from different parts of the world which illustrate this. There is a story that in 900 CE, an Abyssinian herder noticed that his animals were enlivened by eating the red fruit of a tree – the coffee plant. Another legend tells that a Yemeni shepherd named Awzulkernayien discovered the Middle Eastern stimulant khat by watching his goats run wild after chewing the leaves. *Catha edulis* or khat contains cathine and cathinone, which are stimulant compounds similar in effect to amphetamine. The Peruvian Indians have a story that llamas travelling in the high jungle region of the Andes were deprived of their normal diet and sampled coca leaves as an alternative. The coca leaves sustained the llamas and the Indians then copied the behaviour of the animals. Pumas in Peru were seen to eat the bark of *Cinchona* trees when they were ill, and the native Indians thus observed the possible medicinal value of the bark.

The same *Vernonia amygdalina* plant used by chimpanzees for treating worm infestations is used by a number of African ethnic groups in the form of a concoction for treatment of malarial fever, schistomiasis, and amoebic dysentery, as well as for intestinal parasites.

Archaeological evidence of use of herbal remedies by Neolithic hominids and early man

If primates use medicinal herbs, it is likely that early hominins (human ancestors) also did so as part of their survival strategy. Dediu and Levinson have suggested that the last common ancestors of modern humans, Denisovans and Neanderthals dating from about half a million years ago, had some capacity for language, and that this may be related to a mutation in the FOXP2 gene, which is the first gene found that is relevant to human communication.[10] The capacity for language is also linked to the development of suitable vocal anatomy. Language development in hominins would have facilitated communication, including about the use of medicinal herbs and care of the sick.

The use of psychoactive plants is deeply rooted in the traditions of many native communities, so it is impossible to say when they might first have been used. But despite this, it is possible to speculate that their use has great antiquity. For example, Australian Aborigines exploit pituri, derived from a plant of the *Nicotiana* species, by breaking up the leaves and mixing them with ash to form a 'quid' which is chewed. The plant contains nicotine and nornicotine. As the Aborigines have lived in Australia for more than 50,000 years, they may have been using the drug for millennia.[11]

Neanderthals lived in Eurasia between *ca.* 230,000 and 40,000 years ago, with some surviving in Gibraltar until about 26,000 years ago. There is evidence from animal remains at Neanderthal sites showing that they were expert hunters. Dental calculus or tartar, composed mainly of calcium carbonate and phosphate mixed with food debris and bacteria, is the deposit of inorganic salts on teeth. Studies have shown, from analysis of dental calculus, micro-fossils trapped in teeth, and plant remains on stone tools, that the Neanderthals exploited a wide range of plants as part of their diet.[12] This has been confirmed from a study by Sistiaga *et al* of faecal samples from a Palaeolithic site at El Salt in Spain dating to about 50,000 years before present time, which showed that although Neanderthals predominantly ate meat, they also had a significant intake of plant material.[13]

El Sidrón is a cave system formed by weathering in the Asturias region of northern Spain. It stretches into the hillside for a length of 2.5 miles. The remains of at least thirteen Neanderthals have been found in the Ossuary Gallery of the cave, which was discovered in 1994 by cave explorers. The remains have been radiocarbon dated to about 48,000 years old. Chemical and microscopic analysis of material trapped in the dental calculus of five Neanderthal individuals and reported by Karen Hardy *et al* has provided the first evidence of the use of medicinal plants such as yarrow (*Achillea millefolium*) and camomile (*Chamaemelum nobile*) by Neanderthal man.[14] Yarrow flowers are still used in traditional herbal medicines in Spain.

In 1975, Ralph Solecki of Columbia University described excavations at the Shanidar Cave in the Bradost Mountain in northern Iraq, where remains of ten Neanderthals dating from 35,000 to 65,000 years ago were found.[15] Associated with the Shanidar IV male skeleton was evidence of flower pollen from *Achillea* species (yarrow) and *Centaurea* (cornflower), amongst other herbs. Both herbs are still used in Iraq: yarrow for dysentery, intestinal colic, wind and as a general tonic; and cornflower as a diuretic, stimulant, and for fevers. Another herb identified was *Ephedra altissima* which contains ephedrine, an alkaloid that produces amphetamine-like stimulant effects. However, it has subsequently been speculated that the plant material may have been dragged there by burrowing rodents.

Studies of sediments in caves inhabited by early man have been used to infer the prehistoric usage of medicinal plants. Martkoplishvili and Kvavadze investigated Upper Palaeolithic sediments in the Dzudzuana, Satsurblia, Kotias Kide and Bondi caves in Western Georgia.[16] The sediments were dated as being from 36,000 to 11,000 years old. Significant amounts of pollen from *Artemisia annua* (sweet wormwood), *Artemisia absinthum* (wormwood), *Achillea millefolium* (yarrow), *Centaurea jacea* (knapweed) and *Urtica dioica* (nettle) were found. Levels of modern pollen grains of these species were very low, showing that they were not transported long distances and that the levels found were probably due to flowering branches being brought into the caves by the population living there. These plants are still used in popular modern herbal medicine in Georgia.

Dillehay and his colleagues reported in 2010 on excavations of five sites in the Nanchoc valley in Northern Peru.[17] The sites have been dated to about 7,930 years ago. Coca leaves were recovered from the hard-packed floors of the remains of buildings, together with burnt and precipitated calcium from lime. Some of the leaves were agglutinated, indicating that they had been chewed. The leaves were compared with modern coca leaves from the genus *Erythroxylum* and found to be similar. Coca leaves were chewed by the Incas together with lime to release the cocaine. Today the species *Erythroxylum novogranatense* is commercially cultivated in the Ecuadorian and Peruvian Andes.

The hallucinogenic San Pedro cactus *Echinopsis pachanoi* grows in the Andes Mountains at altitudes from 2,000 to 3,000m. It contains mescaline amongst other compounds. It is used in the course of healing ceremonies. Evidence of its use in Peru was found in the Guitarrero Cave in the Callejón de Huaylas valley. Pollen and fossil remains were found at occupation levels dated between 8600 and 5600 BCE. A sample of the cactus was dated to 6800 to 6200 BCE.[18]

There is considerable archaeological evidence for the cultivation of the opium poppy, *Papaver somniferum,* in the Mediterranean and Middle East. Poppy seeds were found in a room under the sediment in Lake Bracciano at the La Marmotta site of an ancient Italian city. The site dates from 7,700 years ago. Poppy capsules were found in small woven baskets in the Cueva de los Murcié-lagos burial cave near Albuñol, in Granada, Spain. These were radiocarbon dated to *ca*. 4,200 years old.[19]

Xie *et al* published a report in 2013 on the investigation of an ancient burial site, the Gumugou Cemetery, in the Xinjiang region of Northwest China.[20] The site is about 3,800 years old. Twigs of *Ephedra* species were found at the site. The herb *Ephedra* (*ma huang* in Mandarin Chinese) is still very widely used as an herbal medicine in China for asthma, fever and headache. *Ephedra* pollen was recovered at the Banpo archaeological site which was discovered in 1953 and is located in the Yellow River Valley just east of Xi'an, in the Shaanxi province of China. The site is about 4,500 years old.

In September 1991, two German hikers discovered a mummified brown corpse protruding from the melting glacier ice near the summit of the 11,808ft Similaun Mountain in the Tyrolean Alps.[21] Near the corpse was an axe with a wooden handle, some string, some chamois fur (an animal now extinct in this part of the Alps) and a long wooden stick.

The corpse was exhumed from the ice and is now preserved in the South Tyrol Museum of Archaeology. It is referred to as the Iceman or Ötzi. In December 1991, tests on pollen samples associated with Ötzi showed that he dated from about 3200 BCE. The Iceman carried with him two pieces of fungus, threaded on leather straps. These were identified as *Piptoporus betulinus* – birch polypore or the razorstrop fungus that grows on birch trees. Some researchers have suggested that the fungus might be used for its pharmacological effects, since bracket fungi were used in ancient Roman and Greek medicine. It has been suggested that since the Iceman had intestinal worms, the fungi could have been used to treat them, but this has been disputed.

In 1921, a Bronze Age wooden coffin was discovered in a burial mound on the Egtved farm in South Jutland in Denmark. On investigation it contained the body of a young girl covered with a woollen rug. A flowering yarrow plant species was found by her left knee, laid so that its white blossom faced the head of the coffin. She is known as the 'Egtved girl' in Denmark. Subsequently, another coffin with a body of a young girl from the Mound People was found in 1935 at Skrydstrup. Beneath the animal hide covering her were found leaves of wood chervil, a medicinal herb. The burial mounds probably date from around 1250 BCE.[22]

Many of the psychoactive herbal products were found as grave-goods buried in tombs or associated with ceremonial places. Thus, it can be argued that these products had a ritual sacred role amongst the beliefs of these societies as part of their communication with the spirit world. Shamanism involves a practitioner reaching an altered state of consciousness, often using psychoactive drugs, in order to perceive and interact with a spirit world and channel transcendental energies into this world. Shamans purported to treat ailments/illness by alleviating traumas affecting the soul/spirit to restore the physical body of the individual to balance and wholeness.

Fermented beverages

Alcohol remains the most popular recreational drug around the world, and has a very long-established use. From the 1970s onwards, archaeologists started to use gas or liquid chromatography in combination with mass spectrometry to analyse organic residues in unglazed pottery sherds from vessels which might have been used to ferment or store alcoholic drinks.[23] The earliest example is from some pottery sherds at the Early Neolithic village of Jiahu in China, dating from 7000 to 6600 BCE, which may have been used for wine. Two ceramic vessels were found at Hajji Firuz Tepe in the Zagros Mountains of Iran, dating from 5400 to 5000 BCE which contained a resinated wine with terebinth or pine resin added as either a preservative or as a medicine. A fully equipped winery dating to about 4000 BCE was discovered in the cave complex of Areni 1 in Armenia, with vats, storage jars and drinking vessels. As we shall see, alcohol becomes one of the most popular solvents used to dissolve medicinal ingredients in the formulation of medicines, particularly in the form of beer or wine.

Mesopotamian medicine

Mesopotamia was an ancient region located in the eastern Mediterranean between the Tigris and Euphrates rivers. It was bounded in the northeast by the Zagros Mountains and in the southeast by the Arabian Plateau. It mostly corresponds to today's Iraq, but it also includes parts of modern Iran, Syria and Turkey.

The earliest written evidence of the use of medicines is from the many thousands of clay tablets inscribed with cuneiform script. The clay was kneaded to mix the dry and wet parts and to remove air pockets. It was then formed into tablets from hand-sized up to 30–40cm square. The wet tablets were inscribed with a stylus commonly made from a sharpened reed, but it could also be made from wood, ivory, metal or bone. The cuneiform signs were from Sumerian, Akkadian, Hittite and other languages. The development of writing was probably influenced by the development, in the fourth millennium BCE, of larger urban centres such as the cities of Eridu and Uruk. One of the earliest Sumerian tablets was found at Nagpur and is about 5,000 years old. It was translated in 1953 by Samuel Kramer and Martin Levey, a chemist from Philadelphia.[24] It contains 12 recipes for drug preparations and references to over 250 medicinal herbs, including the poppy, cassia, myrtle, asafoetida, thyme, henbane and mandrake. In the 1920s, Reginald Campbell-Thompson collected, photographed and translated about 660 cuneiform tablets dating from the seventh century BCE. The translations were published as '*The Assyrian Herbal*' and he identified about 250 herbal drugs used in Assyrian medicine.[25] The tablets were from the library of one of the most prominent kings, Assurburnipal. Assurbanipal or Ashshurbanipal, was king of the Neo-Assyrian Empire from 668 BCE to *ca.* 627 BCE. He was the last strong ruler of the empire, which is usually dated between 934 and 609 BCE. The tablets were copies of much older texts which are some centuries earlier. A photograph of a typical cuneiform medical tablet is shown in Picture 1 in the illustrations.

The practice of medicine combined therapeutic recipes and 'magical' incantations which appealed to the psychology of the patient. Geller[26] has explained that the Babylonian belief system incorporated magic in which illnesses are caused by demons or angry gods. Treatment could be from an exorcist-priest practising from a temple or from an *asû*-physician, who was a layman. The priest derived his power from his relationship to the gods, usually Ea and Marduk. The physician had his relationship with Gula, the god of healing. Treatments were chosen based on previous precedent and the experience of the physician with an earlier use of a medicine.

Plants and minerals were classified in terms of their šiknu, their nature or properties in terms of their medicinal use. The Akkadian texts include lists of both 'simples' and more complex recipes. A simple is a recipe for a single-component drug, whereas the more complex recipes include a combination of a number of herbal and/or mineral or animal ingredients and were probably used to treat a number of conditions.

The *materia medica* of Mesopotamian medicine consisted of a wide range of types of plant ingredients – seeds, fruit, leaves, flowers, branches, grains such as barley, and spices and vegetables. Despite the heroic efforts of Campbell-Thompson, very few of the ingredients can be identified with any certainty. Animal products such as snake-skin, turtle and mussel shells, and mongoose blood were also used. Other components of the products included liquids used as a solvent vehicle for the drugs – water, milk, urine, beer and wine. A variety of dosage forms were used and these will be considered in later chapters of this book.

Egyptian medicine

Nunn has summarised Egyptian history in relation to food and medicine.[27] The beginning of recorded history was under the first king of the First Dynasty, Narmer, in the Early Dynastic Period. During the later dynasties of this period, shipping trade was established which included supply of some drugs. Writing appeared during this era.

An ostracon is a piece of broken pottery. In ancient Egypt these pieces of broken pottery or stone (most often limestone) were used as notepads as they were a cheaper and more plentiful option than papyrus. An ostracon from Deir el-Medina from 1244 during the reign of Rameses II – the third pharaoh of the Nineteenth Dynasty of Egypt, often regarded as the most powerful pharaoh of the New Kingdom – records absences from work. Pa-hery-podjet was recorded as absent 'on certain days for the preparation of medicines.' Thus, Pa-hery-podjet may be the name of the first recorded apothecary/pharmacist.[32] It is thus probable that in antiquity in some periods the role of the physician and the pharmacist were separate.

Medical specialisation had become well advanced by the time of the Old Kingdom and it is considered that many parts of some of the medical papyri were first written during this period. However only later copies have survived. By the Late Period, Greek medicine was challenging Egyptian medicine. The great Hippocratic school was established in Cos from 430 to 330 BCE.

The most important medical papyri were found during the nineteenth century or the early years of the twentieth century. They are listed in Table 1.1.

The Kahun gynaecological papyri, comprising three pages, were discovered by Sir William Flinders Petrie in 1899, near the town of Lehun in the Fayum. They were damaged and have been reassembled for translation. The Edwin Smith papyrus was found in a Theban tomb and put up for sale by Mustafa Agha in about 1860. It was purchased by Edwin Smith in 1862 and donated to the New York Historical Society in 1906 by Smith's daughter. It comprises seventeen pages on the recto side of the papyrus and five on the verso. Another papyrus was bought in 1872 by the Egyptologist George Ebers. This papyrus has 110 pages and contains spells, information on diseases and treatments

Table 1.1: Summary of the important medical papyri.

Title	Where held	Approximate date	Contents
Kahun	University College, London	1820 BCE	Gynaecological
Ramesseum III, IV and V	Oxford	1700 BCE	Gynaecological, ophthalmic, paediatric
Edwin Smith	New York Academy of Sciences	1550 BCE	Surgical
Ebers	Leipzig	1550 BCE	Medical
Hearst	University of California	1450 BCE	Medical
London	British Museum	1300 BCE	Magical
Carlsberg VIII	University of Copenhagen	1300 BCE	Gynaecological
Chester Beatty VI	British Museum	1200 BCE	Rectal disease
Berlin	Berlin Museum	1200 BCE	Medical
Brooklyn	Brooklyn Museum	300 BCE	Snake bite

for various conditions. When Flinders Petrie and James Quibell were excavating the temple tomb of Ramses II at Thebes in 1896, Quibell uncovered a wooden box containing papyri – the Ramasseum papyri. The papyrus Hearst was discovered at Deir el-Ballas in Upper Egypt by the Hearst Egyptian Expedition. It has eighteen pages dealing with urinary tract treatments, blood, hair and snake and scorpion bites. The London papyrus was owned by the Royal Institution and transferred to the British Museum in 1860. It comprises nineteen pages and contains magic spells against swellings, skin diseases, eye diseases and burns. The Chester Beatty papyri were presented to the British Museum by Sir Alfred Chester Beatty, a millionaire philanthropist. Papyrus VI contains eight pages mainly concerned with rectal disease and Papyrus VII contains spells against scorpion stings. The twenty-four-page Berlin papyrus was acquired by Giuseppe Passalacqua in Saqqara (the necropolis for Memphis, the ancient Egyptian capital) and sold to Friedrich Wilhelm IV of Prussia for the Berlin Museum. The Carlsberg papyrus is owned by the Carlsberg Foundation and is housed in the University of Copenhagen. The Brooklyn papyrus deals mainly with snake bites.

Various translations have been made of the papyri. The most complete are in the various volumes of the *Grundriss der Medizin der alten Agypter* published from 1954 to 1973 by the Akademie-Verlag in Berlin. The Ebers papyrus is the main source of knowledge about Egyptian medicine. An English translation of the Ebers papyrus based partly on the German *Grundriss* text by Paul Ghaliounghui of the Academy of Scientific Research and Technology in Cairo was published in 1987.[28] References are given in this book as E or Ebers with a number denoting its listing in Ghaliounghui's book – for example E21 or Ebers 21. A photograph of a section of the Ebers papyrus is shown in Picture 2. This is an asthma remedy where the patient inhaled herbs heated on a brick.

As with Mesopotamian medicine, illness was often felt to be caused by malevolent spirits or powers. These demons could travel on the wind and enter the victim through the mouth, nose, or a break in the skin. Treatments were aimed at ridding the body of these agents. Appeals and prayers to the gods were part of the treatment. The god Re was felt to have devised many of the incantations and the god Thoth with devising remedies for use for treatment. The efficacy of a particular remedy derived from a magical power inherent in the substances in it. The Ebers papyrus includes a number of incantations, such as an utterance to apply a remedy to any part of the body, an utterance to loosen a bandage, and an utterance to drink a remedy.

The Egyptian remedies mentioned in the papyri include mineral ingredients, materials of animal origin, and herbal materials.

A wide range of mineral drugs was used. Natron is a mixture of sodium salts produced by natural evaporation of waters on the land after flooding. It was most commonly used externally, often with a bandage. The Ebers papyrus recommended natron for drawing out pus from a wound. Malachite (a form of copper carbonate) was used in eye preparations and it may have been antibacterial as it released copper into solution. Lapis lazuli (a sodium/aluminium silicate) was imported; its medical use was mainly in ophthalmic products. Galena (lead sulfide) was also used in ophthalmological preparations. Alabaster (calcium carbonate) was used in skin ointments, and yellow ochre (clay containing iron oxide) was used for treating baldness.

Animal and human origin materials were used in about half of the preparations described in the papyri. Honey was a common ingredient and considered to come from the god Re; it was used in both internal and external remedies. It is probably the oldest wound-healing agent. Modern studies of its therapeutic use have shown that it has antibacterial, antiviral, anti-inflammatory and antioxidant activity. It induces the white blood cells (the leucocytes) to release cytokine proteins which begin tissue repair.

Milk was used in many of the compounded remedies, often as a vehicle to dissolve other components or to make them more palatable. The milk of someone who has borne a male child was often used, and indicates that this may have been thought to have some particular properties. Beer was another common ingredient. A remedy for a lung treatment was colocynth and sweet beer left overnight and then drunk over four days (Ebers 21).

Excrement was used from a number of animal species including crocodile, lizard, cat, birds, bats and man. These faecal- or excrement-based medicines are called 'Dreckapotheke' ('dirt pharmacy') in German, and the same word is often used in English texts. These were mostly used in external preparations and for treatments of the eyes. One remedy for treatment of eyes contained lizard dung, a mineral, and a fermentation product of honey (Ebers 370). Another remedy for treatment of a burn was to apply black mud on day one, followed on day two by an application of the dung of small cattle, cooked and mixed with yeast (Ebers 482). A remedy for removal of a thorn was ass dung mixed with vegetable mucilage and applied to the entry wound (Ebers 728).

Various animal fats were used as either the basis for external preparations or as part of the treatment. A treatment for tremor of the head was to mix natron with oil and fat, honey and wax, make it into a mass and apply under a bandage (Ebers 252). One of the most remarkable treatments was one for baldness which consists of a mixture of fats from the lion, hippopotamus, crocodile, cat, snake and ibex (Ebers 465). A remedy for greying of the hair was horn of gazelle, fried with oil/fat and applied to the head (Ebers 458). Fats were also included in preparations to be drunk, for example, goose fat, cumin and milk were included in a remedy to be drunk for conditions of the belly (Ebers 5).

Other animal tissues used include blood from a variety of animals, cow and goat bile, and urine. A remarkable example of the use of blood was the remedy to treat effusions of blood which contained a mixture of blood from the pigeon, Nile goose, swallow and vulture (Ebers 737). A remedy for suffering in half the head (probably meaning migraine) was the skull of a catfish fried in oil and anointed on the head (Ebers 250). Even whole animals could be used – such as the remedy for warding off inflammation, which was a frog fried in oil or fat and put on the skin (Ebers 301). Fresh meat was used as an application for a wound on the first day.

A huge variety of plant ingredients are mentioned in the papyri. These include vegetable and marsh plants, fruit, spices and herbs, and herbal remedy ingredients. For the herbal remedy ingredients there is good agreement between commentators on some of these, but not for other herbs where the interpretation of the Egyptian word is unclear or disputed. Even when there is reasonable consensus, it is not clear whether the word denotes a flower, root, stem, seed or fruit. Nunn has listed over thirty herbal ingredients where there is considerable agreement between commentators. This list includes acacia, barley, bean, bryony, castor oil (*Ricinus*), Christ thorn (*Zizyphus spina-Christi*), cinnamon, coriander, date, emmer wheat, fig, grape, hemp (*Cannabis sativa*), juniper, leek, linseed, lotus, onion, pea, pomegranate, raisin, sycamore fig, tamarisk, willow and wormwood. The products include mixtures to be taken by mouth, eye preparations, skin preparations and products to be placed in the rectum and vagina.

Considering the preparations in the papyri from the exalted viewpoint of the twenty-first century suggests that there is little therapeutic rationale for many of them. But we should perhaps pause before leaping to judgement. For example, one of the most frequently used herbs was colocynth, *Citrullus colocynthis*. This herb occurred all over the Mediterranean and North Africa. It was used in products to be drunk, products for use on the skin, for eye preparations, as a preparation for tremor in a body part, and for vaginal use as part of a contraceptive device. The chemical constituents of colocynth and its pharmacological effects have been reviewed by Al-Snafi, and he has concluded that it has antioxidant, antidiabetic, antimicrobial, anti-inflammatory, analgesic, gastrointestinal, reproductive and other effects.[29] In a study in albino rats by Roy, Thakur and Dixit, petroleum ether extracts of colocynth incorporated into an ointment base were at least comparable to minoxidil 2 per cent solution (the commercial product marketed as Regaine®) in stimulating hair growth.[30]

Haimov-Kochman has reviewed some of the gynaecological preparations described in the papyri and used for reproduction, conception and delivery. He concludes that there is a rationale for many of them.[31] For example, the Ebers papyrus recommends the use of linen soaked in honey and acacia spikes formed into a pessary for contraception. Saponins can be extracted from *Acacia auriculiformis*. Saponins are compounds with soap-like properties that foam when mixed with water. The acacia saponins have been shown to immobilise sperm, and prevent sperm entering the mucus of the uterus to fertilise an egg.

Chapter 2

Hippocrates and Greek Medicine

Medicines in the Greek Bronze Age

The Greek Bronze Age lasted from 2800 BCE to 1100 BCE. It consisted of the Minoan civilisation on Crete and the Mycenean on the mainland. The main site of the Minoan civilisation on Crete was at Knossos, with other sites at Gournia, Mallia and Phaistos. It has been estimated that the average life expectancy on Crete was between 31 and 35 years. Arnott has concluded that the wealthy elite who lived in the palaces at Knossos would have been able to call on a priest-healer whose cures were based on magic rituals, but which might well have been combined with some knowledge of folk-medicine.[1]

Starting in 1894, the British archaeologist Sir Arthur Evans excavated the site at Knossos and discovered many clay tablets 4.5cm to 19.5cm long by 1.2cm to 7.2cm wide. These dated from 1425 to 1390 BCE. They were scored with horizontal lines over which text was written. This script was denoted by Evans as Linear B. Between 1951 and 1953 the architect and amateur linguist Michael Ventris (1922–1956), together with the philologist John Chadwick (1920–1998), discovered that the text was a form of early Greek script and were able to decipher it. Most of the tablets have now been deciphered and they are lists of stores, debts and land transactions. The tablets of medical interest contain the names of various plants, used in food and/or medicine. These are wheat, barley, olives, figs, coriander, sesame, cumin, celery, fennel, cyperus grass, safflower, iris root, linseed, mint, pennyroyal and honey. Garlic and onion have also been found during the excavations. Ventris and Chadwick assumed that these were all food and spices, but they could have also been used in medicine – as they were in the time of Hippocrates. Homer writing in about 750 BCE described in the *Iliad* how Hecamede gave Nestor and Machaon a restorative drink of boiled onion juice, honey and flour of pearl barley.

There is archaeological evidence for the use of opium in the Greek Bronze Age.[2] The method of incising unripe opium poppy heads (*Papaver somniferum*) to produce the opium latex was known in Crete at about 1250 BCE, as shown by the bare-breasted female terracotta figure discovered in 1937 bearing on its head three hairpins shaped as poppy capsules, each incised with vertical notches. Further evidence is provided in the form of a painted decoration on a cylindrical box with a lid from Central Crete, where the painting on the lid shows a bird opening a poppy capsule. This is dated from about 1380 BCE. A famous golden signet ring dating from about 1450 BCE discovered in the acropolis of Mycenae shows a female deity receiving an offering of three poppy capsules. Poppy seeds have been found in excavations at Terynth in Mycenae, showing that it had been cultivated and harvested since about 1300 BCE. Opium contains morphine and would have been used as a sedative and painkiller.

Hippocrates

Hippocrates is one of the most important figures in the history of medicine. He has been called the 'Father of Medicine' for his achievement in establishing medicine as a distinct discipline in ancient Greece.[3] He is credited (rightly or wrongly) with devising the *Hippocratic Oath*, a document which sets out the ethical principles for physicians in treating patients. In its original classic form, the *Oath* began: 'I swear by Apollo the physician, and Aesculapius the surgeon, likewise Hygeia and Panacea, and call all the gods and goddesses to witness, that I will observe and keep this underwritten oath, to the utmost of my power and judgment'. A revised version of the *Oath* is still used in some medical schools.

There is very little direct evidence of his existence and life from contemporary or near-contemporary sources. Plato (*ca*. 424–348 BCE) was one of the founders of the Western tradition of philosophy, together with his teacher, Socrates and his pupil Aristotle. He developed the dialogue form of philosophical writing. His book *Protagoras* is a dialogue between Socrates and the elderly Protagoras. In this dialogue, one of the characters is called Hippocrates, and when he is questioned by Socrates mentions the famous Hippocrates, the physician of Cos. The book *Phaedrus* was written in about 370 BCE. It is a dialogue between Phaedrus and Socrates.

In this dialogue Plato mentions Hippocrates of the Asclepiad family. These are the only contemporary references to Hippocrates.

The best-known account of the life of Hippocrates is from Soranus of Ephesus, a Greek physician of the first and second centuries CE, who practised medicine in the reigns of the Roman emperors Trajan and Hadrian, and who wrote a collection of medical biographies. Soranus' book draws on information from Eratosthenes (*ca*. 276 BCE–*ca*. 195 BCE) who was born in the Greek colony of Cyrene, which is now the city of Shahhat in Libya. Eratosthenes studied in Athens and his work as a writer and poet led the pharaoh Ptolemy III Eueregetes to invite him to become a librarian at the great Library of Alexandria. Within five years he became chief librarian. A modern account of the life of Hippocrates by Jacques Jouanna was published in English translation in 1999.[4]

One of the earliest Greek gods reputed to specialise in healing was Asclepius. Healers and patients invoked his name in prayer and healing ceremonies at home and in temples. However, it is now thought that Asclepius may have been an actual historical figure, renowned for his ability as a healer. Asclepius and his sons, Machaon and Podalirius, are mentioned in Homer's Greek epic poem *The Iliad* written about 750 BCE, but only as men not gods. The family clan of healers known as the Asclepiads claimed to be the descendants of Asclepius and to have inherited a knowledge and mystical power of healing from him. Hippocrates was born on the island of Cos in 460 BCE. Cos is the second largest island in the Dodecanese, 20km from Bodrum in modern Turkey. Hippocrates is said to have been descended from the sons of Asclepius and was part of this noble medical family. According to Soranus, Hippocrates' father was Heraclides, a physician, and his mother was Praxitela.

Hippocrates received his medical education within his family group, and particularly from his grandfather, who was also named Hippocrates. It would have been mainly oral instruction and practical demonstration. After completing his training in Cos, he started his practice as a physician. He married and had three children, two sons and a daughter.

Having achieved fame in Cos, there is a story that he was summoned to the city of Abdera on the Thracian coast to treat the philosopher Democritus, whom the citizens of Abdera thought to be insane. However, he discovered that Democritus was working on a book on madness and was laughing at the folly of man.

After the death of his parents he moved to Thessaly in northern Greece, and practised there, and possibly elsewhere in mainland Greece. But before moving, he married his daughter to his pupil Polybus. During his time in Thessaly he probably trained other students, as he mentions in the *Speech to the Envoy* sending disciples to other parts of Greece during the plague years of 419–436 BCE. The whole of his writing was done after he left Cos.

Hippocrates died sometime between 375 and 351 BCE. His tomb was somewhere between Larissa and Gyrton. After his death his reputation grew very rapidly and there were sacrifices made on his birthday each year.

There are about seventy treatises attributed to Hippocrates. However, they are diverse in their origins and styles, and the dates when written. Some are contemporary with Hippocrates, others much later. The treatises are a mixture of practical handbooks for the physician, lectures, essays, and books intended for a wider public. The whole body of work attributed to Hippocrates and his followers is called the *Hippocratic Corpus*. The *Aphorisms* is perhaps the most famous of the works.

Within the various treatises there are over 250 different medical materials mentioned.[5] These are mainly herbal ingredients, but also oils and fats, milk, eggs, animal horn and sponge.[1] Insects such as the blister beetle, from the family *Meloidae*, are also mentioned. These beetles produce the chemical cantharidin, released when agitated or attacked by predators, as a means to defend themselves and their eggs. It causes irritations and blisters, hence the beetle's name. A variety of minerals such as salt, sulphur, gypsum (calcium sulphate), alum, and pumice are also included, as well as metallic salts and compounds from lead, copper, arsenic and antimony.

Some of the ingredients were either imported or originally came from overseas. Totelin has reviewed Hippocratic recipes.[6] The largest number of the foreign ingredients have the designation 'Egyptian' and include Egyptian acorn, Egyptian alum, Egyptian oil (a type of scented oil), Egyptian perfume, Egyptian salt, and Egyptian bean. Homer wrote about the renown of Egyptian drugs in Book Four of the *Odyssey*, in about the eighth or seventh century BCE, that 'for there the earth, the giver of grain, bears greatest store of drugs, many that are healing when mixed, and many that are baneful; there every man is a physician, wise above human kind …'. Other 'exotic' foreign ingredients included Theban salt, Indian pepper, Libyan leaf and Pontic nut. Attic honey, Thasian wine, Cnidian berry, Cretan ivy, Cypriot ash, Milesian wood and Black Earth from Samos were also among some of the ingredients that came from different regions in Greece.

The list of herbal materials is extensive and comprises cereals, fruit, nuts and vegetables, as well as flowers, roots, bark etc. from various plants. One of the aphorisms attributed to Hippocrates (although it is not actually to be found in any of the treatises in the *Hippocratic Corpus*) is 'Let food be thy medicine and medicine be thy food', suggesting an overlap between the two categories of substances. Touwaide and Appetiti have shown that 40 per cent of the remedies in the *Hippocratic Corpus* are comprised from only forty-four plants.[7] Of these, thirty-three species can also be regarded as food. Today's consumers are increasingly being exhorted to eat so-called 'superfoods' and nutraceuticals or functional foods – that is foodstuffs that provide health benefits in addition to their basic nutritional value. Clearly these ideas have a history dating back to antiquity. The Hippocratic treatise *Regimens*, which probably dates from late fifth century BCE to early fourth century BCE, consists of four books, the second of which is devoted to food ingredients and their properties. The list of foods includes cereals such as barley, wheat and spelt (a primitive wheat); meat, poultry and seafood; eggs, cheese, honey, fruits and vegetables. W. H. Jones's 1931 translation of the introductory section of *Regimens* is as follows: 'I maintain that he who aspires to treat correctly of human regimen must first acquire knowledge and discernment of the nature of man in general… and further the power possessed severally by all of the foods and drinks of our regimen …'

A typical entry in *Regimens* is the following: 'The onion is good for sight, but bad for the body, because it is hot and burning, and it does not lead to stool; for without giving nourishment or help to the body it warms and dries on account of its juice'. Vegetables cited in the *Corpus* include beetroot, cucumber, cabbage, turnips, radish, beans, garden peas, lentils, lettuce, garlic, leeks, onions, rocket, celery, fennel, chickpeas, and wild carrot. Herbs include sage, marjoram, mint, pennyroyal, savory, basil, fennel and dill.[8]

The herbal plant materials include a wide range of flowers, fruits, leaves, bark, and roots. The fruits cited include mulberries, figs, pears, apples, quinces, medlars, almonds, grapes and pomegranates. Some of the plant materials such as squill (an expectorant to reduce the thickness of mucus in the lung) and the opium poppy (painkiller) are still used in one form or another in conventional modern medicine; many more of them are still used in Europe in Traditional Herbal Medicinal Products licensed by the European Union (EU) Member States or unlicensed botanical food supplements.

Wine was used in the *Corpus* as a solvent for other materials, and also to be applied externally to the body. The treatise *Use of Liquids* includes a chapter on the external application of wine, for example, to treat wounds, where it is says that wine can exercise a cooling or hard action. In *Wounds* a poultice made from watercress mixed with wine and crushed flax grains is recommended to connect the edges of a wound. In the treatise *Fractures* it is recommended that dark wine be put on an open fracture. In the treatise *Nature of Women*, a prolapsed womb is treated with dark wine extract of pomegranate. Wine was also used in a number of other recipes for instillation into the uterus. The treatise *Internal Affections* recommends the use of a clyster (now known as an enema) consisting of nitrate mixed with wine, oil and honey to purge phlegm. For dropsy (excess fluid in parts of the body – or oedema), an enema containing wine, honey, oil and leaf sap from wild cucumber was prescribed.

Wine was also used in the form of a vapour bath. In the treatise *Places of Man*, if the uterus ascends upwards and becomes obstructed, it is treated with pleasant-smelling, warming substances such as myrrh or sweet oil (almond oil). Then a vapour-bath of wine is applied, the area washed with warm water and diuretics used to increase the flow of urine and remove excess fluid.

A large proportion of the use of medicines was aimed at evacuation – either upwards as vomiting, or downwards as purgation. In the *Nature of Man*, it is recommended to induce vomiting in the winter because this period causes more phlegm, and evacuate the bowels in the summer. Purgatives were generally employed in treatment. The *Places in Man* says: 'If some disease attacks a person, and the person is strong, and the disease is weak, you may confidently employ a purgative medication stronger than the disease, since if anything of what is healthy happens to get carried off with what is diseased, no damage will result.'

In an era when the average life expectancy was only around thirty years, child-bearing was crucial, and several of the *Corpus* treatises deal with diseases of women, such as womb movements, conception, pregnancy and childbirth. A Hippocratic fertility test was to apply a clove of garlic to the womb, and see the next day if the woman smelt of it through the mouth – if she did she was pregnant. Another pregnancy test in the *Aphorisms* is: 'If you wish to know whether a woman is with child, give her hydromel (honey and water) to drink when she is going to sleep. If she has colic in the stomach she is with child, otherwise she is not.' A recipe in *Diseases of Women* for displacement of the womb to one side is for a drink composed of four blister beetle bodies with five peony seeds, eggs of cuttlefish and seed of parsley mixed in wine. For amenorrhoea (absence of menstrual periods), *Places in Man* recommends direct application of myrrh or sweet oil (almond oil). It also recommends direct application of cow's dung, bull's gall, or anything else which is similar, and 'evacuate downwards with laxative medications that do not provoke vomiting and are mild, in order that purging does not become excessive.' The same treatise suggests that uterine applications can be made by combining the drugs with semi-boiled honey into pessaries, which are wrapped in cloth and allowed to melt.

Some of the Hippocratic treatments combine physical methods with the use of medicines. For example, to correct a prolapse of the uterus, the woman was attached to a ladder by her feet, upside down, and the ladder then raised and dropped to the ground. Then the woman's legs were crossed and tied together and she was left for a day and a night with only some cold barley water to drink.

Totelin has reviewed the 1551 formulations in the *Corpus*. The most frequent dosage form is, as might be expected, oral drinks with 439 recipes.[6] The vaginal/rectal route has an astonishingly high number, with 422 pessaries/vaginal applications, 13 suppositories and 200 enemas. By comparison, there are only 77 ointment formulations and 56 poultices (a soft moist mass spread on a cloth and applied to the skin).

The *Nature of Man* treatise was written by Polybus, Hippocrates' student and son-in-law. It contains the theory of the four humours – that the nature of man consists of blood, phlegm, yellow bile and black bile. The text states in W.H.S. Jones' translation:

'The body of man has in itself blood, phlegm, yellow bile and black bile; these make up the nature of his body, and through these he feels pain and enjoys health. Now he enjoys the most perfect health when these elements are duly proportioned to one another in respect of compounding, power and bulk, and when they are perfectly mingled. Pain is felt when one of these elements is in defect or excess or is isolated in the body without being compounded with the others.'[8]

Particular humours predominate in each of the four seasons. Thus, blood, hot and wet, predominated in spring; yellow bile, hot and dry, in the summer; black bile, cold and dry in the autumn; phlegm, cold and wet in the winter. Good health was considered to be due to a balance (*krasis*) between the four humours. The *Nature of Man* also mentions the theory of elementary qualities – hot, dry, cold and wet. The text says: 'But as a matter of fact, cures are many. For in the body there are many constituents, which by heating, by cooling, by drying or wetting one another contrary to nature, engender diseases; so that both forms of disease are many and the healing of them is manifold.' As an example, in *On Regimen*, the herbal drug called *thymos* (probably a variety of thyme) would be suitable for restoration of *krasis* in a condition where there was an excess of phlegm, presumed to be wet and cold, as the drug would help expel phlegm. However, it was Galen, writing about 600 years later who popularised this theory as to the nature of man and the four elementary qualities. He stated that the ideas he expounded were based on the earlier work of Hippocrates.

The contribution of Hippocrates and his followers to Greek medicine was very considerable. Previously it had been thought that disease was caused by the intervention of gods and demons. Hippocrates proposed a more rational approach in which disease is caused by factors such as the choice of diet, living habits and the changes of the seasons. Treatment consisted of a re-balancing of the four humours. The Hippocratic school gave great importance to taking case histories and the clinical observation of symptoms such as pulse, presence of fever, movement, pains, and excretions.

Aristotle and Theophrastus

Aristotle (384–322 BCE) was born in Stagira of Chalcidice in Macedonia. His father Nicomachus was a physician at the court of Amytas. At the age of 17 he moved to Athens where he studied and taught at Plato's Academy.

Theophrastus (371–286 BCE) was born in Eresos in Lesbos. His father Melantas was local fuller (someone who was involved in the treatment of cloth). As a young man he went to Athens and became a pupil of Plato. After Plato died, Aristotle and Theophrastus left Athens and moved to Mytilene in Lesbos. They began their studies there into natural science – Aristotle into zoology and Theophrastus into botany.[9] After about two years, Aristotle received an invitation from Philip II, King of Macedonia, to act as tutor to his teenage son, the future Alexander the Great. In about 355 BCE Aristotle moved back to Athens and founded the Lyceum.

Under Philip II, Macedonia expanded into the territories of the Paeonians, Illyrians and the Thracians. His son, Alexander the Great (356–323 BCE), extended the territory throughout central Greece, the Persian Empire and part of India. After he died his empire became fragmented. Classical Greece entered its Hellenistic phase with the conquests of Philip and Alexander the Great, and Greek became the common language beyond Greece itself and its culture influenced others.

After the death of Alexander, anti-Macedonian sentiment forced Aristotle to leave Athens into exile in Chalcis. Theophrastus then took over the running of the Lyceum and was its head for thirty-seven years. The school was called Peripatetic as teaching was apparently done whilst walking around the garden with the students.

Theophrastus wrote a considerable number of books. The fourth century CE writer Diogenes Laertius, who wrote a book on the lives of eminent philosophers, credited him with 227 treatises. The most interesting from our point of view are his *Historia Plantarum* (Enquiry into Plants) in nine volumes, and *De Causis Plantarum* (Causes of Plants) in six volumes. Theophrastus is regarded by many as the founder of the science of botany. The two books were not textbooks; they were part of a series of lectures given to students on the botanical research that he had carried out. Aristotle had classified animals and information about them in his *History of Animals*, and he proceeded to explain characteristics of them in a series of books such as *On the Parts of Animals*, *On the Generation of Animals*, *On the Motion of Animals*, *On the Soul*, and in the short text *Parva Naturalia*. Theophrastus used the same model with his two books, *Historia Plantarum* (about the identification of plants and their properties) and *De Causis Plantarum* (about certain common or distinctive characters of plants). The medicinal properties of plants are described in Book IX of the *Historia Plantarum*, and the plants are described elsewhere in this text. Thus, taking the book as a whole it is thought to be the earliest extant herbal in Greek.

Diocles of Carystos was a physician who lived at the time of Aristotle in Athens and wrote on a variety of topics including medicines. It is thought that some of Theophrastus' information derived from Diocles, but there are only fragments available of Diocles' works.

Some of Theophrastus' information came from the *pharmacopōlai* (drug sellers) and *rhizotomoi* (so-called root cutters), although the *rhizotomoi* collected other parts of the plant as herbs, as well as the roots. He records, without necessarily endorsing them, some of the rather bizarre superstitions from the *rhizotomoi* about collecting herbs. For example, he mentions the perils of peony collecting:

'They say that the peony, which some call the *glycyside*, should be dug up at night, for if one does it in the daytime, and is observed by a woodpecker while he is gathering the fruit, he risks the loss of his eye-sight; and, if he is cutting the root at the same time, he gets prolapse of the anus.'

In relation to cutting thapsia (the deadly carrot plant used as a purgative): 'that one should stand to windward and that should first anoint oneself with oil, for that one's body will swell up if one stands the other way'. To collect mandrake, 'it is said that one should draw three circles round mandrake with a sword, and cut it with one's face towards the west; and at the cutting of the second piece one should dance round the plant and say as many things as possible about the mysteries of love.' And that

> 'when one is cutting gladwyn (*Iris foetidissima*), one should put in its place to pay for it cakes of meal from spring-sown wheat, and that one should cut it with a two-edged sword, first making a circle round it three times, and that the first piece cut must be held up in the air whilst the rest is being cut'.

The *Historia Plantarum* includes about forty-three herbal medicinal plants. The first material mentioned is the mandrake. The leaves are mixed with barley meal and applied to wounds in the form of a poultice. The root is used as a remedy for gout and as a sedative. Other herbal materials mentioned include cinnamon, iris rhizome, germander, wood garlic (*Teucrium scordium*), mint, pomegranate, cardamom, black hellebore (*Helleborus niger*) and white hellebore (*Veratrum album*). Some of the herbs mentioned such as scammony (*Convululus scammonia*) as a purgative continued to be used until the nineteenth century. Theophrastus recommends the male fern (*Dryopteris filix-mas*) for expelling the flat worm. Male fern contains filicin (a mixture of substances), the most active of which is flavaspidic acid. Male fern was used until comparatively recently for expelling tapeworms; it has now been replaced by less toxic drugs such as niclosamide.

Nicander of Colophon

Nicander lived in the second century BCE in Clarus, in Asia Minor, which is now Ahmetbeyli in modern Turkey. His family held the priesthood of Apollo. He was a physician who also wrote a number of works in poetry and prose.[10] Two poems have come down to us – *Theriaca*, which was probably written sometime between 241 and 133 BCE, and *Alexipharmaca*.

Theriaca deals in 958 verses with venomous animals and the wounds they inflict, and is the one of the earliest available works on this topic, although it was probably based on an earlier text by the third century BCE writer Apollodorus. *Theriaca* is dedicated to Attalus III, the last king of Pergamon.

Alexipharmaca deals in 630 verses with poisons and their antidotes. The Greek word 'theriake' is derived from therion, a wild or venomous animal. A 'theriac' is an antidote to poisons.

Poisoning from venomous animals and insects was clearly a considerable risk in the Mediterranean at this time, so it was necessary to have a wide range of treatments available. *Theriaca* includes details of fumigations to expel venomous creatures, descriptions of various snakes, and herbal remedies for treatment of bites. One remedy was birthwort (*Aristolochia* species, called 'birthwort' because the herb was used to induce labour) in wine for bites from male and female vipers. The last recipe in the poem was for a general panacea which consisted of twenty-five ingredients mixed with wine to drink.

Chapter 3

Galen and Roman Medicine

The Rise of the Roman Empire

The Roman Republic is dated from the fifth to the first century BCE. During this period, it rose from a regional power to a dominant force in Italy and adjoining countries. Rome had become victorious in the Macedonian and Punic wars by the second century BCE and this was followed by the acquisition of Greece and Asia Minor. By 100 BCE Rome was a Republic and its emperors had acquired the territories of Gaul, Illyria and Spain. During the reign of the Emperor Trajan (53–117 CE), Rome controlled the Mediterranean, Germany, Britain, Asia Minor, the Caucasus and Mesopotamia. The culture, including the practice of medicine, was very significantly influenced by the Greek heritage, as we will see.

Roman Britain (55 BCE to 410 CE)

In 55 BCE, Julius Caesar invaded Britain for the first time. A second invasion followed in 54 BCE. The Romans invaded Britain again in 43 CE under the Emperor Claudius, and after battles against Caractacus in 43 CE and Boudicca in 61 CE, Britain was defeated. Julius Agricola was appointed as the Roman Imperial Governor in 77 CE. When Constantine III was named emperor in 407 CE, he withdrew the remaining Roman legion to go to Gaul. After attacks by the Saxons, Picts and Scots, Roman officials were expelled and Britain became independent in 410 CE.

Aulus Cornelius Celsus

Almost nothing is known about the life of Celsus. He lived approximately from 25 BCE to 50 CE. The writer on rhetoric (public speaking) Quintillian and Pliny the Elder refer to Celsus, so he probably lived at the time of the Emperor Tiberius. Celsus was the Roman author of an encyclopaedia on agriculture, military arts, rhetoric, philosophy, jurisprudence and medicine. Whether or not Celsus was a physician has been disputed, but his writings give clear opinions on treatments and symptoms, include information on patients he knew personally, and he was knowledgeable on the medical writers of his own age and older Greek authorities, particularly Hippocrates. The only part of the encyclopaedia that survives is the eight-part treatise *De Medicina* (On Medicine). Book Two of *De Medicina* was on general pathology, book Three on specific diseases, book Four on parts of the body, books Five and Six on pharmacology, book Seven on surgery and book Eight on orthopaedics. There are references to Hippocrates and also to Diocles of Carystus, Praxagoras, Chrysippus, Herophilus and Erasistratus in the introduction to the text. An English translation of the text by W.G. Spencer was published in 1935 by the Harvard University Press, and it is from this text that details of Celsus' medicinal practice is taken.[1] Celsus' practice was conservative, to observe and watch and let nature take its course if possible.

The text in Book Two of the 1935 English translation includes Celsus' two books on pharmacology and gives detailed information on 156 herbal drugs, about 13 minerals and various animal materials used either as medicines or excipients (substances used with a medicinally active drug as a vehicle or to modify its properties). The text states the properties of the individual medicinal substances when used as 'simples' – used on their own. It also gives a large number of detailed formulations for various types of dosage form containing a mixture of medicinal substances.[2]

The dosage forms listed includes three types of plaste*r – alipe*, which are plasters without grease, *lenia*, which are soothing, and *septa* which are exedent. Other dosage forms are *adurentia* – caustic formulations, *arida medicamenta* – dry formulations used as dusting powders, *cataplasma* – poultices, *catapotia* – pills, *collyria* – eye preparations, *emplastra* – plasters such as pitch plasters and mustard plasters, *enchrista* – liniments and liquid ointments, *gargarizationes* – gargles, *glutinalia* – glues made from animal hides and horns to agglutinate wounds, *malagma* – poultices applied to diseased areas or to draw out pus, *papyrus* – rolled papyrus used to apply a remedy to a fistula, *charta combusta* – papyrus ash used as a caustic treatment for ulcers and putrid wounds and bald patches on the head, *pastillum* – a pastille which could be taken by mouth or applied to the skin, *pessoi* – pessaries administered vaginally for diseases of women, *potio* – a draught (single doses of a medicine) and *unguenta* – ointments.

Details of the properties and uses of individual medicinal substances are given, and some examples of the use of herbal medicines are the following:

Galbanum, oak gall, was used as an astringent especially for inflamed gums.

Gentiana, gentian, was used for stomach disorders and to treat fever.

Hyoscyamus, the nightshade family, was used as a hypnotic, and its bark was used in a poultice for joints.

Lavandula, lavender, was used to treat coughs.

Ligustrum, privet, was chewed to treat gum ulcers.

Lupinum, the lupin, its seeds were used for intestinal worms, and also in plasters for eczema of the scalp.

Mandragora, the mandrake, was used as a sleep inducer, and externally in a heating plaster.

Myrrh was taken as a stimulant, and used externally to treat ear inflammations.

Scammony was used as a drastic purgative, to treat worms and for snake-bites.

Solanum, nightshade, was apparently used to soothe the insane by applying it to the scalp.

Thymum, thyme, was used as a diuretic (to increase flow of urine) and in the form of a gargle for paralysis of the tongue, and for the treatment of angina.

Terebinthus, the turpentine tree, was used to treat dyspnoea (breathlessness).

A wide range of mineral medicinal substances were also mentioned. These included various copper salts, alum, arsenic trisulfide, limestone, chalk, iron oxides and sulphate, lead sulphide (which was used to stop haemorrhages), lead acetate, sodium chloride used in enemas, antimony sulfide used as a caustic agent in plasters and eye ointments, and sulphur used as a pore opener and cleaner, and in a fomentation (cloth dressing) to relieve pain in the limbs. Litharge or lead oxide was used to make lead plasters, and lead plasters were still in use until the twentieth century.

Animal drugs mentioned include lizard dung, blood of pigeon, wood pigeon and swallow, rennet, especially that of the hare, ox-bile, eggs, cantharides (the blister beetle), salamander ash, and sheep's dung.

The text includes several antidotes for bites and stings, or for poisoning, called a 'theriac'. The word is derived from the Greek '*therion*', a wild or venomous animal. A formula given is for Mithridatium. This was one of the first theriacs, and it was developed in the first century BCE by King Mithridates of Pontus, a region on the southern shores of the Black Sea. It contained many ingredients, all mixed into a paste with honey. Mithridates took it daily, the idea being that the body would become so used to these poisons that it would build up an immunity to them and so could not be poisoned. Mithridates was defeated in battle by the Roman general Pompey in 63 BCE. According to Pliny the Elder, the recipe for Mithridatium was then taken to Rome where it was manufactured by the city's pharmacists. By the time Emperor Nero came to power in 54 CE, other ingredients had been added to the original formula. Nero was also worried about poisoning, probably with good reason since his predecessor Claudius was rumoured to have been poisoned by his wife and Nero's mother Agrippina. Nero asked his own physician Andromachus to improve the formula. This theriac, Theriacum Andromachi, contained sixty-four ingredients including viper's flesh. Andromachus also claimed that the theriac would relieve pain, weakness of the stomach, difficulty in breathing, colic, jaundice and dropsy. Both Mithridatium and Theriacum Andromachi were mentioned by Galen in his text on antidotes (see later in this chapter). Between Galen's time and the Middle Ages, Theriacum Andromachi and Mithridatium were mentioned in many medical texts ranging from those of Oribasius in his *Collectorum Medicinalum Libri* in the fourth century up until Niccolo da Salerno in his *Antidotarium Nicolai* in the twelfth century. As we shall see later, theriacs continued to be used until modern times.

Scribonius Largus

Very little is known about Scribonius Largus – his only extant work is the *Compositiones Medicamentorum* and much of what we know about him is inferred from the text.[3,4] He lived in the first century CE and died about

50 CE. His book is dedicated to Caius Julius Callistus who was a freedman of the Emperor Claudius, and who had a senior role in the court. Largus accompanied Claudius to Britain as one of his physicians during the military campaign in 43–44 CE. The book was unusual for the time, in that it was written in Latin not Greek, and is the only such text written before the fourth century. There is no English translation of the full text, but a French translation by Joëlle Jouanna-Bouchet was published in 2016 as *Scribonius Largus – Compositiones Médicales*.[3]

Largus was clearly a general practitioner as he mentions a wide social range of his patients in the text – from a perfume-seller's slave, wounded gladiators and hunters bitten by their own dogs, as well as members of the imperial court. Some of his recipes are endorsed by association with celebrated patients, for example, a toothpowder is associated with Messalina (Claudius' third wife), and eye ointments and poison antidotes with Augustus, the first emperor of the Roman Empire. He mentions some of the sources of some of his information and formulations, citing amongst others Hippocrates and Asclepiades of Bithynia (124–40 BCE), the controversial Greek physician who opposed the humoral doctrine of Hippocrates. Asclepiades believed that particles moved round the body and could cause disease. He advocated gentle treatment, exercise, food, wine, baths and massage.

The list of over 300 'simples' in the *Compositiones Medicamentorum* includes plants, minerals and materials of animal origin. The plant materials derive from flowers, stems, bark, roots etc. They range from absinth to ginger. Opium is included in the list. Many of the plant materials such as aloes, cinnamon, *Sambucus* (elderflower), fennel, ginger, gentian, hyssop, *Hedera* (ivy), *Urtica* (nettle), myrrh, peony, thyme and verbena are still used by medical herbalists and are included in medicines licensed in the UK as Traditional Herbal Remedies.

A wide range of mineral materials was mentioned, including verdigris (copper carbonate), various other copper salts, aluminium silicate, bitumen, cadmium, chalk, iron, litharge (lead oxide), molybdenum, lead, antimony and sulphur.

Animal materials mentioned include cantharides (blister beetle), deer horn, snail, crocodile testicles (recommended as a treatment for epilepsy), propolis (a form of glue and filler made by bees), bull's blood, sponge, dog's faeces, egg yolk and sow's womb.

The text of the *Compositiones* roughly follows a head to toe arrangement for the treatments, starting with headache and going through to a product for gout. Recipes 1–162 are recipes for various diseases, 163–199 are the theriacs (including Mithridatium) and other antidotes, and 200–271 are plasters and poultices.

Dosage forms included in *Compositiones* include decoctions, ointments, plasters, poultices, cerates, papers, enemas, oils, pills and fumigations.

One of the more curious of the treatments used by Largus was to use a live stingray placed on the head of the patient to treat a part of the head which is in pain. As soon as the head goes numb the fish is removed, otherwise the head may remain numb forever. The headache may be permanently cured after one treatment, but he recommended that several electric rays should be obtained in case two or three treatments are needed. This use of an electric treatment anticipates by approximately two millennia the modern therapeutic use of transcranial electrical stimulation to treat various conditions including pain.

Dioscorides of Anazarbus (*ca*. 40–90 CE)

We know little about the life of Pedanius Dioscorides. Galen mentions that he was born in Anazarbus in the Roman province of Cilicia in Asia Minor. Dioscorides himself mentions that he studied pharmacology at Tarsus, where there were teachers of pharmacology and botany. He dedicated his work, the *De Materia Medica* (On Medical Materials) to Arius, one of his teachers. *De Materia Medica* was a five-volume encyclopaedia on medicine and medicinal substances. The text of the book shows that he had travelled widely through Greek-speaking areas of the Roman Empire.[5] He was probably a military physician or attached to the Roman legions as a civilian doctor – he writes in the text of 'my soldier's life'. The book received a ringing endorsement from Galen: 'To me this book appears to be the most perfect of all treatises on materia medica'. *De Materia Medica* became well known through Latin and Arabic translations, and was in use until the nineteenth century. The original version would have been on papyrus rolls, but once these were replaced by codices (made with papyrus or parchment and similar to a modern book), they included illustrations of some of the herbs. With the development of printing there was an intensification of interest and numerous editions of Latin translations were printed from 1478 onwards. The book was also translated into Italian, French, Czech, Spanish, Dutch, and German. In 1655, an English translation was produced by John Goodyer, but not published until 1934. The most recent English translation is by Professor Lily Y. Beck, the third edition of which was published in 2017.[6]

Book I of *De Materia Medica* described spices, oils, unguents and trees. Book II described living creatures, honey, milk, animal fats, grains and vegetables; Book III dealt with roots, extracts, herbs and seeds and Book IV with the remainder of the herbs and roots. The final book, Book V, dealt with wines and minerals. The books are an assemblage of information on just over 1,000 medicinal substances – mainly plants, but about 114 were drugs from animals and 98 from minerals. For plants, the book entries consisted of the name of the plant, its habitat, botanical description, the medicinal uses, any side effects, dosages, harvesting and storage instructions, and non-medical uses. A wide variety of geographic sources are mentioned for the medicinal substances, including Libya, Illyria, Macedonia, Syria, Spain, India, Arabia, the Cycladic Islands, Crete, Turkey and Cyprus.

A wide selection of dosage forms was mentioned in the text. These included decoctions (extracts of the herb), pessaries, suppositories, *acopa* (a soothing or stimulatory liniment), *cataplasma, malagmata* (emollient poultices), *eclegmata* (thick syrups), *catapotia* (pills coated with wax or honey) and a variety of ointments and salves. Some medicines were taken in a range of dosage forms. Myrrh, for example, was used in the form of a little pill for chronic coughs, pains of the side and chest, diarrhoea and dysentery. It was smeared with a liquid astringent for armpit odour and when used as a mouthwash, it strengthened the teeth and gums. It could be dusted on head-wounds to cure them, and it filled out sores in the eyes and cleared trachoma (an infection of the inner surface of the eyelid). Eye conditions were very common, and Dioscorides lists twenty-eight different actions for ophthalmic preparations including swollen eyes, hardening of the eyes, fungus growth on the eyelids, misting of the eyes, black eyes and corrosion of the eyelids.

The text in Book IV on the opium poppy (*Papaver somniferum*) described the collection of the juice from the poppy capsule by scratching round the capsule with a knife and collecting the juice into a spoon. The use of opium as a sedative, analgesic and to treat coughs is described.

Mandragora or mandrake is also in Book IV. Dioscorides described the use of both the leaves and the juice obtained by cutting up the fleshy roots and extracting juice by putting the chopped roots into a press. Dioscorides stated that the juice boiled down with wine, then strained and stored could be used to administer 'to insomniacs, to those in much pain, and to those they wish to anaesthetise either for surgery or cauterization.' This is the first use of the term 'anaesthesia' in medicine, and it was reintroduced in the nineteenth century. Other uses of the mandrake were when compounded with ophthalmic and analgesic medicines, as a pessary to 'draw the menstrual period', and when used as a suppository it acted as a sedative. Mandrake is now known to contain a variety of alkaloids such as atropine, scopolamine, scopine, hyoscyamine and belladonnines. The properties of the mandrake root were celebrated in literature over the centuries. Shakespeare makes references to it in a number of his plays. For example:

> 'Give me to drink mandragora
> That I might sleep out this great gap of time
> My Anthony is away'
> *Anthony and Cleopatra, Act 1, Scene 5*

Book I included the willow, *Salix* species. Dioscorides listed a number of uses for willow leaves and bark. These included the use of the bark mixed with vinegar for removing warts and calluses, and in the form of a decoction for treatment of gout. It was also recommended for dandruff. It is now known that willow contains salicin which breaks down to form salicylic acid, which is still used in keratolytic preparations for warts, corns and calluses, and scaly conditions such as dandruff. Salicin when taken by mouth is an analgesic, although salicylic acid is now more commonly taken in the form of aspirin (acetylsalicylic acid) which breaks down to salicylic acid in the body.

The animal products were from a large variety of land and marine animals, fish, and birds. Following Theophrastus, Dioscorides also mentioned the use of electric rays to treat chronic head pains, and he also stated that when placed on an everted or prolapsed anus, it reverts it to its original position. Many of the animal remedies were for the treatment of bites and stings. For example, dried boar's liver ground up and mixed with wine for snakebites, and stag genitalia ground up and drunk with wine for viper bites. Included in Book II is a section on animal dungs – from cattle, sheep, pigeons, chickens, mice, dogs and lizards. Fresh human dung was recommended for plastering on wounds to keep them from inflammation and to glue them together. Lizard dung was recommended for women to achieve a healthy colouration and a glowing complexion.

The mineral medicinal substances were listed in Book V. They include various earths, ores and salts such as antimony, arsenic sulfide, copper ores and salts, iron ores and salts, litharge (lead oxide), cinnabar (mercuric sulfide), galena (lead sulfide) and sulphur. It is interesting to note the variety of mineral materials used, some of these were to become fashionable in the seventeenth century following the doctrines of Paracelsus.

Galen of Pergamum

Claudius Galenus, known in English as Galen, was born in September 129 CE at Pergamum, a Greek city in what is now eastern Turkey, then part of the imperial Roman Empire. His father was Nicon, a prominent architect and part of a wealthy family. His grandfather was also an architect. A modern biography of Galen, written by Susan P. Mattern, was published in 2013 by Oxford University Press entitled '*The Prince of Medicine: Galen in the Roman Empire*'.[7]

The temple of Asclepius, the Greek god of medicine, stood to the east of the city of Pergamum. It had been founded around 200 BCE. Asclepius was regarded as the most important god and his temple was widely known and revered.

Galen's family was wealthy and the income from the family estates enabled him to practise medicine without charging any of his patients.

His father was well-educated – Galen states that his father 'attained the height of geometry, architecture, logic, mathematics, and astronomy', and he seems to have passed on his love of learning to Galen. Nicon himself taught Galen until the age of about 14 when he became too involved in city politics.

He placed his son's philosophical education in the hands of individuals from different schools of thought – a Stoic, a Platonist, a Peripatetic and an Epicurean. Galen took up the study of medicine from the age of 16. He studied with Satyrus, a sophist. Another of his teachers was Aeschrion, an Empiric, who was very experienced in the use of medicines. Galen also mentions a teacher called Stratonicus, who introduced him to clinical practice and particularly on the importance of the relationship between physician and patient. His training would have been both intellectually based on the teachings of Hippocrates and others, and also involve practical demonstrations and hands-on clinical involvement. The practice of dissection of human corpses was forbidden, but Galen was able to gain experience with animal dissection. He also gained expertise in pharmacology from his teachers and from other local experts. His teacher Satyrus had been taught by an empiricist, Quintus. The empiricists argued that it was not necessary to know how a treatment works as long as it is effective. They emphasised the need for clinical observation of the patient and his symptoms, the effect of medicines, the body etc. This training probably caused Galen to give emphasis to case histories in his writings.

Galen's father died when Galen was 19 and not long after his father's death, Galen left Pergamum to study under Pelops in Smyrna. Pelops had been a student of Numisianus, who had himself been a student of Quintus. Galen visited patients with him, and studied anatomy, pharmacology and Hippocratic medicine. When Numisianus left for Alexandria, Galen followed him. Alexandria was another noted centre of medical education including human anatomy. Leaving Alexandria at the age of 28, Galen returned to Pergamum, where he was appointed physician to the gladiators. He served for four years and was able to devise effective treatments for wounds, suturing them and applying linen dressings soaked in wine. The alcoholic content and acidity of the wine would have been bactericidal, thus preventing infections. In 161 CE, he travelled to Rome, via Palestine and Cyprus, where he investigated some of the *materia medica* produced in places he visited during his journey.

Arriving in Rome in 162 CE, Galen set up his medical practice. He became well-known as a result of his success in treating the philosopher Eudemus, who recommended him to his friends and colleagues in the aristocracy and imperial circles. Galen also carried out public demonstrations of animal anatomical dissections with a running commentary to those interested in medicine, including his friend Flavius Boethus, a former Roman consul. The books he wrote at this time were particularly on anatomy. After four years he left Rome to return to Pergamum.

In 168 CE, Galen received a summons from the joint Roman emperors Marcus Aurelius (121–180 CE) and Lucius Verus (130–169 CE) in Aquileia. A plague, possibly smallpox, was affecting the population there and the two emperors returned to Rome. Galen became friends with Marcus Aurelius and while he was off leading a campaign to wage war against the Marcomanni in Germania, he asked Galen to look after the health of his son and heir, Commodus. During the period of the emperor's absence Galen was also busy researching and writing more books. In 176 CE, Marcus returned to Rome and Galen had an opportunity to treat him. Marcus regularly took a daily dose of theriac, prepared for him by Demetrius his physician. When Demetrius died, Galen was asked to continue to make it for him. It is clear from case histories recorded in his books that Galen was able to treat many other patients, including slaves and peasants when not working for the emperor. Marcus died in 180 CE and Galen continued to treat Commodus when he became emperor.

In 192 CE, a great fire ravaged Rome and destroyed Galen's library of the writings of earlier great physicians and much of his own writing. It also destroyed much of his stock of ingredients and medicinal products. The lost works included '*On the Composition of Drugs by Type*' which had to be rewritten. After the fire, Galen was a very productive author and wrote many more books in his last six years. He is reported to have died at the age of 70.

Galen produced more books in his lifetime than any other author in antiquity. It has been estimated that he may have written 600 treatises, but less than a third of them survive. Between 1821 and 1833, Karl Kühne published an edition of about 122 of Galen's writings – in a Latin translation of Galen's original Greek text with the Greek original and the Latin translation facing it.[8] It consisted of twenty-two volumes totalling over 20,000 pages. From the point of view of this book, some of the key texts on medicines are *De Simplicium Medicamentorum temperamentis et facultatibus* (On the Powers of Simple Drugs), *De Compositione Medicamentorum secundum locus* (On the Composition of Drugs by Part), *De Compositione Medicamentorum per genera* (On the Composition of Drugs by Type), *De Theriaca ad Pisonem* (On Theriac to Piso) and *De Antidotis* (On Antidotes).

Galen defined his theory of the properties of drugs in *On the Powers of Simple Drugs* in terms of the ideas from Hippocratic medicine: the active properties of hot and cold, the passive ones of dry and moist. Each substance is a mixture of active and passive qualities – for example, mandrake was mentioned as a material with wet and cooling properties. Substances were also graded in terms of their degree of heat or cold. Rose water is first degree cooling, opium is fourth degree cooling, and alum is third degree drying.

The first of the four books in this treatise defined Galen's theory of the four humours.

In the text of *On Food and Diet,* translated by Mark Grant, Part Two deals with '*On the Humours*'.[9] The world is made from air, fire, water and earth. Animals and humans are composed of the four humours of yellow bile, blood, phlegm and black bile. The humours are combined with heat and moisture, cold and dryness. Health is characterised by the equality and symmetry of these humours.

Books VI to XI of *On the Powers of Simple Drugs* provided a catalogue of drugs and their healing properties, with Books VI to VIII dealing with herbs and plants; Book IX with earths (such as Lemnian earth and Samian earth) and mineral medicines; and Books X and XI covering animal products, blister-beetles, excrements, and the flesh of poisonous snakes. Book X includes the *Dreckapotheke* – faeces of cows, goats, crocodiles and dogs. This treatise included 440 different plants and 250 other substances.[10] Many of the drugs were suggested as having similar actions and thus being interchangeable if one or the other was not available.

In the treatise *On the Composition of Drugs by Part*, Galen gave an analysis of the use of medicines starting from the top of the patient's head with a recipe for treating hair loss and finishing at the toe with a recipe for gout.[11] As an example, one of Galen's recipes for treating baldness contained *Euphorbia* (spurge), *Thapsia* (deadly carrot), *Laurus nobilis* (bay laurel), *Hellebore* and sulphur in a base of lion and bear fat.

The Villa Romana del Casale at Piazza Armerina in Sicily is one of the most important monuments of the Roman world. It was built in the third and fourth century CE. It covers 3,500 square metres. Throughout the villa are numerous mosaics created by North African craftsmen from Carthage (now a suburb of Tunis) in the third century CE. The corridor of the great hunt is 60 metres long and contains scenes of hunting of many wild animals. All the captured animals are shown being loaded onto carts, then onto ships to Rome. The animals depicted in the mosaics include panthers, antelopes, horses, lions and boars. An elephant being loaded onto the ship is shown in Picture 3. Readers may wonder how Galen obtained fat such as lion and bear fat: this trade in exotic animals provides part of the explanation. Lions and bears were some of the animals fought by the *venatores* (animal gladiators) in the Colosseum in Rome.

On the Composition of Drug by Type was a compendium of dosage forms and administration of medicines; it included four books on plasters, two books on multifunctional drugs, and one book on emollients, purgatives and analgesics. Some of Galen's plaster remedies were based on his experience in treating wounded gladiators at Pergamum.

The Galenic theory of the four humours can only readily be applied to simple medicines. For the compound products consisting of many components such as the theriacs, their efficacy was based on an empiricist knowledge of their usefulness based on either his own experience or the experience of other physicians, such as Dioscorides in his treatise *De Materia Medica*.

Galen was one of the most important physicians in history, and his writings and theories influenced the practice of medicine from Roman times through to the time of the Renaissance and later.

Archaeology of Roman Britain and other parts of Europe

Roman Britain (55 BCE to 410 CE) had a strong military presence as an occupying force. It would have included Greek doctors and other medical auxiliaries – *capsari* – the orderlies or wound dressers, the *medici ordinarii*, a doctor.[12] There were hospitals in the principal sites of occupation – *valetudinarii*. These would have been in charge of a junior medical officer – the *optio valetudinarii*. As well as these, there would have been root-cutters who grew and collected herbs and pharmacists who prepared the medicines. Remains of specific plants have been found from Roman Britain such as celery, poppy seeds, henbane (used as a sedative), rue, cabbage and dock. Excavations at Silchester found traces of *realgar* (arsenic sulfide), which Celsus recommended for treating wounds and ulcerations. In Neuss in Germany, part of the valetudinarium was excavated. They found examples of centaury – used for wound healing, eye conditions and a snake-bite antidote. They also found St John's Wort (*Hypericum perforatum*) used to remove bladder stones and again as an antidote. Plantain was also found – used to treat dysentery.

Artefacts found at various sites include pestles and mortars, and folding balances.[13] Stone plates have been found at Silchester, which may have been used for rolling pills. Another set of artefacts, which have been found at a number of excavation sites, are the collyrium stamps. These are small stone blocks with an inscription cut into the four edges. The inscriptions are usually names of the physician and sometimes the product. The text is in mirror form so that when it is stamped the words are the right way round. The collyria stamp blocks were used to stamp collyria – the medicinal product used as eye preparations. Eye conditions seem to have been quite common and included conjunctivitis, running eyes, scars and swellings. As well as herbs, a range of minerals were used in eye products such as copper carbonate, burnt copper, alum, lead acetate and red lead (lead oxide).

Chapter 4

Avicenna and the Arabian Period

After Galen

In the fourth century CE, the Roman Empire was divided into the Greek East and the Latin West. Constantine reorganised the empire making Constantinople (now Istanbul) his new capital and legalising Christianity. The Eastern Roman Empire was known as Byzantium. When the Western Roman Empire became fragmented and fell in the fifth century, Byzantium survived and flourished. The teachings of Hippocrates and Galen were preserved by a series of Byzantine physicians. These included Oribasius, Aetius of Amida, Alexander of Tralles and Paulus Aegetina.

The Greek physician and writer Oribasius was born in Pergamum in about 320 CE. He studied medicine at the medical school at Alexandria under Zeno of Cyprus.[1] He became the personal friend and physician to the Roman Emperor Julian. After Julian died, he was banished to foreign courts but recalled by the Emperor Valens. His main books were a collection of excerpts from Galen, and the *Collectiones medicae*, a compilation of excerpts from earlier medical writers and from his contemporaries. Oribasius died in about 400 CE.

Aetius of Amida (*ca.* mid-fifth century to mid-sixth century CE) was a Byzantine physician. He was a Christian. His major work was his *Sixteen Books on Medicine* which is a compilation of work from earlier writers such as Oribasius and Galen.

Alexander of Tralles (*ca.* 525 CE–*ca.* 605 CE) practised as a physician in the reign of the Emperor Justinian I (527–565 CE).[2] He came from the city of Tralles in Asia Minor, the son of a physician. His main book is the *Therapeutics* and is a head to toe compendium of diagnosis and treatments for patients.[3] It is partly a compilation of earlier authors, but it includes recipes drawn from his own clinical experience.

Paulus Aegetina (*ca*. 625–690 CE) was born on the island of Aegina, an island south-west of Piraeus, the main port of Athens.[4] He studied at Alexandria, and travelled widely. His main work is the *Medical Compendium in Seven Books* which is a compilation of the work of earlier authors including Aetius of Amida. An English translation of his book by Francis Adams was published by the Sydenham Press in 1844, entitled *The seven books of Paulus Aegina, Volumes I–III*.[1] Paulus recommended the use of frankincense, myrrh, cooked honey and egg white as astringents, and verdigris, pine resin, turpentine, and raw honey to cleanse wounds.

Nestorius was Archbishop of Constantinople from 428 to 431 CE, when he was condemned for heresy by the Council of Ephesus. He retired to his former monastery near Antioch. In 435 CE, he was sent into exile in Egypt. The Nestorians, the followers of Nestorius, fled firstly to Edessa in Asia Minor then to Jundishapur in Persia (modern Iran), where a medical school was established which became the most important centre in the ancient world. There the works of Hippocrates, Galen, Dioscorides, Oribasius and Paulus Aegetina were translated into Syriac. At this medical school, Greek medicine was combined with that from Persia and India.

The Rise of Islam and the Islamic Golden Age

The Arab conquests and the establishment of an Islamic empire began with the prophet Muhammad in the seventh century. In a century of rapid expansion, the empire stretched from India to the borders of China, and included the Middle East, North Africa and parts of Sicily and Spain. Much of this expansion was at the expense of the Byzantine Empire. After Muhammad's death in 632 CE, these empires were ruled by the Rashdun and later the Umayyad caliphates.

Islamic influence originated in the city of Baghdad, which was built by Caliph Al-Mansur in 762 CE. This started the Abbasid Caliphate. Baghdad contained citizens of many races and considerable effort was given to science and the collection and translation of Greek and other literature. In 830 CE, the House of Wisdom was set up to translate and to house imported scientific books.

Abu Zakariya Yuhanna Ibn Masawaih (777–857 CE) is better known by his Western name of Mesue or Mesue Senior. A famous clinician and authority on Galen, he came from Jundishapur to Baghdad to study medicine and was appointed director of a hospital in Baghdad. His student, Hunayn ibn Ishāq ali-Ibādī (808–873 CE), otherwise known in Latin as Johannitius, was born near Baghdad in Iraq. He was a Nestorian Christian who studied medicine at the Jundishapur school and then in Alexandria before being appointed by the Caliph al Mutawakkil to the post of chief physician to the court. He travelled widely in Syria, Egypt and Palestine seeking out Greek manuscripts which he, his son Ishaq, and his nephew Hubaysh then translated into Syriac and Arabic. With his pupils, he translated the works of Aristotle, Hippocrates, Dioscorides, Oribasius, and Paul of Aegetina.

Mohammed Ibn Zakariya Al-Razi (865–925 CE), better known by his Latin name of Rhazes, was born in Rey, near Tehran in Iran.[5] He was interested in music in his early life – he played the lute. But he was unable to make a living from music so switched to alchemy, playing a part in some of the discoveries in chemistry. He is credited with the purification of alcohol and the discovery of sulphuric acid. He wrote some twenty books on chemistry. At the age of 30 he began his medical studies. After these, he was appointed as head of the Muqtadi hospital. He was also asked by the Caliph to design a new hospital. He was a prolific writer, including references to Galen, but criticising him when Galen's views did not correspond to his own clinical observations – one of his books was *Shukuk Ala Alinusor* (Doubts about Galen). Amongst his most well-known books was the *Kitab al-Hawi fi al-Tibb*, known in Latin as the *Liber Continens*, or *The Virtuous Life* in English. This was a twenty-three-volume encyclopaedia on the causes of diseases. One of its volumes is on pharmacology. Amongst his achievements, he described for the first-time smallpox and measles and recommended simple, rather than complex remedies. His investigations included animal studies on new medicines to determine their effects and toxicity before he gave them to his patients. An example of this was giving mercury to monkeys to test its safety. In contrast to the Latin tradition, Rhazes was meticulous in his recording, interpreting and classifying his clinical observations in the form of case histories. This established a more rigorous approach to medicine and enabled differential diagnosis of diseases.

Abu Ali Al Hussein Ibn Abdullah Ibn Sina (980–1037 CE), known as Avicenna, was born in Afshaneh, Bokhara, then part of Persia, but now in Uzbekistan.[6, 7, 8] He was a child prodigy and at the age of 14 he began studies in natural sciences and medicine, before qualifying as a physician at the age of 18 and beginning to practise. His professional practice was with a number of the emirs in Turkmenistan and Persia, but he led a rather troubled life. During all of his life he was a prolific writer on philosophy, metaphysics, theology, alchemy and medicine. He wrote almost 450 treatises. His work *Kitab al-Qanun fi'l tibb* (The Canon of Medicine) was one of the major textbooks used in medicine in the Islamic world and Europe up until the eighteenth century. Volume I was on the basics of medicine, Volume II on pharmacology, Volume III was on disease diagnosis and treatment, Volume IV was on diseases affecting the whole body, while Volume V was on poisoning and toxicology. Volume II of the *Canon* discussed rules for testing medicines and was a landmark in the development of a scientific method for such testing. Avicenna emphasised the need for experimentation.

A translation of Volume I of the *Canon* by O. Cameron Gruner was published in 1970 under the title of *A Treatise on The Canon of Medicine of Avicenna Incorporating a Translation of the First Book.*[9] The Appendix to this translation is an alphabetical list of the simples (single drugs) mentioned in Volume II of the *Canon.* There are approximately 231 medicines mentioned, mostly herbal such as acacia, aconite root, aloes, anise, asafoetida, barberry bark, black hellebore, hemlock, hops, parsley, pepper, nigella, valerian root, wormwood, and ginger. It includes some animal products such as beeswax, bovine bile, bone marrow, buttermilk, honey, lard and whey. The mineral materials include antimony, borax, verdigris (copper carbonate), creosote, gold, green vitriol (ferrous sulphate), iron rust, kaolin, mercury, naphtha, nitre, liquid tar, silver, salt (sodium chloride), sulphur, lead carbonate, and impure zinc oxide.

A variety of dosage forms was mentioned by Avicenna in the *Canon* – including syrups, pills, smoke for inhalation, enemas and ear drops. Opium preparations were applied orally, topically, rectally and intranasally (into the nose). In the chapter entitled *Afion* in Volume II of the *Canon,* Avicenna reviewed opium and its preparation.[10] He recommended its use both as a single ingredient medicine and in combination, for headache, arthralgia, toothache, in labour, and bladder pain. As well as mentioning its use orally or rectally to treat insomnia, he also mentioned its application to treat severe cough.

The Arab healers had access to a variety of medicinal preparations and introduced many into medicine, such as those from India with which they had trade relations. They used aloes (as a purgative), henbane, ginger, saffron, cinnamon, senna etc. Senna is a mild laxative and was available for use instead of the strong purgatives used previously.

The Islamic civilisation eventually went into decline after the invasion in the thirteenth century by Genghis Khan and his Mongol hordes, who entered the Arab peninsula and destroyed universities and killed the learned scholars. The Grand Library of Baghdad was destroyed and with it its books and documents on science and medicine. Survivors of the massacre asserted that the river Tigris ran black from the ink of the books flung into it.

Chapter 5

Medicines in the Medieval World

The Medieval Period

In European history, the Medieval Period began with the fall of the Western Roman Empire and lasted from the fifth to the fifteenth century. The Roman Empire was at its peak during the second century CE but after that was a period of decline of Roman control. In 286 CE, the Emperor Diocletian split the empire into eastern and western halves. The western empire was beset with difficulties as internal problems allowed invaders such as the Goths and Visigoths to encroach. Christianity gradually spread through the empire from the second to the fifth centuries. The Migration Period was between 300 CE and 700, when various populations moved across Europe. The Angles, Saxons and Jutes settled in Britain. In the 430s, the Huns began invasions into Italy, Gaul and the Balkans. New societies were established as new people and leaders filled the gap left by Roman centralised government. Vernacular languages developed from Latin.

The Anglo-Saxon settlement of Britain changed the language and culture from Romano-British to Germanic, with Germanic speakers developing an identity as Anglo-Saxons. The various tribes who invaded Britain brought with them their own *materia medica* and folklore. However, the ecclesiastical structure of the Roman Empire survived the invasions and movements of people and in 597 CE, Pope Gregory the Great sent a mission to convert the Anglo-Saxons to Christianity. This period saw the rise of monasteries, acting as outposts of education and literacy, and preserving many of the manuscripts of earlier classic Latin texts. With the conversion to Christianity, attempts were made to reconcile the pagan rites and superstitions with the new religion – what is called 'syncretism'.

Anglo-Saxon Medicine

Boniface was born sometime between 675 and 680 CE. He went to school at the monastery in Exeter. He joined the Benedictine monastic community at Nursling near Winchester, where he studied Latin grammar and verse. In 716, he was sent to Friesland in Holland and in 718 to Germany, where he became Archbishop of Cologne in 745. On 5 June 754 he was murdered by a 'heathen band'. He is called the Apostle of Germany and was for a time the patron saint of England. Our interest in him is that from his letters, we know that he received letters from England asking for books on simples (herbal and other medicinal substances), and complaining that it was difficult to obtain some of those mentioned in the texts they already possessed. Thus, we know that books on medicinal drugs were available in England as early as the eighth century.

The oldest surviving book on medicine in Old English is a manuscript written in Winchester in about 950.[2] It is a copy of a book written about fifty years earlier, during the reign of Alfred the Great (who lived from 871–899 CE). It is in three parts. The first two parts are called *The Leechbook of Bald*. Bald was the owner of the book and he ordered Cild to write it. The first part of *The Leechbook of Bald* dealt with skin conditions, the second part with internal ones. The third part of the book, *Leechbook III*, is shorter and less sophisticated and belonged to an older tradition of folk remedies and herbal medicine. The *Leechbook* is felt to be an integration of native folk medicine with earlier medical texts in Latin. It has been suggested that the author may have been conversant with the treatises of Alexander of Trelles and Paul of Aegina. The word 'leech' is the name of the Anglo-Saxon medical practitioner, and derives from the word 'laece' meaning to heal. A leech almost certainly prepared his own remedies. A facsimile page from the *Leechbook* is shown in Picture 4.

There are a large number of medicines described in *Leechbook I* and *II*. In *Leechbook I* there are about 300 medicines of which 80 per cent are of plant origin. *Leechbook II* contains more than 250, of which 70 per cent are of plant origin. The most common plants used were ivy, coriander, smallage (wild celery), pennyroyal, hindheal (possibly wood sage), centaury, radish, barley, oak, carline thistle, celandine, yarrow, horehound, onions, garlic, fennel, rue, lupin, plantain, pepper, wormwood, and betony.

Materials of animal origin included the fat and flesh of various mammals, birds and invertebrates. Animal products included butter, milk, cheese, eggs, wool, hair, bone, blood, urine and faeces. The most common urine products used were from goats, cattle, dogs, doves, sheep, cattle, and pigs. Fat from sheep, cattle, goats, pigs, horses, bears, hens, geese and deer were used. Mineral materials included iron and copper salts, mercury, sulphur, tin, salt, nitre, ammoniac and various stones. Some of these ingredients would have been imported, perhaps by Arab traders, for example, pepper and aloes. Details are included in the book of a recommendation from the Patriarch of Jerusalem to King Alfred for a prescription containing scammony (a Mediterranean plant of the convolvulus family whose roots were used as a strong purgative), tragacanth gum, aloes (which came from India, Arabia or Asia) and galbanum gum resin (which came from Syria). Even if these ingredients were available in England at the time, they would have been rare and very expensive.

The *Lacnunga* is a collection of Anglo-Saxon medical texts and charms (incantations against diseases which seem to be of an earlier pagan origin).[3] It was written in a mixture of Latin and Old English. The word *Lacnunga* does not appear in the text of the collection, but it is an Old English word meaning 'remedies'. The main section of the manuscript dates from the late tenth to mid-eleventh century CE, although some of the text is older. Most of the recipes in the *Lacnunga* are herbal salves (ointments and lotions) or poultices, drinks, and soups. The book included a total of about ninety remedies for self-administration, remedies for administration by a healer, veterinary preparations and miscellaneous products which are not specifically for self-administration or use by a healer. Plant materials used included hellebore, groundsel, watercress, beetroot, aloe, pepper, wild lettuce, dill, wormwood, pennyroyal, lovage, lily, wild celery, teasel, rue, thistle, agrimony, betony, fennel, sage, savine (an evergreen juniper plant), tansy, comfrey roots, chervil, mugwort, marjoram, orache, valerian, marshmallow, hazel, couch-grass, mint, chickweed, costmary (an aromatic herb of the aster family), walnut leaves, plantain, water lily, sweet cicely, barley meal, centaury, radish, dock, celandine, madder root, henbane, ground ivy, lupin, yarrow, wood sorrel, willow bark, garlic, frankincense, leek, house leek, elder-bark, shallot, white horehound, sedge, and yellow iris. Animal materials included roe deer marrow, fox fat, hind's milk, cow's urine, hart's fat, goat's fat, bull's fat, ram's fat, calf dung, and cow dung.

Some of the recipes appear to have a psychological function – for example, one of the recipes is a holy drink for fever and all the temptations of the Devil; another is a holy salve. A typical recipe is for the 'best eye-salve' – take bumble-bee's honey and fox's fat and roe-deer's marrow, mix together. The recipe for green salve contained thirty-seven herbs mixed in oil and wax.

An herbal text in Latin was produced in the fourth century. Its authorship was originally attributed to Apuleius of Madura, a Roman poet and philosopher, but this is now doubted. It is known as the *Herbarium of Pseudo-Apuleius*. The oldest surviving version of the text is one in Leiden from the sixth century, but many other copies exist. The text is based on Pliny's *Historia Naturalis* and Dioscorides' *De Materia Medica*. It contained approximately 130 chapters, each dealing with a medicinal plant. Each chapter included a list of the conditions it would treat and recipes incorporating the herb. The book was widely distributed through the network of Benedictine monasteries, which were a major source of information on healing, on cultivation of herbs and the use of medicinal herbs.

The Old English Herbarium is an Anglo-Saxon medical text produced in about 1000 CE and is a translation of the *Herbarium of Pseudo-Apuleius*. There are three versions of the *Herbarium* held in the British Library and one at the Bodleian. A translation of the text into modern English was produced in 2002 by Anne van Arsdall.[4] The translated text includes 185 herbs and the indications for each one. For example, fennel was indicated for coughs and shortness of breath and for bladder pain. Some of the herbs, such as the castor oil plant, *Ricinus communis*, were of Mediterranean origin. However, since between the ninth and thirteenth centuries the climate of England went through what is called the Medieval Warm Period, it is possible that some Mediterranean herbs could have been grown locally.

The Salerno School of Medicine

Benedict of Nursia (480–543 or 547 CE) founded twelve monastic communities at Subacio, Lazio, which is about 40 miles from Rome. He then moved to Monte Cassino in the hills of southern Italy. [5,6] Monte Cassino was sacked by the Lombards in 570 CE, and the monks moved to Rome. This was probably the reason for the expansion of Benedictine monasticism. The south of Italy was a stronghold for the Benedictines with monasteries at Benevento, Gaeta, Capua, Sorrento, Amalfi and Salerno, as well as the great monastery at Monte Cassino. In 597 CE, Pope Gregory sent Augustine to England with forty monks to convert the pagan Anglo-Saxons to Christianity. He instituted a base in Canterbury and a network of Benedictine monasteries was established across the country. England was the site of the first national Benedictine congregations.

In the south of Italy with Benevento and Monte Cassino, a type of Latin learning was established using a form of Latin script known as Beneventan, with texts of Greek books by Dioscorides, Apuleius and Oribasius translated into this script. From the first half of the eleventh century, a group of physicians was established at Salerno, the ancient sea-port near Naples. They had access to the earlier Latin translations from Greek. One Salernitan physician and writer was Alfanus (1015–1085), who lived at Monte Cassino. He became the abbot at Salerno and finally Archbishop of Salerno. He was a skilled translator from Arabic to Latin. The School at Salerno was at its most productive from the eleventh to the thirteenth centuries when it produced translations of works by Pliny, Dioscorides, and others. A key figure in this activity was Constantine the African.

The only account of the life of Constantine is from Peter the Deacon, the librarian at Monte Cassino, and he is known to have forged some records. According to this account, which may not be entirely reliable, Constantine was born in Carthage and studied grammar, medicine, geometry, music and astronomy in Babylon. After this, he journeyed first to India and then Egypt. He returned to Carthage but he was threatened, had to leave and travelled to Monte Cassino and became a monk. His translations were mainly of Arab texts of the Egyptian Abu Jackub Ishak ben Soleiman, otherwise known as Isaac Judaeus. The works were mainly versions of various texts of Galen. Constantine died in about 1087.

Towards the end of the twelfth century, the School at Salerno became a training centre for physicians. It had its own teaching curriculum with works such as the *Isagoge* by Johannitius, and texts from Hippocrates and

Galen. Two influential new texts were produced – the *Antidotarium of Nicolaus Salernitanus* and the *Antidotarium of Matthaeus Platearius*. The oldest version of the *Antidotarium of Nicolaus Salernitanus* contained 115 prescriptions in alphabetical order, but later versions of the text contain up to 175 recipes. Some of the compositions in the Nicolaus of Salerno text were still in use centuries later. The book was used as a textbook in the University of Paris by 1270 and in Montpellier by 1390. It was an official guide in Naples and Sicily and was translated into Spanish, Arabic, and Dutch.

Toledo

Gerard of Cremona (*ca*. 1114–1187 CE) was born in Cremona in northern Italy. Dissatisfied with his Italian teachers, Gerard moved to Toledo, which had been a provincial capital in the Islamic Caliphate of Cordoba and had remained a seat of learning.[7] It had been reclaimed from the Moors by Alfonso VI of Castile in 1085. There Gerard learned Arabic, initially so that he could read Ptolemy's *Almagest*. He became a translator of scientific books from Arabic into Latin. Confusingly, there is another, later, Gerard of Cremona in the thirteenth century, who may have been the author of the translations of medical works such as Avicenna's *Canon* and some of the works of Galen. Gerard's translation of the *Canon* became part of the medical training curriculum at the universities of Bologna, Montpellier in France and Leuven in Belgium.

Physicians in English Religious Houses

Before the Norman Conquest in 1066, certain of the Norman monasteries were centres of study in medicine, and the school at Chartres became well known. The knowledge from Salerno was merged with Norman medicine.[8]

A succession of Norman physicians came to England, including Baldwin, a monk from St Denis who came to be the physician to Edward the Confessor (1003–1066). Edward rebuilt the priory at Deerhurst in Gloucestershire and Baldwin became its first prior. In 1065, he was asked to treat Abbot Leofstan at Bury St Edmunds, and when Leofstan died

Baldwin succeeded as abbot. He continued to be the physician to King Harold during his brief reign in 1066 and subsequently to William the Conqueror, and to William II, the third son of William the Conqueror, king from 1087 to 1100. Baldwin died in 1097.

Faritius was a native of Tuscany and possibly studied at Salerno. He was the most famous physician in England during the reign of Henry I. He died in 1117.

St Alban, a Romano-British citizen was killed for his faith in the third century CE, and became the first British martyr. Churches were established over the site of his grave, and eventually the Abbey Church of St Albans was built. The life of the abbey attracted skilled physicians. Warin (or Guarin) was trained in medicine at Salerno with this brother Matthew, before he became a monk at St Albans and later abbot in 1183. He presided over the medical care of sick monks in the infirmary and also leprous monks and nuns. He died in 1195. The next abbot (from 1195 to 1214) was John of Cella, who had studied medicine in Paris. Two other physicians were on the rolls of the abbey: Master Reginald in the thirteenth century and Thomas who was the personal physician to the Earl of Arundel.

The treatment of persons of rank and influence was not without its problems, as any serious mistake could lead to the death of the patient. This would embarrass the church. There were a series of papal and conciliar pronouncements on the practice of medicine, including the Clermont Council of 1130, which cautioned against the practice of medicine 'for the purposes of temporal gain' and the Council of Tours in 1163, which prohibited monks from practising medicine.

Early hospitals and universities

There are some records of hospitals being established after the Norman Conquest in 1066.[7] In 1077, Archbishop LeFranc established a hospital in Canterbury with two sections, one for men and the other for women, and with separate wooden huts for the lepers. In or near Oxford, a hospital for lepers was founded in 1126 by Henry I. In 1158, a hospital was established in St Giles, Cold Norton near the Priory, and Oxford got a further hospital in 1180, when Henry II founded the St John the

Baptist Hospital in the town. There was a proliferation of monastic hospitals with over 250 existing by 1200 and over 500 by 1350. Many of the hospitals were lazar houses to house lepers, who were isolated from the community, made to wear special clothes and to ring a bell to advertise their proximity. St Thomas' Hospital was started in 1173 as an annex to an infirmary attached to the Priory of St Mary Overie (later to become Southwark Cathedral). St Bartholomew's Hospital was founded in 1123 by Rahere, who was possibly a court jester to Henry I, and later given to the City of London by Henry VIII.

Medicine was being studied in Montpellier by the twelfth century. There were close links to England at a time when the English held Gascony. Amongst its famous teachers and students were Gilbertus Anglicus (Gilbert the Englishman), Raymond Lully of Majorca, Arnold of Villanova, and Bernard de Gordon.

Gilbertus Anglicus was a thirteenth-century physician who was physician to Archbishop Hugo Walter in England, before returning to the Continent.[10] He wrote the *Compendium Medicinae*, a practical encyclopaedia of medicine and surgery in seven books. It included details of about 400 medicinal substances, and a variety of dosage forms – enemas, ointments, pills, electuaries, suppositories, fumigations, plasters and syrups. He regarded all diseases as being hot, cold, moist or dry. A hot headache with a fast pulse was treated with cold remedies, and by avoiding baths and any sexual activity.

Arnold of Villanova (*ca*. 1240–1311) studied medicine and theology at Montpellier until 1260.[11] He then wandered through Italy, Catalonia and France as part doctor, part ambassador. From 1281, he was the personal physician to Peter III of Aragon. His philosophical and religious works were controversial – he claimed that the world would end in 1378 and that the Antichrist would come. Condemned as a heretic, he was imprisoned in Paris on two occasions. He returned to Montpellier and became its master between 1291 and 1299. He was famous as a physician: amongst his patients were three kings and three popes. He became ambassador to James II of Sicily and Aragon, then was called back to Avignon to treat Pope Clement V. A shipwreck in 1311 claimed his life. It is believed that he was the first physician to use alcohol as an antiseptic.

Bernard de Gordon was probably French, the name de Gordon designating the place in France where he originated.[12] In about 1285 he became master in the Montpellier faculty of medicine and it appears he spent his entire career in the city. His most important book was the *Lilium medicinae*, published in 1303. It was divided into 163 chapters dealing with individual diseases including plague, tuberculosis, scabies, epilepsy and leprosy. The authorities he cited were mainly classical, with references to Galen and Hippocrates outnumbering those of Avicenna and other Arab writers. This work was soon copied all over Europe, and printed in Naples in 1480 and in Lyon in 1491.

Universities were created in Italy, Spain, England and France. Oxford University grew rapidly from 1167, after Henry II banned English students from attending the University of Paris. One of the first known lecturers in medicine in Oxford was Nicholas Tingewick who cured Edward I (1239–1307) when he became ill in Carlisle. Amongst the medicines used by Tingewick were oil of turpentine, aromatic flowers for baths, electuaries for digestive disorders (powdered medicine mixed into a paste with syrup or honey), plasters and ointments, oils of wheat, ash and bay, Damascus rose water, wine of pomegranates, and remedies from pearls and coral. The apothecaries bill for the king's treatment was £134 16s 4d.

Spicers and Apothecaries

As mentioned in Chapter 1, an ostracon (pottery fragment used for writing) from Deir el-Medina in Egypt from 1244 BCE during the reign of Ramses II recorded absences from work. Pa-hery-podjet was recorded as absent 'on certain days for the preparation of medicines.' Thus, Pa-hery-podjet may be the name of the first recorded apothecary/pharmacist from antiquity.

In the Arab world, pharmacies became established as early as the ninth century. By the eleventh century, public shops were becoming established in Southern Italy and France where merchants would sell medicinal preparations, herbs and perfumes. In France they were known as épiciers (spicers). Trease[13] has documented various spicers found in both London and the provinces in the late twelfth century. In 1207, a certain

William was appointed as *speciarius regis* (the king's spicer) to King John (1166–1216).

Frederick II (1194–1250) was King of Sicily from 1198, King of Germany from 1212, King of Italy and Holy Roman Emperor from 1220 and King of Jerusalem from 1225. His mother, Constance, was Queen of Sicily and his father was Henry VI (Holy Roman Emperor). Frederick's reign saw the Holy Roman Empire achieve its greatest territorial extent. His 1231 Edict of Salerno (sometimes called the 'Constitution of Salerno') made the first legal separation of the occupations of physician and apothecary. Physicians were forbidden to also work as pharmacists and the prices of some medicines were fixed. This became a model for regulation of the practice of pharmacy throughout Europe.

Chaucer

Geoffrey Chaucer (1343–1400) is considered the greatest English writer and poet of the Middle Ages. His book, *The Canterbury Tales*, is a collection of twenty-four stories about the lives of a group of pilgrims on their way to the shrine of St Thomas Becket at Canterbury Cathedral. One of the pilgrims is the Physician, and he has his own section in the Prologue. An extract reads as follows, in Frank Ernest Hill's 1936 version for modern readers.[14]

> He was a perfect doctor and a true.
> The cause once known, the root of his disease,
> At once he gave the patient remedies.
> For he would have at call apothecaries
> Ready to send him drugs and lectuaries,
> For each of them from the other profit won;
> Their friendship was not something just begun.
> The ancient Aesculapius he knew,
> Haly and Rufus and Serapion too,
> Avicenna, and great Hippocrates,
> Rhazes and Galen, Dioscorides.
> Averroes, Damascene, and Constantine
> Bernard and Gatisden and Gilbertine.

From Chaucer's text we are able to identify some of the key books and the names of the great physicians with which a fourteenth-century physician might be familiar. These are Haly Abbas, whose book *Liber Regalis* was used in Arab countries and was also popular in Europe; Rufus of Ephesus (first century CE) who wrote on dietetics, pathology, anatomy, and patient care; Serapion (of the School of Jundishapur); Avicenna, the author of the *Canon*; Hippocrates; Rhazes; Galen; Dioscorides; Averroes; John of Damascus or Mesuë who translated Greek documents in the ninth century; Constantine the African; Bernard de Gordon who wrote *Lilium Medicinae*; John of Gaddesden who wrote the *Rosa Anglica*; and Gilbertus Anglicus who wrote the *Compendium Medicinae*.

John of Gaddesden (1280–1361) was named after the village of Gaddesden in Hertfordshire where he had a house.[15] He was trained as a physician at the University of Oxford and practised in London. In about 1307, his treatise on medicine *Rosa Anglica* was published. It includes advice on fevers and covers diseases starting at the head and ending with antidotes and remedies. The book includes many quotations from Galen, Dioscorides, Rufus of Ephesus, Haly Abbas, Serapion, Rhazes, Avicenna, John of Damascus, Gilbertus Anglicus, and Isaac. So many of the distinguished physicians quoted are included in the list in Chaucer's *Prologue* to the *Canterbury Tales* that many writers have suggested that John of Gaddesden inspired the portrait of the Physician printed in Chaucer's poem.

Medical and pharmaceutical practitioners

Town records from the fourteenth century in England, which existed in all major cities, show the existence of spicers, spicer-apothecaries and apothecaries.[16] Two guilds (trade group) or 'mysteries' were formed – the Mystery of Grocers and the Mystery of Apothecaries. In London, the grocers and pepperers were all centred within a small area of Cheapside and they came together in a trade group in 1345 called the Fraternity of St Anthony. The term 'grocer' was derived from a new and fashionable word in the English vocabulary, 'grosser', referring to a particular type of merchant who traded in a variety of merchandise. By 1375, the term 'grocer' was well established and they included the apothecaries amongst their number. There was no official formulary for apothecaries to use, but the *Antidotarium Nicolai* was probably widely used.

The apothecary William Waddesdon supplied medicines to Richard II and Thomas Horton was spicer to the royal household in 1394. In the fifteenth century, Richard Hakely and William Godfrey were apothecaries to Henry VI, who was king of England from 1422 to 1461 and again from 1470 to 1471. John Clerc was apothecary to Edward IV who was king from 4 March 1461 to 3 October 1470, and again from 11 April 1471 until his death in 1483. In London, the apothecaries were all members of the Grocer's Company.

However, there was little regulation of the practice of medicine in the fifteenth century and medical treatment was provided by a variety of practitioners – physicians, apothecary-surgeons, barbers and quacks. In 1421, Parliament authorised the Privy Council to make regulations about medical practice to try to restrict it to those who had adequate training. This was the start of formal regulation. But it would not be until the next century that real progress would be achieved.

Early formularies

All of the treatises on medicine mentioned so far in this book were produced by individual physicians based on tradition and their own experience. The texts were based on the ideas of the early physicians such as Hippocrates, Dioscorides and most influential of all, Galen. The original manuscripts of these authors were translated into Arabic by Rhazes and Avicenna and the medicines used were those from Greek medicine supplemented by drugs from India and elsewhere imported by the Arab traders. From the translators in Salerno and Toledo, the Arab texts were translated into Latin and as a result, Greek medicine once again became available to European practitioners.

In 1439, Johannes Gutenberg in Mainz in Germany developed movable type printing. He also invented an oil-based printing ink that was more durable. In just over ten years, printing began across Europe. In 1476, William Caxton set up a printing press in England. This new method of printing revolutionised book production and meant many more copies could be produced and sold to a wider audience than when production was by scribes copying by hand in a scriptorium. As we shall see, the next century saw the beginnings of a scientific revolution of ideas in medicine, and these ideas were rapidly spread in the new printed books.

Chapter 6

Paracelsus, the Alchemists, and their Legacy

Alchemy and the Alchemical Tradition

Alchemy is a tradition of thought that dates back several millennia. In the eighth century, Jabir ibn Hayyān (Geberus) used his observations in his chemical laboratory to introduce some new ideas into the Greek and Egyptian alchemical traditions. Jabir believed that there were eight elements – the classical Greek ones of air, earth, fire, water and aether but also sulphur, mercury and salt.[1]

In the 1140s, Robert of Chester was living in Spain and translated two books from Arabic into Latin. These were the first books in Europe on alchemy: the *Liber de compositione alchimiae (*the Arabic *Book of the Composition of Alchemy)*, translated in 1144, and the *Liber algebrae et almucabola*, the book by Al-Khwārizmī, about algebra, translated in 1145.

Paul of Taranto was a thirteenth-century Franciscan alchemist and author from Italy. His book, the *Summa Perfectionis,* provided a summary of alchemical practice and theory through the medieval and renaissance periods. It included practical chemical operations alongside the alchemical theory. By the end of the thirteenth century, alchemy had developed into a fairly structured system of belief. Adherents believed in theories of Hermes Trismegistus. The alchemists practised their art: they actively experimented with chemicals and made observations and derived theories about how the universe operated. Thus, alchemy was a system of thought that represented an attempt to discover the relationship of man to the cosmos and to exploit that relationship to his benefit.

The series of tracts called the *Corpus Hermeticum* was written by unknown authors in Egypt sometime before the third century CE.[2] They were attributed to a mythic figure called Hermes Trismegistus. These treatises were collected into a single volume and a copy came into the hands of Lorenzo de Medici's agents. Marsilio Ficino (1433–1499), the head of the Academy in Florence, translated the text into Latin.

His translation was first printed in 1463 and many more times over the next century. Adoption of ideas in the *Corpus Hermeticum* was part of an attempt to establish alchemy as an acceptable part of Christian beliefs. As we shall see later in this chapter, the physicians who also practised alchemy were part of a movement that challenged the orthodoxies of Hippocrates, Dioscorides and Galen. The early alchemists with their experimentation were part of the development of chemistry. Early modern alchemists included van Helmont, Robert Boyle and Isaac Newton.

The Reformation

Martin Luther (1483–1546) was a German professor of theology, composer, priest and monk. According to one account, Luther nailed his *Ninety-five Theses* to the door of All Saints' Church in Wittenberg on 31 October 1517. Another account has Luther writing to his bishop, Albrecht von Brandenburg, protesting about the sale of indulgences, and proposing a debate on the issue. In the Catholic Church, indulgences could be purchased in order to reduce the punishment you were owed for your sins. By buying an indulgence for yourself, you would go to heaven and not burn in hell. His letter to his bishop included a copy of his *Disputation of Martin Luther on the Power and Efficacy of Indulgences*, which came to be known as the *Ninety-five Theses*. His proposal for a debate was not in itself a revolutionary act, but his theses did not stay nailed to the church door – copies were soon printed and distributed widely in Germany and Switzerland, and translated and published elsewhere. The Protestant Reformation against the Catholic Church might never have taken place without the access to printing by the followers of Luther.

Phillipus Aureolus Theophrastus Bombastus von Hohenheim

Theophrastus von Hohenheim (1493–1541) is now more familiarly known as Paracelsus. He is one of the most controversial figures in the history of medicine: a social reformer, an alchemist, and not least, a substantial thorn in the side of the medical establishment of his time.[3] But his ideas have influenced the development of both medicine and chemistry.

He was born in Egg, a village close to Einsiedeln, in the Swiss canton of Schwyz. His father Wilhelm was a medical graduate of the University of Tübingen, and was the physician to the town of Einsiedeln and its hospital. Wilhelm's wife died early in their marriage and he was left to take care of the young Theophrastus. But the times were troubled because the Swiss cantons were trying to establish their independence from the Holy Roman Emperor Maximilian in Germany. In 1499, the Swabian War started, with the Swiss fighting the southern German states. As German immigrants, the Hohenheim family had to leave Einsiedeln.

They re-established themselves in Villach in Carinthia, which is now the most southern state in the Alps in modern Austria. Theophrastus was sent to the Benedictine monastery schools at St Paul's in Klagenfurt and St Andrae in Lavantal. In Lavantal, one of his teachers was Bishop Eberhart Baumgarten, who was an alchemist, and who instructed Theophrastus about metals and their transformations.

At the age of 14, Theophrastus went to university. His intention was to study medicine like his father. But students had to first study to obtain a bachelor degree before proceeding to learn medicine. Theophrastus studied at a number of universities – firstly at Tübingen like his father, then to Heidelberg, Mainz, Treves, Cologne and Vienna. For his study of medicine, Theophrastus chose Italy, home to the best centres of the time. In 1512, he set out for Italy, arriving in Ferrara in 1513, where he studied for two years. His education would have been in the orthodox beliefs in the works of Pliny, Galen and Avicenna. It was in Ferrara that he rather immodestly gave himself the name of Paracelsus – literally meaning beyond Celsus, referring to the Roman writer Aulus Cornelius Celsus (25 BCE–50 CE), the author of *De medicina*.

During his lifetime, Paracelsus practised medicine and taught in many cities across Europe. But his controversial views on medicine and religion alienated the orthodox establishment and he was often forced to flee and continue his wandering. Only one of his books, *Die Grosse Wundarzney* (The Great Surgery), was published during his life; others such as the *Neun Bücher Archidoxis*, the *Das Buch Paragranum Aureoli Theophrasti Paracelsi*, the *Von der Frantzösischen kranckheit Drey Bücher* (Three Books on the French Disease [syphilis]), the *Das Buch paramirum*, and the *Astronomia magna* were only published after his death. The *Opus paramirum* was a collection of five books, and the first two books set out to answer the question as to the constitution of matter. Paracelsus asserted that man is composed of three substances – sulphur, mercury and salt. These are not elements as such but qualities which give form to other materials, for example, salt directs to a solid form. In the body, overeating causes salt to convert to fat. Salt is converted to produce perspiration, sores, scabs and pustular wounds, whereas mercury can cause gout, syphilis and depression, and sulphur can cause fever and plague. Paracelsus died in Salzburg on 24 September 1541.

From around 1550, publishers began to take an interest in the manuscripts of Paracelsus' books. Johannes Huser, a physician at Glogau, Silesia (now in Poland) produced the first complete ten-volume edition of his works. Huser's text was translated into Latin in 1658. Once Paracelsus was in print, his ideas spread and became influential, being taken up by Peder Sørensen and van Helmont, and in his book, *Basilica Chymica*, Oswald Crollius wrote about the new chemistry.

Paracelsus felt that the object of chemistry was to prepare medicinal substances, purify them and also to discover new ones. He was the first of the iatrochemists. (*Iatros* is the Greek word for a physician, thus an iatrochemist is a physician who seeks to provide chemical answers to medical conditions). He advocated, for example, the use of antimony trichloride (butter of antimony) and mercuric oxide. Paracelsus was well aware of the toxicity of some of his remedies and knew the doses needed to be controlled carefully. One of his most famous maxims is that 'All things are poisons, for there is nothing without poisonous qualities. It is only the dose which makes a thing poison.'

By mixing sulphuric acid with wine and then distilling it, Paracelsus created a remedy he called 'sweet oil of sulphur'. When he administered this to chickens, they fell asleep but then recovered without any ill effects. He documented that this material took away pain. Paracelsus had made ether, the anaesthetic, but it did not start to come into widespread use until the American William Green Morton first used it for dental surgery in 1846, over three hundred years later.

Petrus Severinus

Peder Sørensen (1542–1602) is better known by his Latin name of Petrus Severinus. He was born in the seaside town of Ribe in Jutland in Denmark in 1542.[4] At the end of the 1550s, Severinus enrolled as an undergraduate in the University of Copenhagen to study natural philosophy – logic, physics and ethics. In 1562, he left to study medicine in France but returned a year later due to lack of funding. He was offered a canonry position as a doctor in Viborg in 1563, which helped him with his medical studies and eight years later, in 1571, he was made physician to King Frederick II, where he remained in post until the king died in 1588. He then attended Frederick's son Christian IV and he became one of his physicians when Christian became king in 1592.

Severinus' major work was his *Idea medicinae philosophicae* published in 1571. This was based on many of the ideas of Paracelsus. Like Paracelsus, he questioned the orthodox Galenic medical theories and believed medicine should rely on the study of nature. He felt that diseases were caused by seeds of foreign matter in an otherwise healthy body, which could take root and grow. He believed in the usefulness of chemical remedies in treating diseases.

Joannes Baptista van Helmont

Joannes van Helmont (1577–1644) was born in Brussels, the youngest of five children. He was educated at Louvain, where he studied philosophy and metaphysics.[5] A wealthy canonship was promised to him if he studied theology but he felt that this was not his calling. For recreation he started to read Mathiolus and Dioscorides, but he felt that herbalism had made no real advances since the days of Dioscorides. He studied medicine and obtained his medical degree in 1599 from the University of Louvain. During his next years he travelled to Switzerland, Italy and England and in 1609 married Margaret van Ranst, a rich heiress. After his marriage, he retired to Vilvorde and spent his time in scientific research and in providing healthcare to the local sick and poor.

Van Helmont was a disciple of Paracelsus, although he questioned some of Paracelsus' ideas. He was also a mystic and an alchemist. He was an enthusiast for experimentation, and is one of the pioneers of early chemistry. In 1615, he published a book in his native Dutch entitled *Dageraad ofte Nieuwe Opkmost der Geneeskunst* (Daybreak or the New Rise of Medicine) in which he challenged the views of the Galenists. Most of his books were collected and edited by his son Franciscus Mercurius, and published in Amsterdam. Joannes's book *Ortus medicinae, vel opera et opuscula omnia* (The Origin of Medicine, or Complete Works) was published in 1648. This was translated into English by John Chandler in 1664 under the title *Oriatrike, or Physick Redefined*.

Van Helmont was the first to understand that air was a mixture of components, which he called gases. He understood that 'gas sylvestre' (carbon dioxide) was given off by burning charcoal and also produced by fermentation.

Oswald Croll

Oswald Croll (1563–1609) was the professor of medicine at the University of Marburg in Germany and chief physician to Prince Christian I of Anhalt-Bernberg. [6] In 1608, he published his major work the *Basilica Chymica*. This was a summary of his studies into chemical medicine based on Paracelsian ideas. The book was both a practical treatise on preparation of chemical medicines and a theoretical guide to their use. It went through numerous translations in many editions into the eighteenth century.

In 1670, a translation by John Hartmann of the *Basilica Chymica* was published. Some of the remedies can be quoted:

'Mercury is the Balsome [balsam] of Nature, in which it is an incarnative virtue, whereby it wonderfully restores and purifies the microcosmick Body infected with Lues venerea [syphilis]. It is a remedy against infirmities caused by putrefaction of humours, and in desperate Diseases, there is not any more found that more speedily yield relief'.

The formula for Elixir Proprietalis of Paracelsus was given – it contained Myrrh of Alexandria, Aloes, Oriental Crocus and Oyl of Sulphur: 'It affects the Breast and Lights and is admirably useful. It draws out divers humors of the Ventricle, Hecticks, Catarrhs and Coughs in Genera – it comforts and cleanses the Breast'. Some of the remedies seem to us in the twenty-first century to be totally bizarre. For example, the Antiepileptick

Confection of Paracelsus contained 'three skulls of Men not buried, that perished by a Violent Death and dryed in the Air, being somewhat grossly pulverisate by retort at first in gentle fire ...'. Milk of Sulphur was stated to be 'preservative in the Apoplexy'; Salt of Tin was 'most efficacious in suffocation'.

The English Paracelsians

Paracelsian ideas began to be circulated in English translations of Paracelsus from the 1570s. There were translations by John Hester and Thomas Tymme. Hester's translation was entitled *A hundred and fourtene experiments and cures of the famous Phisition Phillipus Aureolus Theophrastus Paracelsus* and was published in 1584. In 1585, Robert Bostocke published his *The Difference between the Auncient Phisick and the later Phisick*, in which he mentions the ideas of Severinus.

The English physician Thomas Moffett (1563–1604) had taken his MD in Basel in 1579. He had visited Denmark, met Severinus and become familiar with his works. He published his book on chemical medicine, *De iure et praesentia chymicorum Medicamentorum dialogus apologeticus*, in 1584, which was a defence of Paracelsus and which he dedicated to Severinus. Moffett was an influential physician as a member of the London College of Physicians, and was involved in some of the early work on the preparation of the *London Pharmacopoeia* (see later in this chapter).

Theodore Turquet de Mayerne (1573–1655) was probably the most famous physician in Europe of his time.[7] He was born in Geneva into a Huguenot family. At the age of 14 he went to Heidelberg, and matriculated in 1588. He left Heidelberg in 1591 to study medicine in the University of Montpellier in the Huguenot Languedoc part of France. He took his bachelor's degree in 1594, his licentiate in 1596 and was admitted as a Doctor of Medicine in 1597. When he was examined for his doctorate, he showed his interests in Paracelsian chemical medicine. He moved to practise medicine in Paris, and was appointed a royal doctor. However, there were tensions with the medical faculty in Paris: de Mayerne was a Protestant, he did not have a medical degree from Paris, and his medicine was unorthodox in that he was an iatrochemist. There were repeated efforts made to persuade de Mayerne to convert to Catholicism. In 1606, he had visited England and forged links with English physicians and the royal court. He was invited to stay in England in 1611 to become one of the physicians to James I with an annuity of £400 a year. He was happy to accept as he had been blocked in his career in France and harried to change his religion. De Mayerne was elected to the College of Physicians of London and took a major role in the development of the *London Pharmacopoeia* described later in this chapter. As an alchemical doctor, de Mayerne had a whole range of secret remedies for elixirs and panaceas which he jealously guarded.

Scientific Revolution in Medicine – Vesalius and Harvey

In parallel with the questions raised by Paracelsus and the later alchemical physicians about the validity of the Galenic theory of the four humours, experimental work and observation were also raising questions. In the summer of 1543, an illustrated book on anatomy was published which was a key part of this scientific revolution. It was written by Andreas Vesalius (1514–1564), who was a professor at the University of Padua in Italy.[8] It was called *De humani corporis fabrica* or *On the Structure of the Human Body*. It was more like a notebook than a learned text, and reported the results of Vesalius' dissections on a large number of bodies. The existing teaching on anatomy had been based on various texts of Galen, who had founded his ideas on his dissection of various animals. Vesalius' book contradicted many of the key aspects of Galen's medicine.

William Harvey (1578–1657) was born in Chigwell in Essex.[9] He was educated at the King's School in Canterbury, then at Caius College in Cambridge where he obtained his BA in 1597. He travelled to Padua in Italy and gained his Doctorate in Medicine in 1602. Returning to England he gained the degree of Doctor of Medicine from the University of Cambridge, before travelling to London in search of work. Here he joined the Royal College of Physicians and obtained a job at St Bartholomew's Hospital, where he worked for most of the remainder of his life. He was the physician to James I and subsequently to Charles I. In 1628, his book, entitled *Exercitio de Motu Cordis et Sanguinis in Animalibus*, on the circulation of blood was published in Frankfurt. This was an account of the function of the heart and the circulation. His account contradicted the orthodox Galenic view that the blood passed between the ventricles in the heart through invisible pores. Galen also thought that arteries sucked in air, and when contracting they discharged vapours through pores in the skin. Harvey's discoveries were met with scepticism and abuse by the orthodox Galenic physicians and it took twenty years for his ideas to gain hold.

The Early Formularies and Pharmacopoeias

The first official formularies were produced by individual physicians or groups of physicians for use in their individual cities or city-states to provide a list of officially accepted medicines for use on patients. Tracing the history of the formularies and pharmacopoeias allows us to look at the medicines used by physicians and the type of preparations they used or prescribed for their patients. We can see the influence of the changes in the theories of medicine which influenced the choice of drugs – Hippocratic and Galenic theory of humours, and the alchemists like Paracelsus popularising the use of chemical medicines.

The early texts were based on the prevailing orthodoxies of Hippocrates and Galen. The official guide for the apothecaries of Florence was the *Nuovo receptario compost del famotissimo Chollegio degli eximii Doctori della Arte et Medicina della inclita cipta di Firenze* (New formulary composed for the famous College of Doctors of Arts and Medicine of Florence). It was written by the physician Hyeronymo dal Pozzo and published in 1498, and was unusual in that it was written in Italian rather than Latin. Recipes were given for a wide variety of dosage forms (see Table 6.1).

The Spanish city of Barcelona was next with the *Concordia Pharmacopolarum Barcinonensium* in 1535. This was commissioned by the Archbishop of Barcelona and made official in his diocese. It was written by Bernard Domenech and Ioanne Benedicto Pau.

Valerius Cordus was born in February 1515 at Simthausen, a village between Marburg and Frankenberg. He was educated by his father and in Marburg, where he gained his Baccalaureate in medicine at the age of 16. Afterwards he went to Wittenberg where he studied medicine, pharmacy and pharmacognosy, and he lectured on Dioscorides. Between 1531 and 1543, he made a number of journeys through the Erzebirge, the Thurinerwald and the Harz, in search of plants and minerals. In Leipzig he spent time with his uncle Johannes Ralla, an apothecary. He wrote his *Historia Plantarum* herbal sometime before his death in September 1544 but it was not printed until 1561. The book describes medicinal plants found in Germany and also foreign *materia medica* such as woods, barks, fruits, roots and resins which were imported into Germany. It includes descriptions of about 500 plants, 60 of them new. His best-known work is the *Pharmacorum Omnium Quae Quidem in usu sunt, conficiendorum ratio. Vulgo vocant Dispensatorium Pharmacopolorum*, commonly known as the *Dispensatorium*. This was approved by the Nuremberg physicians and published posthumously. Editions were published in 1546, 1598, 1612 and 1666. It was translated and made official in Venice in 1558, and in Amsterdam in 1592. The *Dispensatorium* contains recipes for theriacs including Mithridatium which contained forty-three separate ingredients and Theriacum Andromachi with sixty-five ingredients. The various compositions were credited to earlier authorities such as Mesue, Gabrielis, Nicolai, Galen, Avicenna, Rasis, Andromachus, Andromachus Senior, Damocratis, Actuario and Bartholomew Montagnanae. The book lists about 215 simples (named single ingredient medicines) comprised mainly of plants, but also some mineral materials such as lapis, red coral, litharge (lead oxide), borax, and animal materials such as viper. It also included petroleum and tar.

Valerius Cordus is claimed to be the first to manufacture ether by the action of sulphuric acid on alcohol, although Paracelsus also made it at about the same time as mentioned earlier in this chapter. This may be the first synthetic preparation of a medicinal substance.[10] However, unlike Paracelsus he did not identify its anaesthetic properties.

The word *pharmacopoeia* is derived from the Greek word 'pharmakon' a drug or remedy, and 'poia' meaning making or preparing. These texts were designed to provide descriptions of substances used in medicine and their compositions, and were meant to provide physicians with a list of officially approved drugs, and apothecaries with details of the products that the physicians would prescribe for patients. The French physician and anatomist Jacques Dubois (1478–1555), also known as Jacobus Sylvius, was the first to produce a book with word *pharmacopoeia* in its title. His *Pharmacopoeia, Libri Tres* was published in Lyon in 1548.

About thirty years later, the cities of Augsburg and Cologne followed Nuremberg with the production of their own pharmacopoeias. The physicians responsible drew on the work of the young Valerius Cordus, but had the advantage of a wider education and training in Italy as well as Germany.

The *Pharmacopoeia Augustana*, the official pharmacopoeia from the city of Augsburg was published in 1564, and was the legal guide for the physicians and apothecaries. It was written by Adolph Occo III, who was born in Augsburg in 1524, obtained his doctorate in medicine in Ferrara in 1549, and in 1563 was appointed city physician and inspector of the apothecary shops. In 1582, he was appointed dean of the Collegium medicorum. Occo III produced five editions of the *Pharmacopoeia Augustana* in the sixteenth century. The next three editions were produced by Raymund Minderer, the city physician of Augsburg, during the seventeenth century. The text contained a wider range of medicinal products than the *Dispensatorium* and was more influential. It continued to be used until the eighteenth century.

The first edition of the book only included information on the medicinal products, and did not include a list of simples. An analysis of the compositions, however, has shown that it included 400 herbal drugs (including 60 flowers, 108 roots, 52 fruits, 16 barks, 13 woods and 19 aromatics), 91 animal products, and 84 mineral products (including 56 metallic simples, 3 earths, 15 stones, and 10 gems). There was a total of 500 simples.

The first edition had 597 compositions, of which 447 were stated to be required to be available in the Augsburg apothecary shops. But one can only wonder how many of them were actually used regularly. For example, there were a huge number of laxative preparations, but an individual physician must have had his own favourite strong laxative and weak laxative products.

The list of some of the products in the 1564 *Augsburg Pharmacopoeia* compared to the 1498 *Nuovo receptario* and the Valerius Cordus's 1546 *Dispensatorium* are shown in Table 6.1.

It rapidly became a matter of local pride for major cities to have their own pharmacopoeias, often dedicated to princes and kings. The 1567 *Ricettario Fiorentina* was compiled under the order of Alexander de

Table 6.1: Comparison of medicinal products in the *Nuovo receptario* with the *Dispensatorium* and the *Augsburg Pharmacopoeia*.

Dosage Form	Number of medicinal products in the texts		
	Nuovo Receptario	Dispensatorium	Augsburg Pharmacopoeia
Waters	2	–	–
Electuaries	–	18	27
Confections	9	5	8
Pills	51	44	40
Powders	19	6	21
Syrups and Juleps	37	42	70
Mels and Oxymels (honey-based products)	9	7	12
Juices	11	5	10
Linctus	12	6	15
Lozenges	35	26	38
Eye Preparations	1	–	12
Decoctions	7	–	24
Oils	60	54	71
Ointments	34	23	37
Plasters	25	15	24
Cerates	–	3	12

Electuaries were medicinal substances mixed with sugar, water or honey to form a pasty mass.

Confections are also mixtures of medicinal substances with sugar.

A julep was a sweet drink containing the medicinal substance.

An oxymel was a mixture of honey and vinegar with the medicinal substance.

Mels included the medicinal substance in a honey base.

Cerates were skin preparations with a viscosity somewhere between an ointment and a plaster.

The Augsburg Pharmacopoeia also included a cassia preparation meant to be given as a clyster – an enema to be injected via the anus as a laxative. Cassia is a spice similar to cinnamon.

Medici, the first Duke of Florence and dedicated to him. In 1583, the first edition of the *Antidotarum Romanum* was compiled by the Collegium Medicum in Rome and dedicated to Pope Gregory XIII.

The London Pharmacopoeia – the first national pharmacopoeia

The College of Physicians of London was founded by six physicians in 1518 with a Royal Charter from King Henry VIII, after Thomas Linacre had organised the petition to establish the college. The Charter gave the college power to grant licences to those qualified to practise medicine, within 7 miles of London. Outside London, the licensing of physicians was done by the bishop for his diocese. One of the earliest statutes was adopted to control medicines in 1540. This gave physicians the right to appoint four inspectors, called 'censors' to search for apothecary wares that were 'defective, corrupted, and not meet or convenient to be ministered in any medicine for the health of man's body.' In 1585, the college discussed the possibility of preparing a pharmacopoeia which would provide an official guide to the apothecaries of London.[1] But this was deemed a 'toilsome task' and the effort was abandoned.

The physicians remained concerned about the quality of preparations available from the apothecaries. It was noted in 1586, that a poor-quality theriac called 'Genoa Treacle' was being sold. They commissioned the apothecary William Besse to make a special theriac formulation to their own recipe. Besse did this and sent them samples for evaluation for odour, taste etc. The composition was then adjusted and it was manufactured on behalf of the college as Theriacum Londinensis (London Treacle). It contained thirty ingredients, including opium. A book published in 1612, entitled *London Tryacle. Being the enemie of all infectious diseases; as may appear by the discourse following,* set out what the anonymous author felt were the virtues of London Treacle. It was said that 'all or most of the ingredients, having singular force against, either inward poysons, or outward venomous bytings or stingings of venomous beasts. Thus, this composition is of wonderful virtue and efficacy ... against all corruption or rottenness, either of humors or spirits.' Later in the text it states 'it is of marvellous force against the Plague, and sweating-sickness Pocks.'

The effort to establish a standard formulary was re-opened in 1589, when the college agreed that there should be 'one definite public and uniform dispensatory of formulary of medical prescriptions obligatory for apothecary shops'. The college agreed that in addition to the normal range of herbs, the formulary should include 'Extracts, Sales (salts), Chemica and Metallica'. The college had therefore accepted that a range of Paracelsian chemicals were needed. However, the work stopped and only briefly resumed in 1594.

In 1617, the apothecaries of London gained their own royal charter. King James I issued a proclamation in 1618, telling the apothecaries what was expected of them, that they should only compound or make any medicine by using the new pharmacopoeia.

In 1616, work restarted on the *Pharmacopeia Londinensis* (the London Pharmacopoeia*)*. Two physicians had a key role in the new book: Thomas Atkins (1558–1635) and Sir Theodore Turquet de Mayerne. De Mayerne's own papers for the book included notes on earlier pharmacopoeias such as the *Nuovo receptario* of 1498 and the *Pharmacopoeia Augustana* of 1564. As mentioned earlier, de Mayerne was a Paracelsian physician and an alchemist, so was able to ensure that chemical remedies such as *Tartarus vitriolatus* (potassium sulfate) and *Mercuris dulcis* (calomel or mercurous chloride) were included in the text. The first edition of the new book was published on 7 May 1618, with the preface written by de Mayerne, although it was not entirely satisfactory and a second revised edition was published in December 1618. The text was in Latin and included lists of the drugs and preparations without any indication of their uses. The preface to the text haughtily stated, 'We, therefore, do not add anything about the efficacy of the medicines. We write this book only for the learned, for the disciples of Apollo and for the welfare, not for the information of the common people'.

The first edition contained 680 ingredients (simples) but the second, December 1618, edition contained 1,190 ingredients. These were mainly plant herbal drugs: 292 from leaves, 144 from seeds, 138 from roots, and 34 from barks. Animal parts or excrements, including dung from man, wolves, mice, sheep, goats, pigeons, horses, hens, swallows, cows and dogs were included in 162 drugs and there were 11 salts and 73 metals and minerals. Many of the ingredients added to the second edition were mentioned by Dioscorides in his *De Materia Medica*. The theriacs included Mithridate, Theriaca Andromachi (Venice Treacle) and Theriacum Londinensis (London Treacle).

The medicinal products in the second December 1618 edition were as listed in Table 6.2:

Table 6.2: Medicinal products in the *London Pharmacopoeia* Second Edition.

Type of Product	Number in the Pharmacopoeia
Waters (both simple and compound)	213
Medicated wines	4
Vinegars	11
Decoctions	8
Wound potion	1
Syrups	90
Honeys and Oxymels	18
Fruit Juices	12
Linctuses	6
Candied plants	64
Conserves and candies	66
Electuaries (including the theriacs)	58
Pills	36
Lozenges	45
Simple oils	38
Compound oils	20
Ointments	54
Plasters and cerates	51
Chemical oils	67
Chemical preparations	19

Some of the preparations that were listed (for example, the waters) were used in making other preparations.

The *London Pharmacopoeia* of 1618 was the first in a series of editions of the book, and have been described in my earlier book *The British Pharmacopoeia: 1864 to 2014*. [11] All editions were written in Latin and so only meant for physicians and apothecaries who were classically educated.

Nicholas Culpeper (1616–1654) was born in Ocklcy on the borders of Surrey and Sussex and sent to Cambridge to study for the church. However, he was more interested in studying the works of the Greek physicians and anatomy. He became involved in an illicit love affair with the daughter of a wealthy family, who unfortunately was killed in an accident when eloping to meet Nicholas to marry him. Leaving

Cambridge, Nicholas went to London where he was apprenticed to Francis Drake, an apothecary, and studied herbal medicine and astrology. He never completed his apprenticeship but started to work as a 'student of physick and astrology'.

The English Civil War (1642–1651) was a series of conflicts between the Parliamentarians (Roundheads) and Royalists (Cavaliers) over how Britain should be governed, and in particular about the powers of the king. Like many of the London apprentices, Culpeper fought on the Parliamentary side in the Civil War, and he was wounded in the siege of Reading. During the Civil War, there was a very active underground press, producing radical Leveller pamphlets and petitions to Parliament. One of the printers was the Cloppenburgh Press owned by Peter Cole in partnership with Richard Overton. Cole commissioned Culpeper to translate the *London Pharmacopoeia* into English to make it more widely available. His translation entitled *A Physical Directory: A Translation of the London Dispensatory* was published in 1649. It was no mere translation, it also included his own, often rather acerbic, notes on the various drugs in the *Pharmacopoeia*, and lists of what he felt were useful drugs that had been omitted. This was an assault on the privileged position of the College of Physicians, as the book had been intended only for use by physicians and apothecaries. *The London Pharmacopoeia* included a list of excreta (*Dreckapotheke*), from man, wolves, mice, sheep, goats, cows and dogs, which were used for a variety of therapeutic purposes. Culpeper's scathing views on these materials was 'As for Excrements, there the Colledg makes shittin work, and paddle in the Turds like Jakes Farmers. I will let them alone, for the more I stir them the more they stink'. Unsurprisingly, the physicians were outraged and his translation was described in the Royalist publication *Mercurius Pragmaticus* as 'by two years' drunken labour hath Gallimawfried the Apothecaries' book into nonsense'. But Culpeper had opened Pandora's Box as far as translations were concerned: all subsequent editions of the *London Pharmacopoeia* were translated by various other authors into English. Culpeper went on to write *The Complete Herbal*, one of the most famous herbals and one of the most popular books in the English language. His other books include *A New Method of Physick, or a Short View of Paracelsus and Galen's Practice; in 3 Treatises. Written in Latin by Simon Partlicius.*

Translated into English by Nicholas Culpeper, Gent. Student in Physick and Astrologie. This was published in 1654, again by Peter Cole. It was an account of alchemical medicine from the Paracelsian view and highly critical of Galenic theory. Culpeper seems to have been happy to write books following both Galenic and Paracelsian views.

During the Great Plague in London (bubonic plague) in 1665–6, the College of Physicians was asked by King Charles II and the Privy Council to provide information on the prevention and cure of the disease. They issued a pamphlet on 25 May 1665 entitled *Certain Necessary Directions as well as For the Cure of the Plague. Set down by the Colledge of Physicians. London.*[12]

The recommendation for treatment was:

'Some may take Garlick with Butter, a Clove, two or three, according as it shall agree with their bodies; some may take fasting, some of the Electuary with Figs and Rue hereafter expressed: some may use London Treacle, the weight of eight pence in the morning, taking more or less, according to the age of the part; after one hour let them eat some other breakfast, as Bread and Butter with some leaves of Rue or Sage moistened with Vinegar, and in the heat of the Summer of Sorrel or Wood sorrel.'

For the richer sort of patient, it recommended:

'The use of London Treacle is good, both to preserve from the Sickness, as also to cure the Sick, being taken upon first apprehension in a greater quantity, as to man two drams, but less to a weak body, or a child, in Carduus (thistle) or Dragon-water.'

The third edition of the *London Pharmacopoeia* was published in 1677, dedicated to Charles II. One important addition was Peruvian bark, which was used for the treatment of fever. Jesuit priests in Peru in the sixteenth century had observed the local population using the bark of the cinchona tree to reduce the shaking caused by severe chills. When Juan Lopez de Canizares, the Spanish *corregidor* (chief magistrate) of Loxa in Ecuador (then part of Peru) was taken ill with an intermittent fever in

1630, the local Indians told him about the bark and how to use it. Seeing its efficacy, the Jesuits sent supplies of the bark back to Spain. In 1639, a Jesuit priest sent some of the bark to Rome and from Italy it reached England and the Netherlands. The bark was taken up by Sir Thomas Sydenham (1624–1689) and became a fashionable remedy. Sydenham also introduced laudanum (tincture of opium) into wide medical practice.

Editions of the *London Pharmacopoeia* continued to be published until the tenth edition in 1851. The College of Physicians of Edinburgh developed their own national pharmacopoeia, the first edition appearing in 1699 as *Pharmacopoea Collegii Regii Medicorum Edinburgensis*. Like the *London Pharmacopoeia* the text was in Latin, until the twelfth edition which was published in English for the first time in 1839. The *Dublin Pharmacopoeia* was first published in Latin in 1802, and the last edition in English in 1850.

The Rise and Fall of the Theriac

As we have seen, one of the early theriacs was introduced into medicine in the first century BCE, developed by King Mithridates of Pontus, who was afraid of being poisoned and created an antidote with many ingredients, which he could take daily to build up his resistance to the individual components in the composition. The composition was further developed by Andromachus, physician to the Emperor Nero. The theriacs rapidly gained a reputation as a universal panacea for many ills: Andromachus claimed that his version would relieve pain, weakness of the stomach, difficulty in breathing, colic, jaundice and dropsy. Galen wrote a number of books on theriacs including *Antidotes I* and *II*, and *Theriake to Piso*. He also quoted a theriac attributed to Apollodorus, who probably lived in the third century BCE, which was meant to counteract the venom of vipers. It consisted of blood of sea turtle, blood of kid, rennet of fawn or hare, and wild cumin.

Theriacum Andromachi was the most famous panacea for all ills. It was recommended to King Alfred the Great (849–899 CE) by Elias III, the Greek Orthodox Church Patriarch of Jerusalem, and the Crusaders took it the Holy Land. In Venice, the Theriacum Andromachi was manufactured in a public ceremony by the medieval apothecaries, and Paris, Montpellier, Madrid, Cairo, Rome, Genoa and Bologna all produced local versions of theriacs. Two eighteenth-century ceramic drug jars for theriacs – Theriacum Mithridatium and Theriaca Londinensis are shown in Pictures 5 and 6.

The physician William Heberden studied at Cambridge, gaining his MD in 1739. He practised medicine in the city and whilst there delivered a series of annual lectures on *materia medica*. One of his lectures was on theriacs, and the text of his lecture was published in 1745 as a ten-page pamphlet entitled *Antitheriaca; an essay on Mithridatum and Theriaca*. Heberden attacked the concept of the theriac, pointing out that the composition of the theriacs had varied greatly over the centuries. Celsus described it as having thirty-eight simples, of which five were removed before Nero's time, but twenty others added, and Andromachus took out six but added twenty-eight more.

According to Heberden, the theriacs 'contained an unreasonable number of ingredients, their contradictory effects even according to the Ancients themselves, the inconsiderable portion of many of them in the quantity of a dose'. The sixth edition of the *London Pharmacopoeia* in 1788 omitted the theriacs.

Having been deleted from the *London Pharmacopoeia* official formulary, it might have been expected that the theriacs would have been relegated to the dustbin of medical history. However, remedies with such an interesting history and reputations gained over nearly two millennia were not so easily extinguished. A theriac was still included in the 1818 French *Pharmacopoeia Gallica*. The 1872 German *Pharmacopoeia Germanica* included a composition entitled *Electuarium Theriaca*, although it only contained twelve ingredients.

In 1832, the Madras Medical Board offered a prize of 500 Rupees for the best dissertation on the treatment of beriberi and rheumatism. The prize was won in 1835 by the assistant surgeon John Grant Malcolmson.[13] A treatment for beriberi was vital as it accounted for half the prison deaths in Madras and it was widespread in the area of the Madras Presidency. Malcolmson found that one treatment being used was called 'treak farook' which was imported by Arab traders into Bombay. The traders told Malcolmson that it came from 'beyond Istamboul via the Red Sea'. When he looked at the leaflets with the product, he discovered that the product was actually the theriac of Andromachus made by John Baptist Sylvestris near the Rialto Bridge in Venice. Unknown to Malcolmson, the pharmacy Alla Testa D'Oro was a well-known pharmacy in Venice and had been producing the theriac since 1605.

Was this the end of the theriac? In 1960, the travel writer Henry Morton was visiting Venice, shopped in the same pharmacy and purchased two small rusty containers of Theriaca Andromachis Senioris, Divinum inventum.[14] It had been made nearly thirty years previously and Morton was told by the pharmacist that it was a general tonic, and was particularly good for intestinal problems and wind.

Society of Apothecaries

The early London apothecaries were members of the Grocers' Livery Company.[15] In 1588, they unsuccessfully petitioned Queen Elizabeth I for a monopoly in making and selling medicines and they became a separate section of the Grocers' Company in 1607. However, their interests were different and as mentioned earlier, the Huguenot apothecary Gideon de Laune, who was the apothecary to Queen Anne of Denmark, petitioned King James I for a charter such as had already been granted to the College of Physicians. Sir Francis Bacon, the Chief Law Officer, was consulted and supported the case. A charter was drawn up, which became official in December 1617.

By 1623, the society had established a laboratory for the manufacture of Galenic herbal remedies. Nicholas Le Fèvre (1615–1669) came to England at the behest of Charles II, and became the Royal Professor of Chemistry and Apothecary in Ordinary to the Royal Household. His book *Traité de la Chymie* was translated into English as *A Complete Body of Chemistry*. This two-volume guide to the manufacture of medicines was dedicated 'to the use of all apothecaries' and used when the Society of Apothecaries established its own chemical manufacturing laboratory in 1671, employing the first Chemical Operator, Samuel Stringer. The Society of Apothecaries' laboratory provided a reliable source of the new, good quality chemical remedies for apothecaries to buy. It also provided teaching to the apothecary apprentices. By 1677 the laboratory was a commercial success producing a profit. The laboratory was funded with further investments from apothecaries in 1702 to become the Laboratory Stock Company. The Chemical Operator in 1676 was a German, Nicolas Staphorst. His catalogue of the preparations which were available was published as the *Officina Chymica Londinensis*. This book is in two halves, the first consisting of an alphabetical list of materials and how they are made; the second is a catalogue of materials in the *London Pharmacopoeia*. The text includes details of chemical medicines from copper, iron, tin mercury, antimony, bismuth, lead, and sulphur. In 1703, the society agreed to supply medicines to the chests of surgeons in the Royal Navy. The society established a new Joint Stock Company and a public shop or warehouse, which would be kept supplied with sufficient variety of medicines for all surgeons in the Royal Navy. The Society of Apothecaries had established what was the first commercial pharmaceutical manufacturer.

Importation of medicines

Between 1550 and 1770, the consumption of imported medicinal materials exploded. Medicines flooded in with other commodities. Wallis has documented that by the 1770s drug imports were about £100,000 per year, fifty times greater than the £1,000 to £2,000 two centuries earlier.[16] Senna, China roots (wild yam), rhubarb, and sarsaparilla were all imported throughout this period. With the increasing operations of the East India Company, there was an increase in import of rhubarb, opium and frankincense. From the eighteenth century the Americas became more important with imports of guaiacum (used to treat syphilis), sarsaparilla (for skin and blood problems) and Peru bark (*Cinchona* bark which made up to 40 per cent of all direct American imports into England). However, most of the medicinal needs of patients will have been met with domestically produced products.

The East India Company was one of the most powerful companies in its time. It was in existence for 258 years from the grant of its charter in December 1600 by Elizabeth I, until 1874. It ran a complex global network and governed populations and territories that far exceeded those in Britain. It had a key role in importation of medicinal substances from Asia and America. Ships' officers on East India Company ships were allowed to do a certain amount of trading on their own account and this included dealing in herbal drugs. There was an official *East India Officers' and Traders' Pocket-Guide in Purchasing the Drugs and Spices of Asia and the East Indies.* [17] This gave an alphabetical list of over 100 substances, from Acacia to Zedoary, with details of where they were grown, the appearance of the crude drug, its smell, taste and whether it dissolved in water. For example, the entry for Aloes (a purgative) reads: 'Aloe Socotrina from the island of Socotora in the Indian Ocean, wrapt in skins. Aloe Hepatica is produced in other parts of the east; the best is usually import from Barbadoes in Gourd Shells, Aloe Caballina – Horse Aloes'. There was another official guide in 1819 for the ships as to which of the ten East India Company warehouses in London particular drugs had to be sent. For example, the following drugs could be warehoused at the London Docks without payment of duty: Balsam Capivi, Peruvian bark, Cantharides, Cochineal, Ginseng, Gum Arabic, Gum Senegal, Indigo, Jalap, Manna, Oils (e.g. Olives, Palm, Salad and Turpentine), Opium, Prunes, Quicksilver (mercury), Rhubarb, Saffron and Senna. Balsam Capivi also known as Copaiba Balsam or Jesuits' resin, was an oleoresin from *Copaifera* tree species growing in South America and the West Indies. It was a stimulant and diuretic.

Access to medicines and medical practitioners

During the seventeenth century, medical help for a sick patient would have come from family and friends, folk remedies, neighbours or charitable clergy, apothecaries, midwives, surgeons and physicians. Ian Mortimer's studies of the mention of 'physick' in probate accounts in the seventeenth century used this as a measure of access to medical services in males with different values of their estates.[18] In 1600, 15–24 per cent of dying patients received some form of medical or nursing assistance; by 1700 this had risen to more than 50 per cent. In his studies, the bulk of medicines or 'physic' were provided by apothecaries, but physicians, surgeons and 'doctors' also provided a substantial amount. Around 30–40 per cent of physicians were licensed by the church diocese rather than the College of Physicians in London. Practitioners were increasingly willing to serve patients in rural areas, to settle in greater numbers in rural areas and to have access to a wider range of medical treatments.

Training of physicians was mainly in the universities. But in the more remote parts of Britain a form of the apprenticeship system still operated with hereditary medical families in Scotland and Wales. The medical members of Scottish Clan Meic-bethad or Clan MacBeth practised medicine from the early fourteenth century to the early eighteenth. Manuscript books used by them include translations into Gaelic of parts of works by Hippocrates, Galen, Averroes, and Constantine. In Wales, the Meddygon Myddfai was a landed family from Carmarthenshire who passed their medical knowledge from father to son. They continued to practise until 1743. Their records are in Welsh and are a mixture of herbal cures, orthodox Galenic medicine and folklore.

Patent medicines

Compounding of patent medicines was a source of income for some of the apothecaries. Gideon de Laune's Pills were sold from his shop in Black Friars. From the late 1600s there was an increasing sale of patent medicines to patients who saw them as an alternative to consulting a physician or apothecary.[19] One of the best-known purveyors was probably Francis Newbery (1746–1818), who had trained in medicine but gave it up before he qualified, in order to concentrate on the patent medicines business he inherited from his father. He had five patent medicines and was reputedly almost a millionaire. Dr James's Fever Powder, which claimed to treat fevers, gout and scurvy, was patented by the English physician Dr Robert James in about 1746. When James died in 1776, his formula was taken over by his manufacturer, Newbery, who continued to advertise it. Nathaniel Godbold (1730–1799) made a fortune from his sales of Vegetable Balsam. Francis Spilsbury (1733–1793) was the owner of Spilsbury's Antiscorbutic Drops (which claimed to treat scurvy) and his widow continued to sell it after his death.

Possibly the most famous of the patent medicines in Victorian times were Holloway's Pills and Holloway's Ointment.[20] Thomas Holloway (1800–1883) was born in Devonport, Plymouth in Devon. He lived in France for a few years in his twenties before moving back to England to set up as a commercial agent in London. His connections with an Italian, Felix Albinolo, who manufactured a general-purpose ointment, gave

Holloway the idea of setting up his own patent medicine business. He started his business in 1837 and advertised his products in newspapers. Holloway's Pills claimed to be able to treat an astounding range of diseases from ague and asthma to worms of all kinds and weakness from whatever cause. The pills contained aloe, myrrh and saffron so would be a mild laxative, but certainly ineffective in treating many of the claimed conditions. Holloway's Ointment was claimed to cure 'Bad Legs, Bad Breasts, Burns, Bunions, Bite of Mosquito and Sand-Flies, Scalds, Chiego-foot, Chilblains, Cancers, Elephantiasis, Fistulas, Gout, Glandular Swellings, Lumbago, Piles, Rheumatism, Sore-throats, Sore-heads, Scurvy, Tumours, Ulcers, Yaws and Sore Nipples.' The fortune generated from the sales of these products enabled Holloway to become a noted philanthropist. He endowed the Royal Holloway College, a college of the University of London, in Englefield Green in Surrey.

Chapter 7

Medicines from Natural Products

s we have seen in Chapter 1, the earliest evidence of the use
of herbal medicinal preparations predates any written record.
Archaeological evidence from analysis of dental calculus in
Neanderthals in the El Sidrón cave system in northern Spain, which
are about 48,000 years old, showed the use of medicinal plants. Written
records on cuneiform clay tablets in Akkadian, Sumerian and Hittite
languages have shown that Babylonian medicine from over 5,000 years
ago included hundreds of drugs in medical compositions and lists of
plants and minerals with claims for their medicinal properties. Herbal
medicines continued to be used as the main remedies until the end of the
sixteenth century when the rationale for their use began to be questioned
by the Paracelsians. Gradually, as we shall see, many of the herbal drugs
were replaced by the active constituents they contained, for example
Peru bark (*cinchona*) was replaced by quinine.

Many of the conventional histories of medicine show the modern
medicinal substances displacing the older herbal drugs. Oliver Wendell
Holmes Senior, the great American physician and essayist (1809–1894)
wrote in 1860 that 'I firmly believe that if the whole material medica,
as now used, could be sunk to the bottom of the sea, it would be all the
better for mankind—and all the worse for the fishes'.[1]

In 1961, the journalist and writer Ritchie Calder (1906–1982) wrote
that 'before 1935 the physician was no better than a medicine man'.[2] The
truth is more complex and more interesting; herbal medicines have not
yet been relegated to the dustbin of medical history. On the contrary,
they have continued to be used over the centuries, in parallel to more
conventional modern medicines, as we shall see later in this chapter.
And natural products are still being investigated by scientists to find
candidates for possible new treatments.

Herbals – documenting plant medicines

Gaius Plinius Secundus, better known as Pliny the Elder (23–79 CE) was a Roman author, naval and army commander and friend of the emperor.[3] Pliny's last work was his encyclopaedia comprising thirty-seven books entitled *Naturalis Historia* (*Natural History*). For his book, Pliny consulted 400 authors including two earlier herbalists, the Greek physician Diocles (fourth century BCE), and Crateuas (*ca.* 100–60 BCE), who had been the physician to King Mithridates VI of Pontus. Crateuas was called 'the rootcutter' by Dioscorides.

Pedanius Dioscorides wrote *De Materia Medica* in about 60 CE.[4] It was divided into five separate parts, each further subdivided into a number of books. The parts of the encyclopaedia dealing with trees, plants and medicaments were Books XII to XXVIII. The original Greek text was translated into Syriac when Greek scholars fled eastward after Constantine invaded Byzantium. It was subsequently translated into Arabic and Persian and became an important part of Muslim medical knowledge. Later it was translated into Latin and became an important source text for writers who followed.

Bartholomaeus Anglicus (*ca.* 1203–1272), otherwise known as Bartholomew the Englishman is believed to have studied at Oxford University. He was a member of the Franciscan order in France.[5] His encyclopaedia, written in Latin, was entitled *De proprietatibus rerum* (On the properties of things). There were nineteen sections to his book; Book Seventeen is on plants (an herbal). Most of his material is drawn from earlier sources – Hippocrates, Dioscorides, Pliny, Avicenna, Macer (who wrote *De virtutibus herbarum*, better known as the *Macer Floridus*) and the Bible. One of Bartholomew's recipes was for a sedative consisting of an extract of *Mandragora* with wine.

Rembert Dodoens (*ca.* 1517–1585) was the son of a city doctor in Mechelen in the Netherlands. After studying at the University of Leuven, he graduated with his licentiateship in medicine in 1535. He travelled widely through Italy, Germany and France before returning to Mechelen to practise as a city physician in 1541. Later he became the personal physician to the Emperor Maximilian II at the Vienna Court. In 1554, he published the *Cruydeboeck*, his herbal in which he described about 1,340 species, some 600 of which were new. He arranged the plants into six groups according to their external physical characteristics. The book contained 715 illustrations, which were added to when a revised version in Latin entitled *Stirpium historiae pemptades sex* was published in 1583. It became a best-seller. Dodoens has been called the father of botany.

John Gerard (*ca.* 1545–1612) was born in Nantwich, Chester. When he was about 17 years old, he was apprenticed to Alexander Mason, a barber-surgeon.[6] In 1569, he obtained the freedom of the Barber-Surgeons' Company and set up his own practice. He established a garden in his home in Holborn and published a catalogue of his plants. In 1577, he started working as the superintendent gardener to William Cecil, the Queen's Lord High Treasurer at his gardens in London and Hertfordshire. He was asked by John Norton, the Queen's Printer, to help with the translation of Dodoens' book *Stirpium historiae pemptades sex*. Dr Robert Priest had been engaged to translate it, but had died before it could be completed. Although Gerard completed the work he had difficulty matching the woodcuts to the plant descriptions and called in the French physician and botanist Matthias de l'Obel to help. He also included some new plants from North America in the text. The book was published in 1597 as the *Great Herball, or, Generall Historie of Plantes* and included details of more than 1,000 plants in 167 chapters. His book was very popular and was a standard reference book for many years.

John Parkinson (1567–1650) was born in Whalley, Lancashire.[7] He was educated by a priest who taught him to read, write and speak Latin, then apprenticed to a prominent London Freeman of the Grocers' Company, Francis Slater. On 16 December 1617, he became a member of the new Society of Apothecaries, swearing his oath before the Attorney General (Francis Bacon), Dr Atkins and Dr Theodore de Mayerne, the King's Physician. As mentioned in Chapter 6 he was one of the apothecaries called in to help with preparing the new *Pharmacopoea Londinensis*. His famous book *Paradisi in Sole Paradisus Terrestris* was published in 1629.[8] The translation of the title in English is *Park-in-Sun Terrestrial Paradise*, so the title is a pun on his name, Parkinson. It was dedicated to 'The Queenes Most Excellent Majestie' and had a foreword by De Mayerne,

Dr Atkins and others. It was one of the first books on horticulture, and its 162 pages detailing almost 1,000 plants with accompanying woodcut illustrations were arranged in three sections: the flower garden, the kitchen garden and the orchard garden.

In 1640, Parkinson published his second book the *Theatrum Botanicum* (*Theatre of Plants*) which was a guide for the apothecaries.[9] The book had 1,688 pages of text, and descriptions of over 3,800 plants. The book was dedicated to Charles I.

We have already mentioned Nicholas Culpeper in Chapter 6. In addition to his translation of the *London Pharmacopoeia*, he published *The English Physitian* in 1652, later renamed as *The Complete Herbal*.[10] This has been one of the most popular books ever published in the English language, and versions of it are still in print. A search on Amazon UK using the search term 'Culpeper Herbal' yielded 142 hits, some of them reprints of his 1652 text, others books based on this text.

Herbals have continued to be published. A popular twentieth century book was that written by Mrs M. Grieve in 1931 entitled 'A Modern Herbal'.[11] This contained 866 pages of text including herbs from Abscess Root to Yarrow. A search on Amazon UK in the Books section using the search term 'Herbal' yielded over 4,000 hits, showing the enduring popular interest in this subject.

Old wine in new bottles – isolation of active constituents from herbal ingredients

Opium was known to the Sumerians, and was also mentioned as a sedative in the Ebers Papyrus. Dioscorides described the method for incising poppy capsules to obtain the juice which is used to form opium.

Friedrich Wilhelm Sertürner (1783–1841) was born in Neuhaus in North Rhine-Westphalia in Prussia (now in Austria). His parents died when he was young and at the age of 16, he was apprenticed to Mr Cramer, the pharmacist in Paderborn. He experimented with extracting opium, then tested the extracts on dogs and mice. In 1805, he isolated a new acid, which he called 'mekonsaure'. But this was inactive when he tested it on stray dogs. Next he isolated an insoluble material with alkali-like properties, and when this was tested in animals it was active.

He called this the *'principium somniferum'*. Later he named it *'morphium'* after Morpheus, the god of dreams in Greek mythology. His findings were published in letters in the *Trommsdorffs Journal der Pharmazie* in 1805 and 1806. However, the publications did not attract any attention. He carried on with his research and showed that the new material was basic and could be dissolved in acids. By trial and error tests in young volunteers, he was able to establish a dose of 15mg as being optimal. In 1817, he published his findings in *Gilbert's Annalen der Physik,* and this time the value of his research was recognised. A French translation of his paper was published with an editorial by Joseph Gay-Lussac, the eminent French chemist and physicist. Gay-Lussac suggested renaming the drug 'morphine'. In 1818, the German chemist Wilhelm Meissner invented the name 'alkaloid' for substances derived from plants where the suffix 'oid' marked that they reacted in a similar way to alkalis.

Morphine was first manufactured as the acetate, and then as other salts, when the Edinburgh physician and chemist William Gregory found a way of making them in a pure form in 1831. Sertürner's work had opened the way to the isolation of other basic (as opposed to acidic) drugs from plant materials. Pharmacists who specialised in the production of drugs from natural products initiated the growth of pharmaceutical manufacture. For example, in 1826 the German firm of H.E. Merck started by extracting morphine and other alkaloids.

François Magendie (1783–1855) worked at the Collège de France in Paris. He is regarded as the founder of the science of pharmacology.[12] He felt that pure substances were required to make the best observations and studied the effect of certain poisons on animal tissues to understand the mechanism of their action.

Pierre Joseph Pelletier (1788–1842) at the Ecole de Pharmacie in Paris began a collaboration with Magendie on the action of drugs. They investigated ipecacuanha which had been used to treat intestinal afflictions and in 1817, they isolated the alkaloid emetine. Joseph Bienaimé Caventou (1795–1877) also worked at the Ecole de Pharmacie with Pelletier. They investigated *Nux vomica* plants, and isolated strychnine in 1818. In 1820, they isolated quinine from *Cinchona* bark.

The following years produced a flood of discoveries of new alkaloids, some of the most important of which are summarised in Table 7.1:

Table 7.1: The discovery of alkaloids.

Year	Source	Alkaloid	Discoverer(s)
1820	Coffee beans	Caffeine	Runge
1826	Barberry	Berberine	Chevalier and Pelletan
1828	Tobacco	Nicotine	Posselt and Reimann
1829	*Etrychnos toxifera* plant	Curarine	Roulin and Boussaingault
1831	Nightshade	Atropine	Mein
1832	Opium	Codeine	Robiquet
1833	Belladonna	Hyoscyamine	Geiger and Hesse
1833	Autumn crocus	Colchicine	Geiger and Hesse
1835	Opium	Thebaine	Pelletier
1860	Coca leaves	Cocaine	Niemann
1873	Calabar beans	Physostigmine	Jobst and Hess

The work on alkaloids was followed by the isolation of other types of drugs.

The glycosides are formed from a sugar molecule and an organic molecule with a hydroxyl group. Some of the glycosides which were discovered in the nineteenth century are listed in Table 7.2:

Table 7.2: The discovery of glycosides.

Date	Source	Glycoside	Discoverer(s)
1828	Foxglove	Digitalin	Dulong
1829	Willow bark	Salicin	Leroux
1842	Garden rue	Rutin	Weiss
1861	Liquorice	Glycyrrhizin	Gorup and Besanez

Digitalin is a mixture of the different glycosides in the foxglove, *Digitalis purpurea*. It was not until 1930 that digoxin was isolated by Sidney Smith from Burroughs Wellcome Laboratories.

The use of willow tree (*Salix*) bark and leaves dates back to Hippocrates in 400 BCE or earlier. Dioscorides, writing in the first century CE, stated in his *De Materia Medica* that the burnt bark mixed with vinegar removes warts and calluses when plastered on them. The juice of the willow leaves and bark when heated with unguent of roses helps treat earaches, their decoction treats gout. *Salix* was included in the *London Pharmacopoeia* of 1618. In 1763, the Reverend Edward Stone wrote to the Earl of Macclesfield, the Lord President of the Royal Society on the use of dried, powdered willow bark in the treatment of agues (fevers). His letter was printed in the *Philosophical Transactions* and is one of the first accounts of a clinical trial.[13] He reported that, 'I have continued to use it as a remedy for agues and intermittent disorders for five years successively and successfully. It hath been given I believe to fifty persons and never failed in the cure.' The French chemist Henri Leroux managed to isolate pure salicin from willow bark in 1829. In 1838, the Italian chemist Raffaele Piria at the Sorbonne in Paris, split salicin into a sugar and another component (salicylaldehyde); he then converted the salicylaldehyde, by hydrolysis and oxidation, to an acid of crystallised colourless needles, which he named salicylic acid. This was a first step to the manufacture of aspirin, which we will explore in the next chapter. A Scottish doctor, Thomas John Maclagan, investigated the use of salicin in rheumatic fever on eight patients in Dundee in 1876 and published an article in the *Lancet*. He described salicin as 'the most effective means yet for the cure of acute articular rheumatism'. Maclagan found that salicin was more pleasant to swallow than salicylic acid.

Some more recently discovered plant derived drugs are listed in Table 7.3.

Table 7.3: Recently discovered plant-derived drugs.

Herbal Source	Active Drug	Therapeutic Use	Notes
Ephedra sinica	Ephedrine	Asthma	Ma Huang, a herb used in traditional Chinese medicine. Ephedrine was made chemically in 1885
Rauwolfia serpentina (Indian snakeroot)	Reserpine	High blood pressure	Marketed in 1954
Chondrodendron and *Curarea* species	Tubocurarine	Muscle relaxant	Marketed in 1942
Vinca rosea (Madagascar periwinkle)	Vinblastine and Vincristine	Anti-cancer	Discovered in the 1950s. Marketed in 1963

Herbal Source	Active Drug	Therapeutic Use	Notes
Taxus (yew) species leaves	Paclitaxel	Anti-cancer	Marketed in 1992 for ovarian cancer
Artemisia annua (sweet wormwood)	Artemisinin	Malaria	Traditional Chinese medicine. Rediscovered in 1971

Drugs from Microorganisms – Antibiotics

Penicillin

The antiseptic substances that a microorganism can produce are called antibiotics. The history of antibiotics dates back to long before the 'discovery' of penicillin by Alexander Fleming in 1928, and its subsequent production during the Second World War (1939–1945). The medical use of moulds dates back to antiquity. Imhotep, the Egyptian scribe, physician, magician and philosopher from about 3000 BCE is known to have treated infections with mouldy bread.[14] Mouldy jams were used in parts of Canada, and mouldy bread was used in Devon and in Kansas, USA. Trace amounts of antibacterial compounds from the moulds would have had a curative effect.

William Roberts (1830–1899) studied at University College, London and also in Paris and Berlin.[15] He was a house surgeon at the Manchester Royal Infirmary, then became Professor of Medicine at Owens College, University of Manchester from 1863 to 1883. In an 1874 paper he wrote:

> 'I have repeatedly observed that liquids in which the *Penicillium glaucum* was growing luxuriantly could with difficulty be infected with Bacteria; it seemed, in fact, as if this fungus played the part of the plants in an aquarium, and held in check the growth of *Bacteria*, with their attendant putrefactive changes.'

We do not know what antibiotic the *Penicillium* mould produced, but Roberts' study was sixty years before Fleming's rediscovery.

In 1899, Emmerich and Löw prepared a substance called 'pyocanase' from old cultures of *Pseudomonas pyocyanea*. They found that it killed *Staphylococci* and the organism responsible for plague: *Yersinia pestis*. Pyocyanase was used quite widely in the early 1900s for diphtheria cases, for eye infections, for injection into abscesses and even for meningitis.

Bartolomeo Gosio (1863–1944) was an Italian medical scientist who studied medicine in Turin and Rome.[16] In 1899, he became Director of the Scientific Laboratory of the Public Health Service in Rome. He isolated a novel antibiotic from a *Penicillium* fungus on mouldy corn. The crystals of antibiotic he had made were active against anthrax bacteria. His findings were forgotten until rediscovered by two American scientists, C.L. Alsberg and O.M. Black in 1912. They gave the antibiotic the name of *mycophenolic acid*. Although the antibiotic was too toxic to use commercially, a chemical derivative of mycophenolic acid (mycophenolate mofetil) is now used as an immunosuppressant to prevent organ rejection in kidney, heart and liver transplant patients.

Alexander Fleming (1881–1955) was a Scottish farmer's son from Ayrshire.[17] He studied at the Kilmarnock Academy and later the Royal Polytechnic Institution in London. For four years he worked in a shipping office but, on receipt of an inheritance from an uncle, was able to study medicine at St Mary's Hospital Medical School. He graduated in medicine and obtained a further BSc in bacteriology. In 1914, he enlisted and served through the First World War as a captain in the Royal Army Medical Corps, returning to St Mary's Hospital in 1918. He became its Professor of Bacteriology in 1928. His area of research was antibacterial compounds as he had witnessed many deaths during the war due to infected wounds. While investigating *Staphylococci* bacteria in 1928, Fleming left a stack of cultures on Petri dishes on a bench in a corner whilst he went away on a family holiday. When he returned, he noticed that one culture was contaminated with a fungus which had destroyed the colonies of the *Staphylococci* bacteria. He grew the contaminating mould, which he identified as a variety of *Penicillium*, and found that it killed a number of infection-causing bacteria. Although he wrote up his work and published it in the *British Journal of Experimental Pathology* in 1929, he was unable to isolate and purify the new compound, which he called 'penicillin'.

Cecil George Paine (1905–1995) was born in London.[18] He qualified as a physician at St Mary's Hospital Medical School in London in 1928. He studied bacteriology under Alexander Fleming before moving to the Royal Infirmary in Sheffield in 1929. At the end of 1930, to the beginning of 1931, he began some trials in patients using cultures of *Penicillium* which he had obtained from Fleming. In an interview in 1986, Paine said that he 'made some brews with the usual meat broths', and filtered them to obtain a penicillin solution. He tried it on babies with gonorrhoeal eye infections and 'it worked like a charm'. A miner with a badly lacerated cornea had a *Pneumococcus* infection. Paine said that: 'We tried penicillin and it cleared up the infection like nobody's business, and they were able to deal with him and he made a good recovery'. This was the first successful clinical use of penicillin.

In 1939, Howard Florey and Ernest Chain at the Sir William Dunne School of Pathology in Oxford started to research how to manufacture and isolate penicillin. Its chemical structure was identified by Edward Abraham in the Oxford team. Shortly after the team published its first results in 1940, Fleming telephoned Howard Florey to say that he would be visiting within the next few days. When Chain heard that he was coming, he remarked, 'Good God! I thought he was dead'. Florey asked British pharmaceutical manufacturers to help produce penicillin, but under wartime conditions they could not help. In 1941, Florey travelled to the US and was able to get help from the US Department of Agriculture research laboratory in Peoria, Illinois. They were able to improve the manufacturing yield by changing to a deep fermentation process. A consortium of twenty-one US companies started the manufacture of penicillin.

The Cocoanut Grove was a nightclub in Boston, Massachusetts, USA. On 28 November 1942, it was the scene of the one of the deadliest nightclub fires in US history, killing 492 people and injuring hundreds more. Thirteen survivors of the fire were among the earliest patients to be treated with penicillin. In early December, Merck and Company rushed a 32-litre supply of the drug, in the form of culture liquid in which the *Penicillium* mould had been grown, from New Jersey to Boston. The patients received 5,000 IU every four hours, a relatively tiny dose, but the drug was crucial in preventing infections in the skin grafts. By 1944, enough penicillin was produced to treat the Allied war wounded. After the war, a range of penicillin-based medicines was developed, such as Penicillin V which could be taken by mouth. From 1954, researchers at Beecham Research Laboratories in the UK started developing a series of semi-synthetic penicillins. Ampicillin and amoxycillin were developed during the 1960s.

Streptomycin

Selman Waksman (1888–1973) was born in Nova Pryluka in Russia – now in the Ukraine. He emigrated to the US in 1910, gained his BSc at Rutgers College in 1915 and his PhD at the University of California in 1918. He joined the faculty at Rutgers in the Department of Biochemistry and Microbiology. He led a team in the 1940s to try and discover new antibiotics. In 1943, one of his PhD students, Albert Schatz, was screening *Actinomyces* soil bacteria organisms for activity against the organism that causes tuberculosis: *Mycobacterium tuberculosis*. Schatz isolated some strains of *Streptomyces griseus* and found that they inhibited the TB organism. He then produced some samples of a new antibiotic – streptomycin, which was used in toxicity studies in animals and in clinical studies in patients. Waksman, as his supervisor, claimed sole credit for this discovery and was awarded a Nobel Prize in 1952. Schatz was understandably aggrieved about the lack of acknowledgement of his role. The detailed history of the discovery of streptomycin is included in the 2012 book by Peter Pringle: *Experiment Eleven: Deceit and Betrayal in the Discovery of a Wonder Drug.*[19]

In 1949, Waksman and H.A. Lechevalier discovered another antibiotic: neomycin.

Tetracyclines

Benjamin Minge Duggar (1872–1956) was born at Gallion, Alabama.[20] He gained his PhD in 1898 at Cornell University and also studied in Germany, Italy and France. By 1944, he had retired from his post as plant physiologist at the University of Wisconsin and worked as a consultant to the US pharmaceutical company Lederle Laboratories in Pearl River, New York, where he researched antibiotics from soil organisms. In 1945, he received a soil sample from Professor William Albrecht at the University of Missouri. From this soil sample he isolated *Actinomyces aurofaciens* which produced a bright yellow antibiotic compound. This was chlortetracycline, the first in a series of new antibiotics – the tetracylines. The new antibiotic was marketed in 1949 as Aureomycin. A team at Pfizer followed up in 1951 with oxytetracycline which was isolated from *Streptomyces rimosus*. Other chemical derivatives of these tetracyclines were manufactured such as demethylchlortetracycline, doxycycline and minocycline.

Anti-tumour antibiotics

In the 1950s, a team of researchers from the pharmaceutical company Farmitalia started investigating anticancer drugs derived from microorganisms. They found a strain of *Streptomyces peucetius* which produced a red pigment. The anticancer antibiotic daunorubicin had been found which was active against tumours in mice. After human trials the drug was approved in 1979. It was used to treat cancers of the blood and bone marrow, such as acute myeloid leukaemia and acute lymphocytic leukaemia. The Farmitalia researchers mutated the strain of *Streptomyces* and produced another related anticancer antibiotic, doxorubicin. This was approved in 1974 and is used to treat many types of cancer in the bladder, stomach, lung, thyroid and others.

Medicines from animal products

In 1891, the English physician George Redmayne Murray (1865–1939) tried out a new treatment for thyroid deficiency – myxoedema.[21] He injected a 46-year-old woman patient with an extract of fresh sheep's thyroid. After three months the patient was dramatically better. He followed this with treatment of further cases. Other physicians tried out an oral thyroid extract, and this became the treatment of choice. In 1914, the American chemist Edward Kendall, working at the Mayo Clinic, isolated the main hormone in the thyroid: thyroxine. It took 3 tons of pigs' thyroid to produce 33 grams of pure thyroxine, so the dry thyroid extract was still used until the 1970s.

The British physician Edward Mellanby (1884–1935) began researching the causes for rickets in 1914.[22] Rickets is a disease of children that causes bow legs – a deformity caused by the bending of soft leg bones as the child begins to walk. He fed dogs a diet of porridge and they developed rickets, and Mellanby was able to treat them by adding cod liver oil to their diet, demonstrating that it was a component in the cod liver oil that prevented rickets. In 1922, the American biochemist Elmer McCollum tested cod liver oil in which the vitamin A had been destroyed, and it still cured rickets. He named the component vitamin D, and in 1936 the structure of vitamin D_3 (colecalciferol) was identified. Calcium and vitamin D_3 is now commonly prescribed for patients with low bone density (osteopenia) or bone weakness (osteoporosis). Vitamin D deficiency has also been associated with a range of diseases such as an increased risk of cardiovascular disease, hypertension, multiple sclerosis, autism, Alzheimer's disease, and rheumatoid arthritis. Colecalciferol (vitamin D_3) is one of the most widely prescribed drugs by general practitioners in Britain.

The term 'diabetes' was coined by Apollonius of Memphis in Egypt in about 250 BCE. Avicenna, in his book *The Canon of Medicine* in 1025 CE, provided a more detailed account of the symptoms of the disease. The English physician Matthew Dobson (1732–1784) identified sugar in the urine of patients suffering from diabetes. He published his findings in 1776 in *Experiments and Observations on the Urine in Diabetics.* [23] In 1889, the role of the pancreas in diabetes was discovered by Oskar Minkowski, who worked with Josef von Mering on the study of diabetes at the University of Strasbourg. They induced diabetes in dogs by removing their pancreas, which showed that the pancreas contained regulators to control blood sugar. In 1921, a Canadian surgeon, Frederick Banting, worked with a student, Charles Best, at the University of Toronto on the extraction of the hormone from the pancreas. They started a programme to prepare insulin concentrates from pancreases from slaughtered cows and pigs. A biochemist, James Collip, helped with the extraction and purification techniques. They treated a young diabetic with the insulin they had obtained and this controlled his diabetes. The US firm Eli Lilly started commercial manufacture of insulin in 1923.

The search for new medicines from natural products

In his 1629 herbal book *Paradisi in Sole Paradisus Terrestris,* the apothecary John Parkinson stated that the 'Foxgloves are not used in Physicke by any judicious man that I know.' In 1775, William Withering, one of the physicians at the Birmingham General Hospital, was driving to see patients in Stafford, when he was asked to stop and see an old woman with dropsy – the oedema and swelling of tissues in the body caused by heart or kidney failure. He found that she had recovered, and she attributed her recovery to a multi-ingredient herbal tea. He felt that her recovery was due to the presence of *Digitalis*, the foxglove, in the tea.

He wrote in his book *An Account of the Foxglove, and Some of its Medical Uses: with Practical Remarks on Dropsy, and Other Diseases*:

'In the year 1775 my opinion was asked concerning a family receipt for the cure of the dropsy. I was told that it had long been kept a secret by an old woman in Shropshire, who had sometimes made cures after the more regular practitioners had failed. I was informed also, that the effects produced were violent vomiting and purging; for the diuretic effects seemed to have been overlooked. This medicine was composed of twenty or more different herbs; but it was not very difficult for one conversant in these subjects, to perceive, that the active herb could be no other than the Foxglove.'

He investigated various parts of the plant carrying out trials using 163 of his patients and found that the powdered dried leaves were more effective than the root or the fresh leaf.[24] In 1785, he published his book., *An account of the foxglove and some of its medical uses; with practical remarks on the dropsy, and some other diseases.* The dried leaf of *Digitalis* was used in medicine until the 1960s.

Another example of a modern medicine derived from plant material is galantamine, which is an alkaloid present in the common snowdrop, *Galanthus nivalis*, the red spider lily, *Lycoris radiata* and the daffodil, *Narcissus pseudonarcissus*. In Homer's *Odyssey* composed in the eighth century BCE, the god Hermes gives Odysseus 'a black root, but milk-like flower' called 'moly', which Hermes tells Odysseus will make him immune to the sorceress Circe's drugs. The description supports identification as the snowdrop. In 1947, two Russian chemists, Proskurnina and Areshkina discovered an alkaloid in a *Galanthus* species which they named galanthamine.[25] It was found, in 1960, that this inhibited acetylcholinesterase, the enzyme which breaks down acetylcholine, one of the nervous system transmitters in the muscles and brain. In 1982, it was realised that the drug might be useful in treating Alzheimer's disease where it had been found that the levels of acetylcholine in the brain of patients were too low. During the 1990s, a process was developed to extract what was now known as galantamine from daffodil bulbs. Growing trials began in Wales in 2006 and they are now grown there commercially in the Black Mountains, although there is also a chemical method of synthesis. The product was launched to treat Alzheimer's disease in 2000 in the US and Europe.[26]

Herbal plant materials continue to be investigated to develop new medicines. In 1966, M.E. Wall and M.C. Wani were screening natural products for anticancer drugs and isolated camptothecin from the bark and stem of *Camptotheca acuminata* (the Happy Tree), a tree which grows in China. The herbal material was used in traditional Chinese medicine. The chemists made some derivatives of camptothecin: Irinotecan was marketed in 1996 to treat colon cancer and small lung cell cancer, and topotecan in 2007 to treat ovarian cancer and lung cancer.

David Newman and Gordon Cragg from the Natural Products Branch of the US National Cancer Institute in Frederick, Maryland have produced a number of reviews of natural products as a source of new drugs. Their latest covers the period from 1981 to 2010. They found in the area of cancer from the 1940s to 2010 that 48.6 per cent of drugs are natural products or derived from natural products.[27] They concluded that overall, natural products 'play a dominant role in the discovery of leads for the development of drugs for the treatment of human diseases.'

In the United States most herbal products ('botanicals') are promoted as dietary supplements. But two have received a full approval from the Food and Drug Administration. The first is Veregen, a product approved in 2006, which is derived from green tea, for treatment of genital and perianal (around the anus) warts. The other is Mytesi, a drug approved in 2012, which is extracted from the red bark sap of the South American croton tree and used to treat diarrhoea associated with the use of anti-HIV drugs.

Continued use of traditional herbal medicines in the twenty-first century

According to the WHO document *Traditional Medicine Strategy 2014–2023*, in many developing countries, traditional medicines play an important role in meeting the primary health needs of the population.[28]

Over 100 million Europeans are currently users of traditional and complementary medicines, with one-fifth regularly using them. There has been an increase in self-health care as consumers become more active about their health.

In the early twentieth century, the use of herbal drugs declined as the alkaloids, glycosides and other pure substances replaced them. However, the herbal medicines continued to be used by herbal medicine practitioners and became increasingly sold in over-the-counter remedies for customers as part of the growth of what is called 'complementary and alternative medicine' (CAM). Examples of CAM include homeopathy, acupuncture, osteopathy, and chiropractic as well as herbal medicine. The main European markets for herbal medicinal products are Germany, France, Poland and the United Kingdom.[29] In 2014, €1,084 million was spent in Germany (retail prices) on self-medication herbal remedies, followed by France with €610 million in 2013. The French Syndicat National de Compléments Alimentaires (Synadiet) estimated the French market to be even larger at €1.48 billion in 2014.[30] The UK market was estimated to be £485 million (€668 million), and the Polish market at €600 million. A review of ten UK consumer surveys on the use of herbal medicines in 2013 found that 37 per cent of the population used herbal products.[31] The UK market is mainly composed of multi-herb products, while other countries prefer single herb products. The largest commercial producers of herbal ingredients are France, Austria, Poland, Romania, Bulgaria and the United Kingdom. The growth of the national markets is being driven partly by the increase in the number of elderly consumers in the population.

In 2013, 17 per cent of the European population was 65 or over; by 2050 it will be about 30 per cent. Health issues, which will be targeted by herbal product manufacturers in this increasingly elderly population, include the menopause, muscles and joints, memory and learning. Many of these customers think that 'natural products' have fewer side effects compared to conventional medicines.

One popular group of products is the herbal teas – or to be strictly correct, the tisanes. Product indications for these include relaxation (lemon balm), digestion (fennel), and sleeping difficulties (valerian).

Regulation of herbal medicines in Europe

In the European Union there are two parallel systems operating for official regulatory control of herbal products. The first is for herbal products that make claims to treat a medical condition. One method is for a company to apply for an approval for a marketing authorisation, with detailed references to the scientific literature on that ingredient to show that it is recognised as safe and efficacious. The other way is for it to apply using the simplified Traditional Herbal Medicinal Product registration scheme that was introduced in 2004 by European Directive 2004/24/EC. This simplified procedure needs evidence of the quality of the product but in terms of safety and efficacy, it is only necessary to show that the product has been used medicinally for at least thirty years, including at least fifteen years in the European Union. From 2004 until December 2016, a total of 1,719 products were registered in one or more EU countries using the traditional use scheme. The UK had granted 348 (355 by 2018); Germany, 285; Poland, 215; Austria, 209 and Spain, 100 registrations.

Some of the most popular herbal ingredients in approved Traditional Herbal Medicinal Products in the UK are shown in Table 7.4.

The table lists the numbers of authorisations by the UK Medicines and Healthcare Products Regulatory Agency by 2018. Many of these individual authorisations allow a number of different brands of the same product to be sold under different names by supermarkets, health food stores, mail order companies etc.

In addition to these traditional herbal medicinal products, some products have obtained a full authorisation by submitting full data on quality, safety and efficacy. These include eleven products containing senna to treat constipation. Again, the individual authorisations allow different brands of the same product to be sold under different names by different sellers. Similarly, there are full authorisations for capsicum skin products for relief of pain.

Many of the herbal materials used in UK traditional herbal medicine products were included in the 1618 *London Pharmacopoeia*.

The other possibility for marketing an herbal product is as a food supplement, but without making any specific medicinal claims. The

Table 7.4: Most popular herbal ingredients used in UK traditional herbal medicines.

Drug Name	Botanical Name	Number of UK Traditional Herbal Medicinal Product authorisations in which included	Typical use
Valerian	*Valeriana officinalis*	54	Sedative
Echinacea	*Echinacea purpurea*	37	Cold and influenza relief
St John's Wort	*Hypericum perfoliatum*	28	Anti-depressant
Passion flower	*Passiflora incarnata*	24	Sedative
Hops Strobile	*Humulus lupulus*	21	Sedative
Milk Thistle	*Silybum marianum*	15	Indigestion and upset stomach
Black Cohosh root	*Cimicifuga racemosa*	15	Relief of symptoms of the menopause
Dandelion	*Taraxacum officinale*	15	Diuretic
Senna leaf/pods	*Cassia senna*	6	Laxative
Capsicum	*Capsicum* species	3	Pain relief applied to skin

Based on data on authorisations supplied by the Medicines and Healthcare Products Regulatory Agency (MHRA). Reproduced with permission of the MHRA under the terms of the Open Government Licence (OGL) v3.0.

health claims are much vaguer and might read for example, 'contributes to the maintenance of normal blood pressure' or 'contributes to the maintenance of healthy skin.' Belgium, France and Italy have established a list of plants authorised in food supplements, some with maximum levels and safety warnings. This is the so-called BELFRIT list which now comprises approximately 1,000 botanical ingredients.[32] Between 2004 and December 2016, Italy had only granted twelve traditional herbal medicine registrations, Belgium twenty-eight and France thirty-three. It is therefore clear that most herbal products in these countries are being marketed as food supplements, not medicines.

The European Medicines Agency is responsible for regulation of medicines in the European Union. It has established a Committee for Herbal Medicinal Products. Its role is devising EU monographs covering the therapeutic uses and safe conditions of well-established and/or traditional use for herbal substances and preparations; and drafting an EU list of herbal substances, preparations and combinations for use in traditional herbal medicinal products. At the time of writing (April 2019); there were 341 herbal substance monographs each including information on the use of the herb, the type of dosage form in which it is used (tablet, ointment, etc.); the therapeutic indications, dose and method of administration; contra-indications, interactions, undesirable effects, and pharmacological properties. Ninety-five of the herbal materials which were in the May 1618 *London Pharmacopoeia* are included in the European Medicines Agency's Committee on Herbal Medicinal Products listing, with approved indications. Thus, the distinguished commentators at the end of the nineteenth century and early twentieth century who wrote obituaries for herbal medicines were premature – herbal medicines are still in very wide use. To adapt a quotation from Mark Twain, the rumours of their death were exaggerated.

However, despite the centuries of use of many traditional herbal medicines, it is still reasonable to ask the question as to whether they really work, even for the more restricted medical claims allowed today. The European Medicines Agency's Herbal Medicines Committee monographs review the toxicological studies in animals, the clinical data in patients for the herbal materials, as well as information on the active constituents of the herbal materials and their pharmacological properties. There is therefore some evidence for the claims made for them. Some, of course, have been accepted as conventional medicines. Senna tablets containing standardised amounts of the senna glycosides are used routinely by doctors to treat constipated patients.

The gold standard for evaluation of any drug is a randomised, placebo-controlled clinical trial in a large number of patients. A number of reviews have been carried out on the efficacy and safety of some of the most popular herbal remedies applying this gold standard approach.

The physician Edzard Ernst was born in Germany in 1948. His father and grandfather were both physicians. He qualified in 1978, and during his education received training in acupuncture, herbalism, homeopathy, and spinal manipulation. He was the first Professor of Complementary Medicine at the University of Exeter, and has reviewed the data on CAM from an evidence-based medicine viewpoint. He is well known for his disagreement with the Prince of Wales on homeopathic medicines. In medicine, the findings of several single, independent clinical studies can be brought together in a meta-analysis, using statistical methods to calculate an overall effect. In 2002, Ernst published an overview of the risk and benefit of some of the most commonly used herbal drugs, by doing a meta-analysis of the placebo-controlled trials carried out on these drugs.[33] St John's Wort (*Hypericum perforatum*) is now used mainly as an herbal antidepressant. It contains hypericin and hyperforin, which are thought to be the main active constituents. Ernst concluded from his review that St John's Wort has an excellent safety profile and is superior to conventional antidepressants in mild to moderate depression. However, problems can occur when it is taken with other medications. He concluded that there was no such clear evidence for ginseng for any condition. He felt that the trial data for echinacea for respiratory infections was not fully convincing. He felt that the herb 'saw palmetto' was efficacious in short-term trials for symptoms of prostate enlargement (in older men the symptoms may include frequent urination, trouble starting to urinate, weak stream, inability to urinate, or loss of bladder control). He concluded that kava was efficacious for short-term treatment of anxiety.

Bent and his colleagues from the Osher Center for Integrative Medicine at the University of California carried out a meta-analysis of the data on valerian for sleep.[34] This showed some of the difficulties in looking at different clinical studies on traditional herbal products, where the products are not standardised in terms of their active ingredient content or dose. They concluded that valerian may improve sleep quality, but that it was not possible to draw firm conclusions.

Chapter 8

The First Synthetic Drugs

Early synthetic drugs

As mentioned in Chapter 6, the first synthetic medicine was ether. A collection of manuscripts written by the physician Valerius Cordus was published by his editor Conrad Gesner in 1561, seventeen years after Cordus had died. This collection included the manuscript of *De Artificiosis Extractionibus* which recorded the synthesis in 1540 of 'sweet oil of vitriol' [ether] from alcohol and sulphuric acid. He wrote:

> 'Equal parts of thrice rectified spirit of wine [ethanol] and oil of vitriol [sulphuric acid] are allowed to remain in contact for two months, and then the mixture is distilled from a water or sand bath. The distillate consists of two layers of liquid, of which the upper one is oleum vitrioli dulce verum.'

Ether was also mentioned in the writings of Theophrastus von Hohenheim (Paracelsus) in the 1540s, but this was not published until 1605.[2] He tested ether by feeding it to chickens in their food. He wrote: 'Moreover it possesses an agreeable taste; even chickens will eat it, whereupon they sleep for a moderately long time and reawaken without having been injured.' The anaesthetic properties of ether were disregarded for a couple of centuries, as we shall see later in this chapter in the section on anaesthetics.

From the early nineteenth century advances in chemistry made it possible to synthesise a range of chemicals, some of which were used as medicines.

Chloral hydrate

Chloral hydrate was discovered in 1832 by the great German chemist, Justus von Liebig (1805–1873), at the University of Giessen, when he reacted chlorine with ethanol (alcohol). The French physiologist Claude Bernard found that it acted as a sedative,[3] and it was marketed by the German pharmaceutical industry mainly as a psychiatric medication. Its use was common in asylums and hospitals until the Second World War (1939–1945). Chloral was the original 'knock-out drops' or 'Mickey Finn' used to surreptitiously dose unsuspecting victims. Notable users of chloral have included the artist Dante Gabriel Rossetti, who was addicted to chloral with whisky chasers; the German philosopher Friedrich Nietzsche, who used it regularly; and Marilyn Monroe, who died of an overdose of chloral and pentobarbital.

The early painkillers and fever treatments

Acetanilide

In the 1880s, Professor Adolf Kussmaul at the University of Strasbourg was trying to find treatments for intestinal worms.[4] One possible treatment was to use naphthalene. His two assistants, Arnold Cahn (1815–1885) and Paul Hepp, found that the batch of chemical compound had no effect in a patient infected with a variety of worms but it did reduce fever. Later they found that there had been a mistake and the drug with which they had been supplied was acetanilide, not naphthalene as they had thought. They published the discovery of the use of acetanilide in 1886 and called the drug 'Antifebrin'. It was marketed by a company called Kalle from near Frankfurt. This company was taken over by Hoechst in 1908 (Hoechst is now part of Sanofi-Aventis).

Phenacetin

As a dyestuff manufacturer, Bayer needed to find a use for nitrophenol, which was a by-product of the manufacture of Benzazurin G blue dye. The Bayer Research Director, Carl Duisberg, challenged his team of chemists to find a use for nitrophenol. One of the chemists, Oscar Hisberg, found he could make a compound which treated fevers and was also a painkiller. This was acetophenitidine. It was marketed in 1887 as Phenacetin and it became one of the most sought-after painkillers and treatments for fever. One popular combination product was APC tablets, which contained aspirin, phenacetin and caffeine. Phenacetin was marketed until the

1980s when it was found to cause kidney cancers in animals. It was then withdrawn in many countries and replaced by paracetamol. Phenacetin is broken down in the body to paracetamol.

Amidopyrine (Phenazone)

When Emil Fischer (1852–1919) became professor at the University of Erlangen, he invited Ludwig Knorr (1859–1921) to join him and work as his research student. In that time, during his search for quinine-related compounds, Knorr discovered the chemical compound phenazone. As another quinine-related compound, kairin, had shown analgesic and antipyretic properties, Knorr and Fischer asked the Hoechst pharmacologist Wilhelm Filehne (1844–1927) to check unmethylated and methylated phenazone for their pharmacological properties. Knorr patented the compound in 1883. Filehne later suggested the names Höchstin or Knorrin for the substance but Knorr telegraphed from his honeymoon that his version of the name, Antipyrine, was not to be changed. In the 1960s this drug was withdrawn as it had been found to cause a blood disorder: agranulocytosis, where the number of white blood cells are reduced.

Acetylsalicylic Acid (Aspirin)

We have already mentioned the use of salicin and salicylic acid in Chapter 7. Because the salicylate medicines were very irritant to the stomach, other derivatives were investigated. The first person to describe the synthesis of acetylsalicylic acid is believed to be the Frenchman, Charles Gerhardt (1816–1856).[5] In 1853, he did this by reacting the sodium salt of salicylic acid with acetyl chloride. He called his impure compound acetosalicylic anhydride. Pure acetylsalicylic acid (aspirin) was first obtained by an Austrian chemist, Hugo von Gilm, in 1859, by reacting salicylic acid and acetyl chloride. Other chemists repeated this synthesis in 1869, but in the meantime, in 1860, the German chemist Herman Kolbe was able to manufacture salicylic acid from phenol, thus avoiding the need to extract it from willow bark or from the meadowsweet plant *Spirea ulmaria*.

The German firm of Friedrich Bayer & Co was founded in 1863 to manufacture dyes. The company wished to expand into the pharmaceutical market and it set up a new division to make and market new medicines. They had already marketed Phenacetin and subsequently hired the young chemist Felix Hofmann (1868–1946) to work in this area. In 1897, Hofmann synthesised his first sample of acetylsalicylic acid and tested it on his own father. Hofmann recorded that

'the fortuitous cause for the introduction of acetylsalicylic acid was the request by his arthritic father for salicylic acid in a form which did not induce vomiting, because after prolonged use he could no longer tolerate it. Thereupon FH searched through neglected preparations of salicylate derivatives which had been synthesised for other purposes long ago and had them tested. Thus, acetyl salicylic acid, aspirin, was chanced upon.'

Carl Duisberg, the head of Bayer Research, gave the drug to outside pharmacologists and physicians to test. The tests were positive and the pharmacologist at Bayer, Heinrich Dresser, published a paper on it, but without mentioning Hofmann. In 1899, the drug was marketed in powder form and in 1900 a tabletted preparation was marketed in Europe and the USA with the trade name of Aspirin tablets. During the 1920s it was marketed for pain associated with neuralgia, lumbago and rheumatism. Aspirin is still one of the most widely used drugs.

Anaesthetics

Joseph Priestley (1733–1804) was a pioneer with his studies on the production and properties of gases. In 1772, he published an account of the way in which he 'diminished' nitric oxide by subjecting it to a mixture of iron filings and sulphur. He called this new gas 'dephlogisticated nitrous air'. This was the first production of the gas nitrous oxide.[7] Priestley discovered oxygen, which he called 'dephlogisticated air' in 1774.

In 1799, Dr Thomas Beddoes set up the Pneumatic Institute in Bristol for the manufacture of gases and the treatment of the sick. Humphrey Davy (1778–1829) was appointed as its superintendent. Davy prepared gases and experimented with them by getting his friends to inhale them. In 1800, he published the book entitled *Researches Chemical and Philosophical concerning Nitrous Oxide and its Respiration*. In the book, Davy described the effects of nitrous oxide on a painful wisdom tooth. He wrote: 'on the day when the inflammation was most troublesome, I breathed three large doses of nitrous oxide. The pain always diminished.' He concluded that 'nitrous oxide in its extensive operation appears capable of destroying physical pain. It may possibly be used with advantage during surgical operations in which no great effusion of blood takes place.' Despite this recommendation, nitrous oxide was only used for many years for recreation, where balloons were filled with the gas at parties and given to guests to inhale and become intoxicated. It was known as 'laughing gas'.

In December 1844, the American showman, Gardner Quincy Colton, organised a 'Grand Exhibition of the Effects Produced by Inhaling Nitrous Oxide' in Hartford, Connecticut. A local dentist, Horace Wells (1815–1848), attended, became interested and tried it on himself. Wells successfully used it on some of his patients before approaching John Collins Warren, a surgeon at the Massachusetts General Hospital in Boston, who arranged a public demonstration on a dental patient in December 1845. However, the gas bag was removed too early and the patient cried out in pain before the tooth was removed. Wells was discredited and returned to Hartford a bitter and humiliated man. Gardner Quincy Colton continued his public demonstrations of nitrous oxide, and after seeing his show at the 1868 Paris International Exhibition, the gas was introduced to England by Thomas Evans, an American dentist. Evans and Colton used the gas at the London Dental Hospital and other hospitals. The addition of oxygen in nitrous oxide/oxygen apparatus in the 1890s made the procedure safer and more accurate. This anaesthetic agent is still in use today.

William Thomas Green Morton (1819–1868) attended the Baltimore College of Dentistry but left without gaining his diploma. However, he settled down and trained in dentistry with Horace Wells in Hartford, before moving to Boston to set up practice. He met chemist and geologist, Charles Jackson, who later maintained that it was he who suggested to Morton the idea of using ether anaesthesia in dental extractions. Wells demonstrated the use of ether anaesthesia at the Massachusetts General Hospital in October 1846, when a surgeon removed a tumour from the neck of a patient named Edward Abbott. Morton made strenuous efforts to gain recognition for his discovery and news of the advent of painless surgery soon spread worldwide. It became a medical sensation and many different ether inhaler devices were devised.

Chloroform was synthesised in 1831 by three separate people at around the same time: Dr Samuel Guthrie discovered 'chloric ether' in his own laboratory in Sackets Harbor, Jefferson County, New York; the German chemist Justus von Liebig discovered 'carbon chloride'; and the French pharmacist Eugène Soubeiran made what he called 'ether bichlorique'.[7] It remained a chemical curiosity for some years. In the US it was used in the form of an alcoholic solution as a carminative – to induce the expulsion of excess gas from the stomach and intestines. The Scottish surgeon James Simpson (1811–1870) was keen to find a method to operate on his patients without pain so in 1846 he attended a demonstration by Robert Liston of ether anaesthesia in a surgical operation to amputate a leg. However, there were questions about the safety of ether and he started to look at other possible anaesthetic agents. In 1847, he was visited by his friend David Waldie, who worked as a pharmacist at the Apothecaries' Hall in Liverpool. Waldie mentioned to Simpson the possible use of 'chloric ether'. Simpson found a sample locally and tried it out on family and friends. A local manufacturing chemist, Duncan Flockhart and Company, agreed to supply Simpson with chloroform. That same year he tried it out in an obstetric case, Jane Carstairs. He administered it onto a rolled handkerchief which was placed over her mouth and nostrils. The treatment was successful and Jane's second baby was born. He used chloroform on a variety of patients, then wrote a paper for the *Lancet* for the 21 November issue on his experience with his first thirty patients. In addition, he produced a pamphlet entitled '*On a New Anaesthetic Agent, More Efficient than Sulphuric Ether*' and this was advertised on the front page of the *Scotsman* newspaper. By the end of the month it had sold more than 1,500 copies. There was an immediate demand for chloroform from all over England and Scotland. The news of the successful use of chloroform for anaesthesia spread rapidly, and other surgeons began to use it. It became the anaesthetic of choice. In 1853, chloroform was administered to Queen Victoria for the birth of Prince Leopold and again, in 1857, for the birth of Princess Beatrice.

Glyceryl trinitrate and other organic nitrates

Glyceryl trinitrate or nitroglycerine was discovered in 1846 by the Italian chemist Ascanio Sobrero (1812–1888), who worked in Paris with the famous French chemist Theophile-Jules Pelouze.[8] They made nitrocellulose (guncotton) from cotton, then started to look at simpler molecules to make nitrated derivatives to use as explosives. Before turning their attention to glycerol they used mannitol to make the explosive nitromannite. Sobrero named this new glycerol compound pyroglycerine, and was able to demonstrate its remarkable power as an explosive. He also remarked on its pharmacological properties, in that a minute quantity placed on the tongue produced a violent headache. Sobrero's laboratory was visited by Alfred Nobel who realised the commercial potential of nitroglycerine, and went home to Sweden to develop a new class of explosives which could be used to achieve controlled detonation.

Amyl nitrite had been synthesised in 1844, by the French chemist Antoine-Jérôme Balard. Its properties were studied by the English chemist Frederick Guthrie, who remarked that 'one of the most prominent of its properties is the singular effect of its vapour, when inhaled, upon the actions of the heart.' He showed its properties to colleagues in Edinburgh, including Dr Arthur Gamgee. Gamgee began conducting experiments with amyl nitrite on colleagues, including Thomas Lauder Bruton (1844–1916). Bruton started his own research and in 1867, published in the *Lancet* the first report of the use of amyl nitrite in treating a 26-year-old man who suffered from severe chest pains from angina every night. Amyl nitrite relieved the pain, but the effect was only short-lived.

In 1858, there was a controversy in the *Medical Times and Gazette* about the therapeutic properties of nitroglycerine. Mr A.G. Field had experimented on himself and described the effects. Letters from other physicians followed, disputing the dose to be used. William Murrell (1853–1912) was a London physician and familiar with Bruton's work. He began treating angina patients with nitroglycerine in 1878. He published his findings on his trial in thirty-five patients (twelve males and twenty-three females), in an article in the *Lancet*. He reported on four cases with angina who were successfully treated with drops of a 1 per cent solution of nitroglycerine taken in water. Within four years nitroglycerine was regarded as the remedy for angina pectoris. The solution used by Murrell was regarded as inconvenient and he asked the British pharmacist William Martindale to prepare a more suitable preparation. Martindale prepared one hundredths of a grain (650 micrograms) nitroglycerine tablets in a chocolate base. These were included in the official formulary, the *British*

Pharmacopoeia in 1885, and were the first official tablets. Other longer-acting nitrates have since been included in modern medicinal practice – such as isosorbide mononitrate, isosorbide dinitrate and pentaerythritol tetranitrate.

Salvarsan

The origins of syphilis as a disease are unknown. One theory is that it was carried to Europe by the returning crews of Christopher Columbus' ships. Many of the crew members later joined the army of King Charles VIII of France in his invasion of Italy in 1495 and the first recorded outbreak of the disease in Europe occurred in 1494–5 in Naples, during this French invasion. Because it was spread by French troops it was known as 'French disease' or 'French Pox'. From Italy, the disease swept across the rest of Europe. It was a venereal disease, often spread by sailors and soldiers during sexual contact with local prostitutes. The pustules of the disease could cover much of the body. The term 'syphilis' was coined by the Italian poet Girolamo Fracastoro in 1530. Various treatments were used over the years. Mercury was the most common treatment and it had been advocated by Paracelsus. It was applied in various ways, taken by mouth and also applied as an ointment to the affected parts. The most common treatment was with calomel (mercurous chloride). The dose was such that it caused the patient to salivate, which was considered to help expel the disease. Side effects of the treatment included loose teeth and ulcers of the gums. Another popular treatment was with guaiacum. Because guaiacum came from Hispaniola in the West Indies (the island now divided between the two nations of Haiti and the Dominican Republic) where Columbus had landed, it was felt that this might be a cure for the disease, as Nature would surely have provided a cure where a disease originated. By the beginning of the twentieth century, the Special Advisory Board for the Army Medical Service in Britain recommended a more or less continuous course of mercury by mouth for one and a half to two years, in the form of Grey Powder (a powder containing 38 per cent of mercury incorporated into chalk). Mercurial ointment was given in a six-week course rubbed in for 20–30 minutes daily. In 1905, the organism which caused syphilis was discovered by the German zoologist

Fritz Schaudinn (1871–1906) and the dermatologist Erich Hoffmann (1868–1959) working in Berlin. This was the corkscrew-shaped bacterial Spirochaete organism called *Treponema pallidum*.

Paul Ehrlich (1854–1915) is one of the founding fathers of modern medicine. He was born in Upper Silesia in Germany and trained in medicine at the Universities of Breslau, Strasbourg, Freiburg-im-Breisgau and Leipzig.[9] In 1890, Robert Koch appointed Ehrlich as director of a new Institute for Serum Research and Testing in his Berlin Institute for Infectious Diseases. Ehrlich's Institute was moved to Frankfurt in 1899 and renamed the Institute for Experimental Therapy. Since the parasite family of *Plasmodia* organisms which includes the malaria pathogen which can be stained with methylene blue, he thought this dye could possibly be used in the treatment of malaria. He treated two patients at the city hospital in Berlin-Moabit; their fever subsided and the malaria plasmodia disappeared from their blood. Ehrlich had obtained methylene blue from the company Meister Lucius & Brüning AG (later renamed Hoechst AG), which started his collaboration with this company.

Before the Institute of Experimental Therapy had moved to Frankfurt, Ehrlich had already resumed work on methylene blue. After the death of the wealthy banker Georg Speyer, in his memory, his widow Franziska Speyer endowed the Georg-Speyer House, which was built next door to Ehrlich's institute. As director of the Georg-Speyer House, Ehrlich transferred his chemotherapeutic research to the new building. He was looking for an agent which was as effective as methylene blue, but without its side effects. He started screening the activity of hundreds of compounds against *Trypanosoma* infections. Atoxyl or aminophenyl arsenic acid was an arsenic compound that had been synthesised in 1859 by the French biologist Pierre Antoine Béchamp. It had been used in high doses to treat African sleeping sickness, but there was a risk of blindness as it had the potential to damage the optic nerve. Between 1907 and 1909, a number of workers had investigated atoxyl in treating syphilis, with favourable results. But again, there were issues with toxicity. Ehrlich and his chemist Alfred Bertheim started making different derivatives of atoxyl and screening them in mice. Bertheim had been able to show that the original chemical structure assigned to atoxyl was incorrect and once the correct structure was known, they could set about producing chemical modifications of it. In 1909, Ehrlich was joined by a young Japanese scientist, Sahachiro Hata (1873–1938) from the Institute for Infectious Diseases in Tokyo. One compound tested was arsphenamine (Compound 606). Initially the tests on it were negative, but Hata retested it and found that it could cure syphilis in infected rabbits. The animal experiments showed that it was safe, so it was administered in clinical trials to patients with syphilis. Ehrlich and Hata reported the discovery of arsphenamine and its encouraging results on 19 April 1910 at the Congress for Internal Medicine in Wiesbaden. This led to a large number of requests for samples of the drug for testing by other investigators. Hoechst marketed the drug as Salvarsan, 'the arsenic that saves'. The drug needed careful preparation before it could be administered; it was insoluble and needed to be diluted in a basic solution. In 1914, a new arsenical compound was discovered: Compound 904, or neoarsphenamine. Much more convenient to use, it was marketed as Neosalvarsan. Neoarsphenamine was used to treat syphilis in patients until the discovery of penicillin, as detailed in Chapter 7.

Part of the legacy of Paul Ehrlich is the establishment of a method of discovering new medicines by developing experimental animal models for testing new compounds, screening a wide range of chemical compounds, then testing promising candidate compounds in animals, before doing clinical trials in patients.

Sulphonamides

Paul Ehrlich had started looking at dyes which bound selectively to microorganisms as potential therapeutic agents. Other investigators followed up this idea to try to find treatments for bacterial infections.

Gerhard Domagk (1895–1964) was born in Brandenburg in Germany. He graduated in medicine at Kiel University in 1921. In 1927, he was made director of research in experimental pathology and bacteriology at the Farbenfabriken-Bayer Laboratories in Wuppertal-Elberfeld.[10] The two chemists, Fritz Mietzsch and Joseph Klarer, began to synthesise a range of azo dyes for testing by Domagk. Bayer was part of I.G. Farben who dominated the market for synthetic dyes, so facilities were readily available. Domagk began testing of the compounds in mice infected with streptococci. One red dye investigated was chrysoidine where the chemists replaced a hydrogen atom with a sulphonamide group. They called the new compound prontosil. Mice infected with lethal doses of streptococcal and staphylococcal infections recovered when treated with prontosil. Domagk published his results in 1935. The substance was successfully tested in patients with erysipelas (a skin rash) and puerperal fever (also known as childbed fever, a bacterial infection of the female reproductive tract following childbirth or miscarriage). In 1935, the French medicinal chemist Jacques Tréfouël at the Pasteur Institute in Paris working with his wife, chemist Thérèse Tréfouël, and pharmacologists Daniel Bovet and Federico Nitti, conducted research on prontosil. They argued that since chrysoidine was not active against streptococci, it must be the sulphonamide part of the drug substance which was the active part of the molecule. They split off the sulphonamide part, which they named sulphanilamide, and found that it was indeed active against streptococcus. The group also showed sulphanilamide's effective action against other types of bacteria. Sulphanilamide was a known compound not protected by patents and could thus be marketed by anyone. Domagk was nominated for the Nobel Prize in 1938 and this was awarded in 1939. However, since Hitler had forbidden any German from accepting a Nobel Prize he was forced to decline. He eventually received his Nobel gold medal in 1947.

During the next ten years, chemists made many more sulphonamide drugs. One of them was sulfapyridine which was discovered in 1937 by May and Baker. It was known as M&B 693. The sulphonamides were the first effective treatment for bacterial infections.

In December 1943, after attending the Teheran conference with Franklin D. Roosevelt and Joseph Stalin to finalise the strategy for ending the war against Nazi Germany, Winston Churchill became ill and pneumonia was diagnosed.[11] He was given tablets of this new antibiotic (M&B 693; sulfapyridine). He recovered and wrote 'This admirable M&B, from which I did not suffer any inconvenience, was used at the earliest moment and after a week's fever the intruders were repulsed.'

Beta-blockers

In 1878, the Cambridge physiologist John Newport Langley (1852–1925) suggested the idea of a substance in the tissues in the body with which a medicinal substance such as atropine might form a compound. It was not until 1905 he was able to call this a 'receptive substance', based on the actions of nicotine and curare on muscles. Paul Ehrlich changed this name to a 'receptor' in 1900, so that it better described the interaction between the chemicals and cells.[12]

But there were conflicting ideas as to how drugs acted, and the concept of receptors was largely a theory. In the 1920s and 1930s, the physiologist and pharmacologist A. J. Clark developed a mathematical theory to explain how drugs interact with the receptors on the cells. Clark became Professor of Materia Medica in Edinburgh in 1926 and he explained the antagonism between the neurotransmitter acetylcholine and quaternary ammonium salts by the two substances competing for a receptor. In 1948, Raymond Ahlquist from the Department of Pharmacology at the University of Georgia School of Medicine published a paper on his investigations into compounds like adrenaline and their ability to reduce the tone of muscle in the uterus. He was looking for compounds which might reduce period pains. He found that there were two types of adrenergic receptors at which the neurotransmitter passes on messages from the nerves to the muscles and named them alpha and beta receptors.

The firm Imperial Chemical Industries (ICI) was formed in 1926 from the merger of the four largest companies in the British chemical industry. In 1936, the Dyestuffs Group began to carry out pharmaceutical research following on the ideas of Gerhard Domagk at Bayer in Germany. ICI began recruiting biologists in 1937 and as soon as the Second World War broke out, the company moved onto a war footing. 'Atabrine' was a Bayer drug used to treat malaria, and ICI started to manufacture it under its generic name of Mepacrine when it became unavailable from Germany. The company also became involved in the manufacture of penicillin. In 1942, the profits made from sulphonamides and antimalarial drugs led to the creation of ICI Pharmaceuticals. Work was started on the development of drugs to treat hypertension – high blood pressure – in 1951 and the new research centre at Alderley Park was opened in 1957.

James Black (1924–2010) was born in Uddingston, Lanarkshire.[13] He trained in medicine at the University of St Andrews School of Medicine, then worked as a lecturer at King Edward VIII College of Medicine in Singapore. He joined the University of Glasgow Veterinary School in

1950 and established a laboratory looking at physiological problems, particularly cardiovascular disease. Black's father had suffered from angina and had died from a heart attack. When Black approached ICI for a research grant in 1958, they promptly recruited him to work on their coronary artery and high blood pressure projects. The chemists at ICI began making a series of compounds based on dichloroisoproterenol, (DCI) which had been developed by Eli Lilly, and which was the first in a new class of compounds. Pronethalol was synthesised in 1960 and was marketed by ICI in 1963 under the trade name of Alderlin. It was effective in treating angina and some heart arrhythmias. In 1963, Black left ICI. He paid tribute to the work of Ahlquist in developing the theory of two kinds of receptors. He wrote 'Now there is no doubt that the theory of two receptors had a powerful influence in directing the studies of clinical investigators once suitable agents, such as propranolol, became available.' ICI continued to develop beta-blocker drugs and in 1967 propranolol was launched under the name of Inderal, and this was used to treat hypertension as well as angina and heart arrhythmias. In 1970, practolol was launched under the name Eraldin. Eraldin sold well, but by 1974 it had been found to cause blindness in some patients and was withdrawn. ICI had to compensate many patients for what was called 'practolol dry eye'. By 1975, ICI had alternative compounds and atenolol was launched in 1976 as Tenormin.

Black was also interested in developing compounds which would block the histamine receptors in the gut. When ICI was not interested, he left and joined Smith, Kline and French's new Research and Development Department. He worked there until 1973 and developed his second major drug, cimetidine, which was sold under the trade name of Tagamet, and which, for a time, became the world's biggest selling prescription medicine. Black was knighted in 1981 and was awarded the Nobel Prize in Medicine in 1988 together with Gertrude Elon and George Hitchings for their work on drug development.

Chapter 9

Modern Medicines Development

In Chapter 7 a summary was given of how the active ingredients were extracted from natural products – herbal materials, fermentation products, and animal products. These continue to be major sources of new medicines. Chapter 8 included a description of how the first synthesised medicinal chemicals were designed to be similar to natural products such as quinine. The early painkillers were then developed as by-products by German dyestuff manufacturers, such as Bayer, before they became fully fledged pharmaceutical manufacturers. These first chemical medicines were largely developed by 'hit and miss'. The receptor theory explaining how drugs act on the tissues in the body led to the development of drugs such as beta-blockers in the 1960s and 1970s.

Serendipity in drug discovery

The English politician and writer Horace Walpole, writing in 1754, coined the word 'serendipity' after a Persian fairy tale where the Three Princes of Serendip were 'always making discoveries, by accidents and sagacity, of things which they were not in quest of'.[1] Making happy but unexpected discoveries, such as that made by Alexander Fleming with penicillin, has enabled a number of important medicines to be developed. However, it was essential in each case for the importance of a chance observation to be recognised and followed up. As Louis Pasteur said in 1870, 'In the fields of observation chance favours the prepared mind'. Thomas Ban, the Emeritus Professor of Psychiatry at Vanderbilt University in Tennessee, has provided a review of some of the examples of serendipity in drug discovery.[2]

British Drug Houses was founded in 1908 as a wholesaler for private chemists. It expanded into chemicals during the First World War and then subsequently into pharmaceuticals. In 1945 it was trying to produce penicillin but its liquid culture was often contaminated with other bacteria which destroyed the antibiotic. The chemists at British Drug Houses were trying to develop a compound to inhibit microorganisms that break down penicillin. One known compound was phenoxetol. The Czech physician Frank Berger (1913–2008) was asked to work on this project. A number of phenoxetol-related compounds were prepared and when Berger tested them, he found that a class of compounds, the α-substituted ethers, were what he called 'tranquillising' when given to mice, rats or guinea pigs: they made the muscles relax and the animals sleepy. One compound was mephenesin which Berger found was the most potent and the safest. Mephenesin was marketed as a muscle relaxant to use with anaesthesia. In 1947, Berger moved to the University of Rochester in Minnesota, USA. Two years later, he moved to work as the research director at Wallace Laboratories, part of Carter Products. Mephenesin's disadvantage was that it was a short-acting medicine, so Berger started a programme to produce a series of compounds related to it. One longer-acting compound was meprobamate. A trial at a Mississippi hospital showed that it was an effective tranquilliser. The drug was marketed as Miltown by Wallace and as Equanil by Wyeth. By the late 1950s it was the most widely used prescription medicine in the US.

Minoxidil was developed in the late 1950s by Upjohn (which later became part of Pfizer) to treat ulcers. In trials using dogs, the compound did not cure ulcers but proved to be a powerful vasodilator (it widened the blood vessels). It was then tested as a treatment for high blood pressure. These studies resulted in the FDA approving minoxidil tablets under the trade name Loniten in 1979. Before the approval, when Upjohn received permission from the FDA to test the new drug, they approached Charles A. Chidsey at the University of Colorado School of Medicine. He conducted two clinical studies; the second study showed unexpected hair growth as a side effect. Puzzled by this side effect, Chidsey consulted Guinter Kahn and they discussed the possibility of using minoxidil for treating alopecia (hair loss). Kahn and his colleague Paul J. Grant obtained a certain amount of the drug and conducted their own independent research, apparently without notifying Upjohn or Chidsey. The two doctors had been using an experimental 1 per cent solution of minoxidil in several alcohol-based liquids. In August 1988, the drug was approved in the US under the trade name Rogaine® for treating baldness in men. It is sold in Europe under the name Regaine® as a solution and a scalp foam. Thus, a drug for hypertension turned out to be a treatment for hair loss.

Another example of serendipity in drug discovery is the drug now used to treat male erectile dysfunction (the inability to develop or maintain an erection of the penis during sexual activity): sildenafil.[3] In the mid-1980s Pfizer had a very active research programme of cardiovascular research. One approach was to try to develop compounds to treat angina by inhibiting the enzyme phosphorodiesterase (PDE). Five subtypes of phosphorodiesterase were discovered: PDE-1 to PDE-5. One of the compounds developed was sildenafil, which inhibited PDE-5 and showed good vasodilatory effects. When it was tested in clinical trials it was generally well tolerated and at moderate to high doses reduced blood pressure. Some volunteers in the trials reported headaches, flushing, indigestion and muscle aches. Others also reported erections of the penis as a side effect. However, the drug had a short half-life in blood so would have to be administered several times a day for angina, and it also interacted with nitrates used for treatment of angina. Thoughts therefore turned to erectile dysfunction as a possible indication for the drug, since it inhibited PDE-5 (an enzyme that breaks down cGMP, which regulates blood flow in the penis). It required sexual arousal, however, to work. In 1993, trials were started in healthy men with no cardiovascular disease but with erection problems. Sildenafil was found to be effective in a wide range of patients, including those with diabetes, multiple sclerosis and spinal injury. An efficacy of over 70 per cent was seen in all trials. The company marketed sildenafil under the trade name Viagra in 1998. Thus, a drug developed to treat one condition had a 'side effect' which enabled it to be used for another condition – a real case of serendipity.

The first blockbuster drug – cimetidine

In 1963, James Black was hired by Smith, Kline and French Laboratories in Welwyn Garden City to work on compounds to treat stomach ulcers. The production of gastric acid is stimulated by histamine, and it was felt to be worthwhile to study drugs which would counteract the effects of histamine by acting as an antagonist.[4] Black asked the team of chemists led by C. Robin Ganellin to make compounds which might block one of the two types of histamine receptor: the H2 receptor. Between 1964 and 1968 they synthesised about 200 compounds chemically related to histamine. In 1970, the first active compound, burinamide, was discovered, but it had to be injected to work as it was not well absorbed when given by mouth. Another compound which was active in the animal studies was metiamide. However, metiamide caused agranulocytosis – a depression of the infection-fighting white cells in the bone marrow. Because metiamide contained a thiourea group which was thought to cause toxic effects, other compounds that did not contain this chemical group were investigated. Cimetidine was synthesised in 1972, which did not cause agranulocytosis and when tested in clinical trials in patients, relieved the symptoms of stomach ulcers and promoted healing. The drug was marketed in the UK in 1976 and in the US in 1977. By 1979, it had been marketed in over 100 countries under the trade name Tagamet. In 1986, Tagamet sold over $1 billion, becoming the first blockbuster drug (the definition of a blockbuster drug is that it sells over $1 billion in one year).

During the development of cimetidine, the Smith Kline and French chemists and biologists had to consider which parts of the chemical molecules they were developing were essential for blocking the H2 receptor to give the drug its activity in treating stomach ulcers, and which parts of the molecule might give unwanted toxicity. This is known as the study of Structure-Activity Relationships (SARs).

Lock and key theory of drug-receptor action

In 1894, the German chemist Emil Fischer (1852–1919) suggested that how well an enzyme works on the substance on which it acts is based on the two components exhibiting complementary shapes that fit together like a 'key in a lock'. This simple 'lock and key' idea can also be used to describe the interaction between a protein on a tissue and a small chemical molecule such as a drug, where the 'lock' described the protein structure of the receptor and the 'key' the drug.[5] In such systems, it is essential that the 'key' fits well into the keyhole (the receptor) for the pharmacological effect to take place. Keys that are too small, too large or with incorrectly positioned notches and grooves, will not fit into the lock.

Current methods of medicinal chemical discovery

If we consider the receptor system as the target for discovery of new medicines, by the 1980s, instead of carefully synthesising each new chemical candidate in turn using simple equipment, automation had been introduced. Instead, libraries of thousands of chemical compounds had become commercially available, which could be screened for activity.[6]

Combinatorial chemistry has been used since the 1990s to provide large numbers of chemical molecules by chemically linking individual building blocks, which can then be screened for activity as medicines. Using robotics, combinatorial chemistry can enable companies to produce over 100,000 new compounds per year. The approach often used is to attach a chemical starting material onto a solid support such as an insoluble polymer, then carry out a series of reactions on it. The final product is then purified and removed from the solid support.

The evaluation of these thousands of compounds for activity has also been automated using high-throughput screening (HTS) with robotics, data processing and control software, and detector systems. A key component for HTS is the microtiter plate – a small container, usually plastic, which has within it a grid of small open depressions called wells. The wells could contain the different chemical compounds in solution together with a protein or cells of some sort. Measurements are taken of the cells or protein to see how they alter under the influence of the different candidate drug molecules. If a compound produces the desired effect it is called a 'hit'. In addition to cells or proteins, in some cases intact living organisms such as nematodes or zebrafish have been used.

But have all of these advances in automation led to an increased rate of drug discovery? The evidence is equivocal.

Pharmacogenomics and personalised medicine

Patients have a highly variable response to particular medicines. Some will respond well, others hardly at all. Some will show significant side effects, some none. The differences are due to each person's molecular and genetic profile. One example is that many Japanese can only tolerate drinking alcohol in very small amounts since they become easily intoxicated. This is due to a deficiency of the enzyme alcohol dehydrogenase, which breaks down alcohol in the body.[7] Another example was found when African American soldiers were taking the antimalarial drug primaquine. Many of them developed an acute anaemia. This was found to be due to a deficiency of the glucose-6-phosphate enzyme which is essential in providing energy to the red blood cells through the metabolism of glucose.[8]

The study of the effect of genetic differences on the way in which medicines act and are broken down in the body is called 'pharmacogenomics'. This new science enables the treatment to be tailored to the disease and the individual patient, in what is called 'personalised medicine'. Some examples of how genetic information can be used to best treat patients are given below.[9]

Trastuzumab was approved in 1998 and marketed as Herceptin for treatment of breast cancer. It is a genetically engineered monoclonal antibody – see Chapter 10 for more details of these products. About 25–30 per cent of breast cancer patients produce more epidermal growth factor receptor-2 protein (HER-2). Trastuzumab is approved for use in breast cancer patients whose tumours produce more HER-2, so patients have to be tested before treatment is started.

BRAF is the gene responsible for the production of B-Raf protein, which sends signals in cells to direct their growth. In some cancers there is a mutant form of this gene. About 60 per cent of patients with melanoma cancer have a mutation of the BRAF gene, and 90 per cent of those have the mutation called V600E. In 2012, a drug called vemurafenib was marketed as Zelboraf. Vemurafenib only works in people who have been tested as positive for the V600E BRAF mutation, so all patients need to be tested before this treatment is started.

Clopidogrel was approved in 1998 and marketed under the trade name of Plavix. It is used to treat patients at risk of heart attack and stroke. It is broken down in the liver by CYP2C19 enzyme into the active medicinal chemical. About 23 per cent of Occidental and Asian patients are less able to break the drug down – they are poor metabolisers. These patients are more at risk of dying, having a heart attack or a stroke.

Tamoxifen blocks the action of the hormone oestrogen and is used to treat and prevent some types of breast cancer. It is broken down in the body by the liver CYP2D6 and CYP3A4 enzymes into active drugs such as afimoxifene and endoxifen. Eight per cent of the population have no CYP2D6 enzyme activity and about 50 per cent of the Occidental population have decreased CYP2D6 activity. In these women there will be lower levels of the active medicines and they need to be treated with a different type of medicine to tamoxifen.

Warfarin was marketed in the 1950s as an anticoagulant to prevent clots being formed in the blood vessels or lungs. It is often given to stroke patients. The levels of warfarin in the blood are monitored by a clotting test on a blood sample and expressed as the International Normalised Ratio (INR). If the INR is too high there is a risk of bleeding. Warfarin is broken down in the body by the CYP2C9 enzyme in the liver. The major genetic factors which affect the variation in response to warfarin are variants of this CYP2C9 enzyme. In the US the data sheet for warfarin tells the prescriber how to adjust the dose of warfarin based on this patient genetic information.

Drug Repurposing

It takes about 12–15 years to develop, and approval must be obtained from the regulatory authorities before a new drug can be marketed. The whole development process has been estimated to cost between $1 and $2 billion on average. It therefore makes sense to look at some of the old medicines that have already been developed and tested to see if they might be suitable for a new use. There may be 9,000 old medicines that are no longer covered by a patent and which could be considered for possible new uses – what is called repurposing.

One of the most striking examples of drug repurposing is thalidomide. This medicine was marketed as a safe sedative in the 1950s by the German company Chemie Grünenthal. By the early 1960s severe side effects had been seen with the drug, firstly peripheral nerve damage, then the appearance of severe malformations in children born to mothers who had taken the drug. It caused an estimated 10,000 children to be born with birth defects in 46 countries – limb malformations, and defects of the eyes, ears, kidney and heart. It was taken off the market in all countries and it stimulated the development of the official regulatory systems to control the safety of medicines in Europe, the US and elsewhere. In

1965, it was discovered that thalidomide was effective in treating one of a number of conditions, including leprosy – erythema nodosum leprosum. Patients with this condition have crops of painful, red skin nodules with symptoms of fever and general malaise. It also involves other body systems and organs. In 1994, it was seen that thalidomide could stop the formation of new blood vessels from existing ones – what is called angiogenesis.[10] Angiogenesis is part of what drives cells to grow uncontrollably in the bone marrow of patients with myeloma. Thalidomide is now used to treat myeloma cancer patients.

Bupropion was first developed as an antidepressant and approved in the US in 1989. It was subsequently discovered that it was effective in stopping smoking, in conjunction with motivational support. Smoking cessation is the only indication for the drug in the UK and Australia.

Duloxetine was an antidepressant which found a new use. It was developed for use in stress urinary incontinence – this is a condition in which patients have accidental leakage of urine during physical exertion or activities such as coughing, sneezing, laughing, exercise or lifting. At low doses it is used for this condition, and at higher doses it is used for major depression, generalised anxiety and the nerve pain associated with diabetes.

Tretinoin is one of a class of medicines called the retinoids, and it is used for the treatment of severe acne. It is now also used as a treatment for a cancer of the white blood cells – acute promyelocytic leukaemia.

Chapter 10

Biologicals, Biotechnology, Biopharmaceuticals and Biosimilars

Thishis chapter is about biological medicines: those which contain one or more medicinal substances made from a biological source, such as living cells or organisms. Some of the materials, such as insulin or growth hormone, are present in the human body naturally. Most of them are proteins that are much larger and more complex than conventional small molecule medicines, and will contain thousands of atoms. They use complex manufacturing techniques. The word 'biopharmaceutical' is also used to describe a pharmaceutical product manufactured using biotechnology methods such as those involving live organisms.

Vaccines

Smallpox

Smallpox is believed to have originated in Africa in about 10000 BCE and spread to India via Egypt. Smallpox was reported in China in about 1100 BCE. It was introduced into Europe between the fifth and seventh centuries. It has been estimated that during the twentieth century it was responsible for 300–500 million deaths and 10 per cent of deaths worldwide over the last 1,000 years.

Smallpox was a viral disease. It had an incubation period of about two weeks. The first symptoms were headache, sore throat and vomiting. This was followed by the appearance of a pink rash, which gradually spread to the face, abdomen and limbs and grew into itchy blisters. The blisters scabbed over after about a week before dropping off, leaving scarring. There were two strains of the virus, *variola major* which was often deadly, and *variola minor* which was a milder infection.

The earliest attempts to prevent the disease used a process called variolation. This involved taking a sample of pus from a smallpox blister from an infected person and introducing it under the skin of another individual. This seems to have been done for centuries in China, India and parts of Asia. Traders introduced the practice into Turkey. If the person being variolated was lucky, they were treated with the mild form of smallpox. About 2 per cent of people being variolated died from the treatment. This compared to the mortality rate of 30 per cent for untreated people during an epidemic.

Lady Wortley Montagu (1689–1762) introduced the process of variolation to Britain. She was the wife of the British ambassador to Turkey and had seen the process carried out by the local women using pus from a smallpox blister. She was impressed and had the embassy doctor Charles Maitland variolate her son. The Montagus returned to England in 1718. In 1721, during a smallpox epidemic, she asked Maitland to variolate her daughter. She persuaded Queen Caroline, wife of King George II to have some of the royal children variolated, and the practice became fashionable. In 1757, an 8-year- old boy named Edward Jenner was variolated with smallpox; he developed a mild case of the disease but was then immune to any further infection.

Benjamin Jesty (1736–1816) was a farmer on the Upbury Farm in Yetminster in Devon.[1] He was married with four sons and three daughters. It was known in the farming community that milkmaids and other farm workers who contracted cowpox were immune to smallpox infections. Jesty and two of his servants, Ann Notley and Mary Reade, had been infected with cowpox. When an outbreak of smallpox arrived in Yetminster in 1774, Jesty took the decision to infect his wife and two eldest sons with cowpox. He travelled with them to a neighbouring farm and using a needle, transferred pus from an infected cow's udder to the arms of his wife and sons. Although exposed to smallpox over the next years his sons did not catch smallpox. Jesty extended his practice of vaccination to others, including a local lady called Abigail Brown.

Edward Jenner (1749–1823) was born in Berkeley, Gloucestershire.[2] When he was 5, he was orphaned and was brought up by his elder brother. At the age of 13 he was apprenticed to Daniel Ludlow, a surgeon in Sodbury, near Bristol. In 1770, he became a student at St George's

Hospital in London, and a pupil of John Hunter, the surgeon, before returning to Berkeley to practice medicine as a country physician in 1773. For many years Jenner had heard stories that dairymaids were protected from smallpox if they had suffered from cowpox. His first experiment to confirm this was in May 1796, when he found Sarah Nelms, a young dairymaid, who had cowpox lesions on her arms. He used pus (lymph) from the lesions to inoculate an 8-year-old boy, James Phipps. The boy felt unwell for a couple of days but recovered. In July, Jenner inoculated the boy with matter from a fresh smallpox lesion. No disease developed and Jenner concluded that the boy had been protected from smallpox. In 1797, Jenner sent a short communication to the Royal Society describing this experiment, but his paper was rejected. Jenner continued his trials of cowpox and in 1798, having added some more cases, he published a pamphlet entitled *An Inquiry into the Causes and Effects of the Variolae Vaccinae, a disease discovered in some of the western counties of England, particularly Gloucestershire and Known by the Name of Cow Pox*. Jenner called his new procedure 'vaccination' derived from the Latin words for cow – *vacca*, and for cowpox *vaccinia*. Seeking more volunteers for vaccination, Jenner went to London. Although his quest was unsuccessful, others became interested in his work. Dr William Woodville, who was the physician to the Smallpox and Inoculation Hospitals in London, was one of the most practised inoculators and he and Jenner supplied lymph to others. The use of vaccination spread rapidly in England, and by 1800 it had reached other European countries. Jenner received honour and public recognition for his work, and was given two parliamentary grants of £10,000 and £20,000.

In 1805, farmer Benjamin Jesty was invited to London by the Jennerian Society. He came, accompanied by his son Robert. He was presented with a pair of gold-mounted lancets and his portrait was painted by Mr. M.W. Sharpe. A long testimonial was also presented to him acknowledging that he had been the first person to inoculate using cowpox, over twenty years before Jenner's experiments.

The vaccination of all children within three months of birth was made compulsory under the 1853 Vaccination Act. The 1867 Vaccination Act made Poor Law guardians responsible for the control of vaccination. Vaccinators were paid 1 to 3 shillings per child vaccinated in a district.

The pus (lymph) from infected lesions on cows was often infected with other organisms. In 1932, the official monograph in the *British Pharmacopoeia* required it to be treated with glycerol to reduce the numbers of living bacteria. By the 1950s the vaccine was produced using membranes of chick embryos in eggs inoculated with vaccinia virus.

There was a smallpox outbreak in south Wales in 1962. Some 19 people died and 900,000 were vaccinated after a traveller from Pakistan arrived in Cardiff and was diagnosed with the disease. The authors of this book were both working in south Wales at the time and were among those vaccinated.

In 1967, the World Health Organization began a global campaign to eradicate smallpox. On 8 May 1980, the World Health Assembly announced that the world was free from smallpox.

Animal vaccines

Galen had postulated that disease was caused by miasma, a form of 'bad air' emitted by rotting organic matter. Miasma was considered to be a poisonous vapour or mist with particles from decomposed matter (*miasmata*). The Italian physician Girolamo Fracastoro proposed in 1546 in his book *De Contagione et Contagiosis Morbis* (*Infectious and Contagious Diseases*) that diseases are caused by transferable seed-like entities (*seminaria morbi*) that transmit infection by direct or indirect contact.[3] However, the orthodox miasma theory held sway over the germ theory until the work of Louis Pasteur and Robert Koch.

Animal diseases also killed hundreds of animals in the nineteenth century, and caused starvation in the human population where outbreaks occurred. Fowl cholera in chickens and anthrax in sheep were common. Scientists began to study diseases in animals to try to develop vaccines which could be used.

Louis Pasteur (1822–1895) was born in Dole in the Jura in France.[4] He received his Batchelor of Letters degree from the Collège Royal de Besançon in 1840, then studied at the École Normale Supérieure in Paris, graduating in 1845 with a licencié ès sciences. He became briefly professor of physics at the Dijon Lycée in 1848, then professor of chemistry in Strasbourg. In 1854, he became dean of sciences at the University of Lille. Here he carried out his studies on fermentation and showed that the growth of microorganisms was responsible for the spoiling of milk, beer and wine. He moved to Paris as director of scientific studies at the École Normale Supérieure in 1857, and in 1863 became professor of geology, physics and chemistry at the École Nationale Supérieure des Beaux-Arts. From 1867 until 1888 he was director of the physiological laboratory at the École Normale Supérieure and it was during this period that he began work on chicken cholera (in 1879). In 1876, Henri Toussaint had shown that the causative organism was a bacterium. Pasteur cultured the bacterium in a variety of different nutrients to try to find one where the virulence of the organism was reduced. At one point he went on vacation, leaving his assistant Charles Chamberland to carry on making cultures. However, Chamberland also went on holiday and one culture was left to grow. When he returned a month later, he injected the culture into chickens, and although it made them sick, it did not kill them. He subsequently inoculated the chickens with a virulent culture and they survived. Pasteur concluded that he had made the chickens immune to the infection by injecting them with a weakened culture of the bacterium, concluding that this weakened bacterium could be used as a vaccine, and that this method might be used for other microorganisms.

Robert Koch (1843–1910) was born in Clausthal, in Germany.[5] He trained in medicine at the University of Göttingen, then served as an army doctor during the Franco-Prussian War. After the war he moved to Wöllstein in present-day Poland as district medical officer. While practising as a physician he began studying anthrax, a disease of animals and man. Koch was able to show the life cycle of the anthrax bacillus from spores in soil to the rod-like structures seen in the blood, lymph and spleen of infected animals. This was confirmation of the germ theory and showed the role of contagious bacteria in disease.

In 1881, Pasteur found that growing anthrax bacilli at 42°C made them unable to produce spores and argued that he had thus weakened them, providing the basis for the preparation of a vaccine. He was challenged to make a demonstration of his vaccine and so carried out a public demonstration on sheep, goats and cows. This was successful. However, in 1985, when Pasteur's laboratory notebooks became publicly available, it became clear he had used heat and potassium dichromate to kill the bacteria, rather than weaken them.

Human vaccines

Pasteur carried on his investigations into other diseases. In the 1880s, working with Émile Roux, he developed a rabies vaccine from the spinal cord of a rabbit that had died from the disease. He found that if the spinal cord was dried it weakened the disease-causing organism. In 1885, Pasteur tried out his vaccine on dogs, then on Joseph Meister, a 9-year-old boy who had been bitten by a rabid dog. The treatment was successful and Pasteur became a public hero. In 1886, he treated 350 people, only one of whom developed rabies.

There are now a number of types of vaccine: live attenuated (weakened) vaccines; killed vaccines; toxoid vaccines – where the toxin (poison) secreted by the organism is deactivated by exposing to heat or formaldehyde treatment; subunit vaccines – where the part of the organism that causes the strongest response to the disease (the antigen) is isolated and purified; and polyvalent vaccines – where the vaccine works against multiple strains or subspecies of organism. Some examples of each type are given in Table 10.1:

Table 10.1: Examples of different types of vaccine.

Type of vaccine	Examples of the type of vaccine
Live attenuated vaccines	Chickenpox, measles, mumps, rubella, shingles, yellow fever and oral polio vaccine
Killed vaccines	Hepatitis A, rabies
Toxoid vaccines	Diphtheria, tetanus
Subunit vaccines	Anthrax, hepatitis B
Polyvalent vaccines	Human papilloma virus, influenza, meningococcal, pneumococcal and polio

Antitoxins

Emil von Behring (1854–1917) was born in Harsdorf, West Prussia. He took his medical degree at the University of Berlin in 1878.[6] He served as a military surgeon in the Army Medical Corps until 1889 before joining Robert Koch as an assistant at the Institute for Infectious Diseases in Berlin. The institute was a centre for bacteriological research, where F. Loeffler had described the diphtheria bacillus and Kitasato Shibasaburō had discovered the tetanus bacillus. Working with Kitasato in 1890,

Behring injected a toxin from the diphtheria and tetanus bacilli into animals, then showed that the animals were protected against cultures of the living organisms. In addition, he showed the serum from an animal treated with the toxin could be used to treat an animal against an attack of the disease. He called the name of the substance in the serum of the immunised animal an 'antitoxin'. This method could be used to develop a means to immunise patients. Using a more modern terminology, Behring and Kitasato had discovered antibody molecules in the blood of immunised animals, and had shown that the antibodies could neutralise the toxins from tetanus and diphtheria infections. In 1901, Behring was awarded the Nobel Prize for medicine for his work on diphtheria serum therapy. For medical use in treating human infectious diseases, antitoxins are still sometimes produced by injecting an animal with toxin; the animal, most commonly a horse, is given repeated small doses of toxin until a high concentration of the antitoxin builds up in the blood. The resulting highly concentrated preparation of antitoxins is called an antiserum.

Antibodies

Paul Ehrlich was the first to use the term 'antibody' in a text entitled *Experimental Studies on Immunity* published in 1891. An antibody is a protein produced by the immune system to fight outside invading substances.[7] Since the enemy-invading substance actually triggers the production of antibodies, these invading substances are called 'antigens' – 'anti' being short for antibody, and 'gen' meaning 'producer'. The Hungarian physician Ladislas Deutsch coined the term 'antigen' in 1899. In the 1920s, the American immunologist Michael Heidelberger and the Canadian-American physician Oswald Avery found that antigens could be precipitated by antibodies and they went on to show that antibodies are made of protein.

In 1951, Henry Kunkel, an immunologist working at the Rockefeller Institute in New York was investigating the blood of myeloma cancer patients. He found that the malignant plasma cells produced only one antibody, and this was different to the normal plasma cells which produced a wide range of antibodies. During the 1970s, work started on creating a hybrid cell, or hybridoma, by fusing human B cells, a type of white blood cells, with mouse myeloma cells. These hybridoma cells would be capable of secreting antibodies with a known antigen specificity. In 1974, Cesar Milstein and George Kohler working at the Medical Research Council Laboratory of Molecular Biology in Cambridge created a hybridoma which produced large amounts of antibodies. They created an immortal cell line capable of producing an endless supply of identical antibodies. The antibodies were called 'monoclonal antibodies' since they came from a single hybrid cell. They announced their discovery in a paper in the journal *Nature* in 1975. Kohler and Milstein were awarded a share in the 1984 Nobel Prize for physiology or medicine for their discovery.

Monoclonal antibodies have developed into a standard treatment for some diseases and examples of some of the marketed drugs are given in Table 10.2:

Table 10.2: Monoclonal antibodies approved for use in medicine.

Name of drug	Type of drug	Condition(s)
Infliximab	Anti-inflammatory	Rheumatoid arthritis, Crohn's disease
Adalunimab	Anti-inflammatory	Rheumatoid arthritis, Crohn's disease
Tocilizumab	Anti-inflammatory	Rheumatoid arthritis
Secukinumab	Anti-inflammatory	Psoriatic arthritis
Basiliximab	Anti-inflammatory	Rejection of kidney transplants
Daclizumab	Anti-inflammatory	Rejection of kidney transplants
Omalizumab	Anti-inflammatory	Allergic asthma
Gemtuzumab	Anti-cancer	Myeloid leukaemia
Ipilimumab	Anti-cancer	Melanoma
Rituximab	Anti-cancer	Non-Hodgkin's lymphoma
Trastuzumab	Anti-cancer	Breast cancer with HER2 over-expression
Bevacizumab	Anti-cancer	Colorectal cancer
Cetuximab	Anti-cancer	Colorectal cancer
Natalizumab	Other	Multiple sclerosis

Recombinant DNA (rDNA) technology

Living organisms can be used to manufacture chemicals. We have already seen in Chapter 7 that *Penicillium chrysogenum* mould was used to produce penicillin, *Actinomyces aurofaciens* to produce chlortetracycline etc.

The main organisms used to manufacture biological medicines are bacteria and yeasts. Cells from mammals such as Chinese hamster ovary (CHO) cells or baby hamster kidney (BHK) cells are also used.

In the early 1970s, Herbert Boyer from the University of California in San Francisco and Stanley Cohen from Stanford University began to work together on genetic engineering of cells, so that the genetic information in the DNA in the cell came from more than one species.[8,9] Cohen was working on plasmids: small DNA molecules within a cell, physically separated from the DNA in the chromosome. Plasmids are most commonly found as small circular, double-stranded DNA molecules in bacteria and yeasts. The chromosomes are big and contain all the essential genetic information for living under normal conditions, but plasmids usually are very small and contain only additional genes that may be useful to the organism under particular conditions. Cohen had found a way to transfer a plasmid from one organism into another, giving it different properties. Boyer was working on restriction enzymes which allowed him to use them like scissors to snip the DNA in the plasmid to allow an extra gene to be incorporated, and then for the plasmid to be repaired. Using this technique, Boyer and Cohen were able to introduce genes from the toad *Xenopus* into bacteria. Cohen went back to his academic work, but Boyer set up a company, Genentech Inc. in San Francisco in 1976 with an investor, Robert Swanson, to begin to produce medicines using this genetic engineering technology.

In 1923, Eli Lilly in the US started producing insulin for treating diabetes by extracting it from the pancreas of cows. Later, the Danish company Nordisk manufactured it from the pancreas of pigs. In 1978, Genentech produced biosynthetic 'human' insulin in *Escherichia coli* bacteria using recombinant DNA techniques. They licensed the process to Eli Lilly and the first human insulin was sold from 1982 onwards. All insulin used in the US for treating human patients is now genetically engineered material, not from cows or pigs.

Example of some of the important drugs produced using recombinant DNA technology are given in Table 10.3:

Table 10.3: Important medicines produced using recombinant DNA technology.

Type of product	Drug	Condition
Hormone	Insulin	Diabetes
Hormone	Somatotropin	Growth failure in children
Hormone promoting formation of red blood cells	Erythropoietin	Anaemia associated with kidney failure, HIV infection, cancer
Blood coagulation factor	Factor VIII	Treatment of haemophilia A
Blood coagulation factor	Factor IX	Treatment of haemophilia B
Clot-buster drugs	Alteplase, Reteplase	Heart attack
Interferon	Interferon alpha-2b	Hairy cell leukaemia, hepatitis B and C, cancer
Interferon	Interferon beta-1b	Multiple sclerosis
Enzyme	Dorsase alpha	Cystic fibrosis

Biosimilars

When conventional small molecule chemical medicines come off patent, other companies can get approval for similar products using the same active ingredient drug. These are called 'generic' products.

Biological medicines contain highly complex drugs and because they are made from a biological source, and use a complex manufacturing process, they are more variable. When biological medicines come off patent, other manufacturers produce copies of them. These copies are very similar to the original product which is already approved. It will have been shown to work in the same way as the original (have the same efficacy) and be as safe. These medicines are called 'biosimilars' and are not considered to be a generic equivalent to the original product. The European Union (EU) through its European Medicines Agency has pioneered the requirements for approval of biosimilars, and has imposed rigorous criteria for their approval to market them. The EU approved the first biosimilar in 2006, the growth hormone somatotropin. Since then it has approved another forty-six biosimilars.

Biological medicines are a major cost to national healthcare systems such as the UK's National Health Service. Eight out of the top ten medicines in terms of cost in England were biologicals as shown in Table 10.4:

Table 10.4: Top 10 medicines at list price prescribed or used by the NHS in England in 2017/2018.

Name of Medicine	Category	Condition treated	Cost in £ millions
Adalimumab	Monoclonal antibody	Rheumatoid arthritis, Crohn's disease, ulcerative colitis	494
Aflibercept	rDNA	Wet age-related macular degeneration (AMD)	366
Etanercept	rDNA	Rheumatoid arthritis	220
Infliximab	Monoclonal antibody	Rheumatoid arthritis	200
Rivaroxaban	Chemical	Prevention of blood clots	183
Apixaban	Chemical	Prevention of blood clots	182
Trastuzumab	Monoclonal antibody	HER-2 positive breast cancer	164
Ranibizumab	Monoclonal antibody	Wet age-related macular degeneration (AMD)	154
Rituximab	Monoclonal antibody	Cancer	154
Lenalidomide	Monoclonal antibody	Multiple myeloma cancer	147

Biosimilar drugs are cheaper and therefore offer healthcare systems substantial savings.[1] According to NHS England, switching to the latest biosimilars for infliximab, etanercept and rituximab saved the organisation £210 million in 2017–18. The highest cost drug available on the NHS in 2017–18 was adalimumab (Humira, made by AbbVie) and this came off patent in October 2018. Competitors are now able to bring their own versions of this drug to the market at lower prices.

There are a further eighteen biological products coming off patent by 2023. These include the monoclonal antibody products trastuzumab, alemtuzumab and bevacizumab. When patients are switched from the originator product to a biosimilar they will be given information and guidance. In some cases, such as the drug adalimumab, where the drug is self-administered by patients using a special auto-injector syringe device, this method could alter when the biosimilar product is introduced. Any changes will need to be explained to the patient.

Part Two

History of Dosage Forms

Chapter 11

Introduction to Dosage Forms

The public talks about paracetamol being taken for the relief of mild to moderate pain, or hydrocortisone being applied for the treatment of skin disorders. However, it is a tablet containing paracetamol or a cream or ointment containing hydrocortisone that is actually used. Hardly any active ingredients are used without some preliminary treatment or mixing with other ingredients to give a manufactured medicine. So, a physician does not prescribe a 'drug', he prescribes a medicine – a syrup, a tablet, capsule, injection or inhaler.

The form of a medicine (tablet, cream etc.) is known as the dosage form, and the other ingredients with which the active ingredient is mixed are called excipients. The mixture of active ingredient and excipients is called the formulation. Formerly, excipients were referred to as 'inactive ingredients' to contrast them from the active ingredient, but this is misleading. Whilst excipients cannot give an active ingredient an activity it does not inherently possess, the use of inappropriate excipients can reduce or, in extreme cases, even abolish the pharmacological effects of the active ingredient.

The primary aim of the formulator must be to ensure that the active ingredient can carry out its intended therapeutic effect by reaching its target in the body and remaining there in sufficient concentration for an adequate length of time. Though formulators in earlier times would not have used these terms, it would have been their aim too, using the knowledge and skills then available to them.

There would be three key decisions to be made.

a) The choice of dosage form.
b) The choice of excipients.
c) The choice of manufacturing process.

When making these decisions, the following considerations are borne in mind:

1. All ingredients in the medicine, both active ingredient(s) and excipients, must comply with legal standards for their quality, safety and efficacy.
2. The medicine must contain, within strict limits, the correct amount of active ingredient.

The medicine should, if possible:

3. offer long-term stability;
4. encourage compliance by the patient i.e. the medicine is used in accordance with the instructions of the prescriber and manufacturer; and
5. be cost-effective in production and use.

The choice of the type of medicine to be used in conjunction with a given active ingredient is a key decision. Though formulation science has made major advances in recent years, the basic principles governing the choice of dosage form have been known for centuries. The range of dosage forms available is very large. One hundred and three different dosage forms have been the subject of monographs in *The British Pharmacopoeia* from 1864 to 2018, and this total does not, of course, include those dosage forms that had already become obsolete before 1864. The popularity of different dosage forms has changed over the years. But it is important to put these into a historical context.

The nineteenth century was a period of unprecedented change in Western Europe and the US. Using Britain as an example, at the beginning of the century, the state had a predominantly agrarian economy. The majority of the population, then totalling about 10 million, lived in small towns or villages, with the bulk of the male population being employed in agriculture or trades related to it. By the end of the century, most of the population, by now totalling about 38 million, lived in cities or large towns, with the male population being involved in manufacturing of some kind. A range of factors – political, social and economic –

contributed to this change, but undoubtedly a major influence was a series of events now known as the Industrial Revolution, a term first used in the Anglophone world by the economist Arnold Toynbee (1852–1883). Before this, all wooden or metal artefacts were made by human manual labour, perhaps with animal, wind or water assistance, using tools that had been essentially unchanged for centuries. Output was limited by the physical capabilities of the human operator, and there was an unavoidable variation between individual items.

A key development was the invention of the steam engine. Thomas Newcomen invented the first commercially successful steam engine in 1712, and this was significantly improved by James Watt in 1781. If a steam engine is connected to a piston, a rotating motion can be obtained, which in turn can be connected to a machine, usually by a rotating shaft or driving belt. The first impact of this was felt in the textile manufacturing industries where inventions such as the Spinning Jenny by James Hargreaves and the Spinning Mule by Samuel Crompton increased the output of cotton thread and cloth by an enormous margin, steam power replacing the manual efforts of thousands of individual workers. However, human labour was still needed, and workers flocked to these sites of industrial activity, usually from the countryside.

Soon mechanisation spread to virtually all other aspects of manufacture and large-scale production in a relatively small number of manufacturing sites was now feasible. Another consequence of mechanisation was that the product achieved a previously unattainable degree of uniformity, and this in turn demanded that standards for the product had to be established. The standardisation of the thread in screws, nuts and bolts, established by Joseph Whitworth in the 1840s, is an everyday example of this.

If production of a given item was concentrated in only a few sites, then those items had to be transported economically to the ultimate user, and the road system of the time could not cope with it. The steam engine provided a solution to this problem too. When the boiler was connected to a set of wheels, a means of propulsion resulted, leading to the railway system.

By the end of the nineteenth century, machines were available to replace hand-made artefacts, and medicine manufacture was no exception.

There was a gradual decline in the number of preparations made by hand in favour of those whose manufacture could be mechanised. The dramatic increase in the use of tablets and the decline in pill usage are good examples.

As in other applications of mechanisation, the output of many individual producers, many of whom were pharmacists, was replaced by relatively few industrial sites, giving rise to the pharmaceutical industry as we know it today. The pharmacist of the time had acquired his knowledge after a long period of apprenticeship and training, and some of these skills were no longer required. This in turn had a profound effect on pharmaceutical practice and education.

Another factor that had a profound influence on medicine manufacture was the development of organic chemistry, particularly in Germany. In the mid-1850s, the majority of medicines were based on materials of vegetable origin, as they had been for centuries. The active ingredient had to be separated from a mass of vegetable matter by a process of extraction. There were a large number of liquid extracts in the 1864 and 1885 editions of *The British Pharmacopoeia*. For convenience, the liquid extracts were often concentrated to give dry extracts.

In the early part of the nineteenth century, chemical techniques were developed to isolate and purify the active ingredients and determine their chemical structures. A good example is the alkaloids contained in opium (as mentioned in Chapter 7). Whilst it might not have been economically worthwhile or even possible to synthesise these substances, given chemical knowledge at that time, those that could be isolated could be modified chemically in the hope of obtaining a more active or less toxic substance. A good example was the isolation and identification of salicylic acid as the active ingredient of willow bark and the changing of the structure by a simple chemical reaction to give acetylsalicylic acid, otherwise known as aspirin. Aspirin was followed by other anti-inflammatory agents of related structures. These substances were almost invariably solids of high purity, which could then be incorporated into solid dosage forms, of which the tablet and the hard shell capsules are good examples.

The target organ

The choice of dosage form is governed by the location of the target for the active ingredient. Dosage forms exist for application to all body orifices, and if no suitable orifice exists, one can be created with a needle in the form of an injection. There are also dosage forms that do not need an orifice, but can be applied to the intact skin. Targets may be external, on the skin or mucous membranes such as the buccal cavity (the cheek cavity), eye, larynx, nose, rectum or vagina. A direct application to the target is feasible using an appropriate dosage form such as a topical preparation (ointment, cream etc.), lozenge, eye drops, suppository or pessary. It must be borne in mind that a direct application might not be the most effective route of administration.

If direct application is not possible, then an indirect route to the target can be employed. This is usually through taking by mouth and swallowing. The target might be in the gastrointestinal tract itself, but in the majority of cases, the target is elsewhere. The active ingredient is released from the dosage form and absorbed through the gut wall into the blood, in which it is transported via the circulatory system to all parts of the body that the blood itself can reach. The target may be a specific organ, or it might be widespread throughout the body, such as the blood vessels themselves. It may not even be an anatomically distinct organ, but, for example, be an enzyme system, distributed throughout the body. Knowledge of the precise sites of action of active ingredients has increased enormously in recent years.

All other factors being equal, the oral route is preferred. Humans have been using the oral route since birth, and ingestion by mouth delivers the active ingredient to the gastrointestinal tract, which has evolved to be an effective organ of absorption.

Time-dependent effects

If an active ingredient that is to be absorbed into the blood is administered in a dosage form, and the blood concentration is then measured against time, a graph which basically resembles Figure 11.1 is obtained. Note that in the figure, no units are given for time nor concentration.

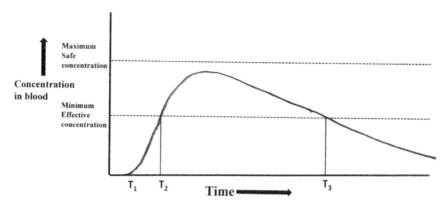

Figure 11.1: Blood concentration vs time curve after administration of a dosage form.

Initially there is a lag time (T_1) between the time of administration and the time which the active ingredient can be detected in the blood. The duration of the lag time is entirely dependent on the route of administration, the physical properties of the active ingredient and the formulation of the dosage form.

If the active ingredient is administered by intravenous injection, then the lag time is very short; just the time that blood takes to travel from the site of injection to the site where the analytical sample is taken. Where the active ingredient is administered by mouth, it must first be released from the dosage form, then dissolve in the gastrointestinal fluids before it can be absorbed into the blood system. Some dosage forms are designed to release the active ingredient rapidly, others not. Contrasting examples are the hard shell capsule, the tablet and the pill. The duration of the lag time for the hard shell capsule is governed by the time the shell takes to dissolve, usually a few minutes. The tablet can be formulated to give a rapid release of the active ingredient, and most pharmacopoeia specifications for the quality of tablets include a maximum *in vitro* disintegration time under precisely controlled conditions. The active ingredient will usually be released as solid particles, and the speed at which these dissolve in the gastrointestinal contents is governed by their solubility and the rate at which they dissolve: the dissolution rate, which is often a function of the surface area of the particles. However, in contrast, it had long been accepted that some pills required a prolonged period before their contents were released, and some were known to pass through the gastrointestinal tract and emerge unchanged in the faeces.

As soon as any of the active ingredient is absorbed, it will begin to be excreted, either directly or via a metabolic pathway. Initially, the rate of absorption will be greater than the rate of excretion, and so the concentration of active ingredient in the blood will increase. Thus, the rate of increase will be governed by the difference between the absorption and the excretion rates. At some time (T_2), the concentration will exceed the minimum effective concentration.

As the amount of unabsorbed active ingredient falls, so the rate of increase in the blood concentration is reduced until a maximum is reached. After this point, excretion predominates and so the blood concentration begins to fall until a time (T_3) when it drops below the minimum effective concentration. The fall continues until the concentration in the blood is effectively zero.

The shape of Figure 11.1 can be modified by formulation techniques, particularly with oral dosage forms such as the tablet. Normally it is desirable to reduce the lag time as much as possible, but in some cases this may not be so. For example, the active ingredient might be unstable in the acidic environment of the stomach, and so some or all of the 'dose' might be broken down before it can be absorbed. It is therefore sensible to prolong the lag time so that the dosage form leaves the stomach for the small intestine in an unchanged state. Formerly this technique was known as enteric coating, but the term gastro-resistance is now preferred. This usually involves coating the dosage form with a substance that is insoluble in strongly acidic conditions but begins to dissolve as the pH rises. In the 2018 edition of *The British Pharmacopoeia*, of the 456 monographs involving tablets, 14 are described as gastro-resistant.

Another area where formulation techniques are important is the extension of the time over which the minimum effective concentration is achieved. One way of doing this is to increase the amount of active ingredient in each dosage unit. However, this approach has limitations. Firstly, there is the possibility that the maximum safe concentration might be exceeded. This depends on the relationship between the minimum effective concentration and the maximum safe concentration, often called the therapeutic index. Secondly, there is a limit to the amount of active ingredient that each unit can contain. Thus, there are not many tablets intended to be swallowed whole that contain more than 500mg of active ingredient, and similarly hard shell capsules rarely contain more than 300mg. Dosage forms containing more than these amounts may be so large as to make them difficult to swallow.

An alternative approach is to formulate the dosage form so that the blood concentration does not reach a peak followed by a decrease, but rather a plateau (ideally horizontal) is achieved for a prolonged time. Prolonged release is usually achieved by coating the dosage form or by creating a non-dissolving matrix from which the active ingredient diffuses into the gastrointestinal contents. In the 2018 edition of *The British Pharmacopoeia*, of the 456 monographs involving tablets, 38 are described as prolonged-release.

There are some circumstances when oral administration cannot be used. It may be that the recipient is unable to take in oral medicines after some forms of surgery ('nil by mouth'), is unconscious or requires a constant level of active ingredient.

In some cases it is not possible to administer the active ingredient orally by reason of its chemical structure. The gastrointestinal tract presents a hostile environment, since its function is to break down foodstuffs into smaller chemical entities that can be absorbed. The stomach is strongly acidic and, like the less acidic small intestine, secretes enzymes that can attack many types of chemical bonds. Though this environment has evolved to break down food, it will also react in the same way to molecules of the active ingredient. Good examples of active ingredients containing a protein structure include insulin, which cannot be administered orally and is usually given as a subcutaneous injection (though other routes avoiding the gastrointestinal tract have been investigated in recent years). With recent advances in the science of monoclonal antibodies, more active ingredients with a protein-like structure have become available, and like insulin, they cannot be administered orally.

A further factor which may impinge on dosage form selection is the speed of response required.

Oral administration, as shown in Figure 11.2, of a solid dosage form such as a tablet or a pill firstly requires that it disintegrates. The tablet is a solid with a low porosity and the liquid contents of the gastrointestinal

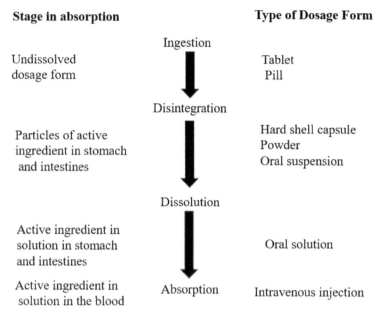

Figure 11.2: Speed of availability of drug from some dosage forms.

tract must penetrate it before the tablet can break up into its constituent particles. This can be quite a prolonged process, and often excipients that aid penetration need to be added. These are called disintegrating agents.

Once the particles of active ingredient are liberated from the dosage form, they must dissolve, as the active ingredient can only be absorbed in a liquid form. Active ingredients administered as a powder or suspension are already in a dispersed state. The dissolving process (or dissolution) can also be prolonged. The aqueous solubility of the active ingredient is measurable but it must be borne in mind that the nature of the liquid in the gastrointestinal tract changes, particularly in relation to its pH. This means that if the active ingredient is an acid or a base, its solubility will change as the pH of its environment changes.

The major site of absorption is the small intestine, and so the active ingredient must be in the dissolved state before it leaves the small intestine, otherwise it will not be absorbed to a significant extent and will be excreted. It may be necessary to accelerate dissolution, and this can often be achieved by reducing the size of the solid particles.

Disintegration and dissolution factors need not be considered if the active ingredient is given as an intravenous injection.

Compliance and convenience

In general, the discoverer of the active ingredient will have determined its optimum amount, the frequency of the dose and also the probable route of administration. Thus, a dosage regimen can be established to which ideally the patient should conform. This is termed compliance.

The formulator must always be aware that ultimately the medicine will be consumed by the patient, and the choice of dosage form and its formulation must bear this in mind. Firstly, the route of administration must be considered. The oral route is the most common from the point of view of patient convenience, but if the site of action of the active ingredient is directly accessible such as the skin, then a dosage form suitable for that route is chosen. The quantity of active ingredient to be administered at any one time must also be deliberated. As examples, if an active ingredient is to be administered via the lungs as a pressurised inhaler, or to the eye as eye drops, then the dose cannot be more than a few milligrams. Larger doses of up to several hundred milligrams would normally be delivered by the oral route, as it is only dosage forms such as the tablet or capsule that can accommodate such amounts.

Factors affecting compliance and the consequences of non-compliance need to be considered, particularly with dosage forms that in themselves do not encourage compliance. If non-compliance seriously affects the patient's health, then he/she is more willing to accept some inconvenience. For example, using an injection causes the patient more inconvenience than using an oral dosage form, but if the active ingredient is inactivated in the gastrointestinal tract, then that inconvenience would usually be tolerated as an alternative to the life-threatening consequences of non-compliance.

Another way to encourage compliance, particularly with oral dosage forms, is to consider its organoleptic properties – those which affect the senses, the taste, smell, texture and visual appearance.

Many active ingredients have an unpleasant, often bitter, taste. For this to be detected by the taste buds under the tongue, the active ingredient must be in solution, and so an obvious technique for masking taste is to prevent the active ingredient from dissolving. With solid dosage forms, this is relatively easily achieved. Tablets can be coated, usually with a thin polymeric film that does not dissolve until after the dosage form has been swallowed. Capsules, either hard shell or soft shell, essentially use the same taste-masking technique, in that the shell takes a few minutes to dissolve, by which time the taste buds have been bypassed.

With liquid dosage forms, the challenge is more difficult; one solution is to incorporate a sweetening agent in the formulation. Traditionally this would have been sucrose, but is now more likely to be a synthetic sweetener such as saccharin, acetosulfame potassium or aspartame. These are many times sweeter than sucrose, but have no calorific value. Neither do they contribute to dental caries.

A flavour may also be added. Though the name implies that the sense of taste is involved, the taste buds are relatively non-discriminating. Rather it is the sense of smell. The reader should consider the following common statement, 'I have a heavy cold; I cannot taste my food.' An infection with the common cold virus does not affect the taste buds, but does affect the olfactory organs situated in the nose. Any 'flavour' must contain one or more volatile substances that can be detected by the olfactory organs. Thus, a more correct statement would be, 'I have a heavy cold, I cannot smell my food.'

If a flavour is used, then the colour of the medicine must 'match' the flavour i.e. the sense of vision is also involved. Thus, a strawberry-flavoured preparation must be coloured red, and a medicine containing a banana flavour coloured yellow. Tests have shown that failure to match taste and colour can have a detrimental effect on compliance.

The selection of an appropriate dosage form and of the formulation of that dosage form are key components of any treatment with medicines.

Chapter 12

Products Taken by Mouth

This chapter deals with the range of medicines taken by mouth, so it includes both liquid medicines and the solid dose forms – the powders, pills, tablets, capsules, cachets etc.

LIQUID MEDICINES

Early history of liquid medicines

The earliest written recorded accounts of the use of medicines in man are in the cuneiform tablets from Mesopotamia written in Sumerian, Akkadian or Hittite. These date from around 2000 BCE or earlier. The medicinal ingredients mentioned were taken either on their own, ground and mixed in a liquid, or drunk with a liquid. Typical liquids were beer, milk, honey and oil.

The medical records of the ancient Egyptians were included in the various medical papyri as detailed in Chapter 1. These show a larger diversity of different medicinal dose forms. The Ebers papyrus from 1550 BCE comprised 877 prescriptions and remedies.[1] It mentioned draughts (single doses of medicines), electuaries (a powdered drug made into a paste with honey or syrup), linctuses (syrupy preparations typically used to treat coughs), mixtures and syrups. The recipes included the active drug, ancillary ingredients to disguise the flavour and a liquid vehicle to carry the other ingredients and allow a suitable measurement of the volume for a dose. The liquid vehicles used included beer, wine, honey, oil and milk. Campbell has shown that the active drugs were ground to a fine powder and that valuable or potent drugs were mixed in a liquid so that they were evenly distributed for dosing.[2] Liquid medicines were used to treat diarrhoea, as antispasmodics, as laxatives, as diuretics to increase the flow of urine, and to treat worm infestations.

Many of the medicinal ingredients described by Dioscorides in his book *De Materia Medica* written in the second half of the first century CE were used in the form of liquid medicines. The first entry in Book I of *De Materia Medica* is the iris, and Dioscorides states that the roots are drunk in hydromel (honey diluted with water) to induce sleep and cure colic; when drunk with vinegar they help those bitten by wild animals; and when drunk with wine they stimulated menstruation. Spignel herb (also known as baldmoney) ground up with honey was recommended for chest rheums (fluid on the lung). Dioscorides recommended storage of liquid medicines in silver, glass, horn or earthenware vessels. The common liquids in which the drugs were dissolved included water, vinegar, wine, and honey.

Distillation of decoctions of herbal drugs

The seventh and eighth centuries CE saw the beginning of the Arab physical sciences. Jabir Ibn Hayyan (721–815) was a prominent alchemist and is credited with the introduction of some basic chemical equipment and discovery of many chemical substances.[3] His invention of distillation equipment led him to the discovery that boiling wine produced a flammable vapour. This led Rhazes (865–925) to discover alcohol. Al-Kindi (801–873) wrote a book entitled *Book of the Chemistry of Perfume and Distillations* which included recipes for perfume oils and aromatic waters. Avicenna (980–1037) is credited with the invention of the cooling coil which allows the vapours produced by boiling liquids to be condensed and collected.

Hieronymus Brunschwig was born in about 1440 in Strasbourg. He trained to be a surgeon but his main achievement is his two books on distillation. The first, in 1500, was known as the *Kleine Distillierbuch* (*Little Book on Distillation*); the second, in 1512, was known as the *Grosses Distillierbuch* (*Large Book on Distillation*). The latter book contained seventy-nine woodcut pictures of furnaces and apparatus used for distillation. Distillation became increasingly used in the preparation of aromatic waters for use in medicines. Book illustrations of apothecaries' shops nearly always contained distillation apparatus. An illustration is shown in Picture 7 of the distillation apparatus at the Hospices de Beaune in France.

Liquid medicines in the early official formularies

In the sixteenth century, three German cities introduced defined lists of simple and compounded medicines. The first was *the Pharmacorum Omnium Quae Quidem in usu sunt*. This was written by Valerius Cordus and became the official formulary of Nuremberg, to be used by the city physicians in treating their patients. It included compositions that were credited to earlier writers such as Mesue, Nicolai, Galen, Avicenna, Rhazes, Andromachus and Andromachus Senior. About thirty years later, the cities of Augsburg and Cologne followed with their own formularies. The *Augsburg Pharmacopoeia* appeared in 1564 and was probably the most influential of the German formularies. It included confections, decoctions, electuaries, lohochs, mels, oxymels, robs (fruit pulps), syrups and theriacs. The electuaries were powdered drug mixed with honey to make it palatable. Confections were soft solids made by mixing powdered drug with liquid to form a smooth paste and lohochs were thick syrupy medicines usually against a cough, now more commonly called a linctus. The decoctions were solutions of vegetable drugs made by boiling the substance in water. Mels were honey based and oxymels were mixtures of honey, water and vinegar. The book included four theriacs, the antidote to poisons and remedy for a wide range of conditions. The theriacs included Mithridatium, Theriaca Andromachis Senioris (theriac of Andromachus Senior) and Theriaca communis from the *Pharmacopoeia Augustana*.

It is difficult to deduce from these official formularies what medicinal products the practising physicians used to treat their patients, since the formularies invariably had a number of products that were used for the same purpose and from which the physician could choose the ones he preferred to use. For example, there were many different laxative products. However, the first edition of the *Augsburg Pharmacopoeia* marked with an asterisk all products to be kept on hand in the Augsburg apothecary shops.[4] This gives us an insight into the type of preparations that the Augsburg physicians wanted to use. This list included 26 electuaries, 113 confections, 78 syrups and juleps, four robs (fruit pulps), 12 lohochs and 10 decoctions. Juleps were drinks made with a sugar syrup; the word 'julep' is still used today in the name of the 'mint julep', which is a bourbon cocktail with sugar and fresh mint. The list included forty-one oils, some to be used for preparations meant to be swallowed and others for use in ointments and other uses.

The *Pharmacopoeia Londinensis* of 1618 drawn up by the College of Physicians included a variety of liquid medicines. There were 178 waters (some would have been given to patients as such, others would have been components in various mixtures as flavours or to add different drugs) and 35 compound waters (which had several ingredients). There were 4 medicated wines, 8 decoctions, 90 syrups, 18 melita and oxymels, 12 fruit pulps, 6 linctuses and 101 electuaries with or without opium. The 1653 translation and commentary on the *Pharmacopoeia Londinensis* by Nicholas Culpeper entitled *The London Dispensatory* contained a long list of Simple Distilled Waters made from fresh roots, flowers and buds, fruits and of 'parts of living creatures'.[5] Another list was of Simple Waters Distilled being digested beforehand and prepared from various roots, leaves, flowers, and berries. A final list was of Spirits and Compound Distilled Waters made from mixtures of various herbal materials. An example of a compound distilled water was Gentian Water Compound, used to prevent pestilential fevers, to ease pains in the stomach, and, Culpeper said, was 'excellent good for the yellow jaundice'. Culpeper says that it was prepared as follows:

'Take of Gentian, roots sliced, one pound and a half, the leaves and flowers of Centaury the less, of each four ounces; steep them eight days in twelve pound of white wine, then distill them in an Alembick'.

Liquid medicinal products prescribed in the eighteenth and nineteenth centuries

We are faced with a difficulty, when considering the large number of liquid medicine preparations included in the editions of the *London Pharmacopoeia*, to try to find what physicians were actually prescribing. The Wellcome Library has an account book of an unnamed apothecary from Odiham in Hampshire for the period 1774 to 1782.[6] An extract from some of the patient records from this book gives some indication of the type of products he prescribed:

Mrs Bullock of Dogmansfield (1774–1775): 20 potions (all purgatives), 12 mixtures, 6 drops.

John Chitty at Hook (1772–1779): 1 embrocation, 8 powders, 10 potions, 3 mixtures, 2 salts, 1 senna, 2 plasters, 1 ointment, 2 draughts.

The Right Honourable Wellbore Ellis (Member of Parliament for Petersfield), (1773–1774): 14 powders, 14 mixtures, 14 draughts, 5 ointments, 1 potion, 7 drops, 2 enemas, 1 oil.

Mrs Gregory in Town (1774–1775): Ophthalmic water 8, mixtures 20, draughts 6, ointments 3, lotions 10, embrocation 1, plasters 2, drops 1, enemas 1, garglc 1.

Mr Richard Raggett, the sawyer in the Biny (1775): 1 powder, 1 mixture, 1 potion, 2 drops, 1 salt, 5 pills,

The Wellcome Library also has the Apothecary Prescription Book from the 1770s for Edward Batt, a surgeon/apothecary and Augustine Batt a surgeon, who practised in Witney in Oxfordshire.[7]. Typical patient records were:

Mr Webb, carpenter (1774–1779): 10 mixtures, 12 draughts, 3 waters, 13 ointments, 1 liniment, 2 powders, 1 plaster.

Mr Benth Fisher (1774–1783): 11 mixtures, 11 draughts, 4 powders, 1 plaster, 2 applications

Mr Rowles Finstock (1774–1775): 9 mixtures, 1 pill, 1 potion, 1 powder, 1 drop

Mr Rutter Westend (1774–1775): 17 draughts, 19 mixtures, 1 plaster, 1 oil, 1 decoction

Mrs Poulton, Frayley (1774–1775): 6 mixtures, 1 ointment, 4 plasters, 1 drop, 8 draughts, 1 electuary, 1 water.

Girls in the bridewell prison (1774–1775): 7 mixtures, 22 ointments, 27 pills, 4 elixirs, 1 drop, 7 electuaries, 2 manna, 2 salts, 2 powders, 2 oils, 1 plaster. [The ointments were mainly mercury ointments used to treat syphilis].

Elixirs were flavoured syrups. The word elixir derives from two Arabic words: *al* and *iksir*. An early elixir was the Elixir Proprietalis which Paracelsus recommended as enabling the user to live as long as Methuselah. This elixir contained myrrh, aloes and saffron. It does not appear to have done much for Paracelsus, who died at the age of 47.

For both the apothecary accounts from Odiham and the Batt family prescription records, it is clear that most preparations given to patients were liquid products – mainly mixtures and draughts. Draughts were single doses of a product, for example, a laxative for a patient who was constipated. If the problem recurred the patient would be given another single dose. The patient took the entire contents of a vial containing the draught so it was an accurate dose. However, draughts were more expensive than taking a dose from a multidose mixture. Cooley wrote in 1856 that when the dose was to be repeated, the mixture had become more popular than draughts except amongst the higher classes.[8] In many hospitals and dispensaries, the patients had to take in their own bottles, many of which were not convenient for a draught. *The Pharmaceutical Journal* of 1870 recorded that patients frequently took in old jam jars and empty British wine bottles, 'with the same bottle making alternate pilgrimages to the public house and the dispensary'.[9]

As mentioned in the preface to this book, by the second half of the nineteenth century, multidose mixtures were the main method for a patient to receive the medicine. Lewis's Chemist in West Street, Ware, Hertfordshire dispensed seventy-six items during one year in 1854–5. Thirty-one of these were mixtures (40 per cent), and twenty-four were pills (33 per cent).[10] There were no draughts. In the period July to December 1899 the same pharmacy dispensed 171 items, 118 of which were mixtures (69 per cent), and again no draughts.[11]. Armitage Dispensing Chemist in Blackheath dispensed 296 prescriptions in one year in the period 1899 to 1900.[12] One hundred and ninety-one items of these were mixtures (64.5 per cent), and only one draught (0.33 per cent).

By the middle of the nineteenth century, the range of liquid medicines to be taken by mouth had shrunk drastically from the hundreds of products in the first editions of the *London Pharmacopoeia*. The *British Pharmacopoeia* of 1864 included a mere nine confections, thirteen decoctions, fourteen syrups, seven mixtures and seven medicated wines.

Even if we include products which were widely prescribed but not in the pharmacopoeia, the range of products is limited. The 1883 first edition of *The Extra Pharmacopoeia of Unofficial Drugs* by William Martindale and W. Wynn Westcott included the more commonly prescribed products as well as the official ones, and had seven confections, fifteen decoctions, nineteen mixtures, ten wines, one linctus, twelve elixirs and thirty-four syrups. The products were much simpler than in the earlier editions of the *London Pharmacopoeias*, in the main having only one or two active ingredients. Some typical mixtures were Amyl Nitrite Mixture for treatment of seasickness, Chalk Mixture for dyspepsia, Croton-Chloral Mixture for neuralgia of the throat, various iron salt mixtures for anaemia, Oil of Sandalwood Mixture for gonorrhoea, and Chian Turpentine Mixture for cancer of the female organs. Morphine Linctus was used for treatment of coughs. The elixirs were flavoured syrups with alcohol, which added to their popularity.

One issue with all of these multidose liquid medicines was the method of measurement of the dose using household spoons. The doses were often given in tablespoons (about 15ml), but teaspoons (about 5ml) and dessert spoons (about 10ml) were also used. However, these could vary considerably in volume, so glass medicine measures were also sold. Controversy about the accuracy of dosage was to continue until well into the late twentieth century. In the 1970s, an NHS 5ml standard spoon was specified by British Standard 3221, but this did not prevent controversy about its accuracy.

Patent and proprietary medicines

Alongside the official medicines in the eighteenth and nineteenth centuries, there was a considerable market in proprietary products making improbable claims to treat a wide range of diseases. Consumers would be enticed to buy these by the extravagant newspaper advertising.[13] Many of these were liquid medicines. One of the most popular was Daffy's Elixir, sold from the eighteenth century, which claimed to cure the 'Stone, Gravel, Convulsions, the Gout, Rheumatism, Cholic, Dropsy, disorders peculiar to Women and Children, Consumption (tuberculosis), the Piles, Fever, Agues, Fluxes, Spitting of Blood, Pain in the Breast, Limbs, Joints etc.' Thomas Wakley (1795–1862) was a surgeon by training but moved into medical journalism and founded the *Lancet*. He campaigned against quackery and exposed the ingredients of the proprietary nostrums such as Daffy's Elixir – which contained senna. Another product was Bateman's Pectoral Drops sold as giving immediate 'Ease in all Colds, Coughs, Agues, Fevers, Fluxes, Pains of the Breast, Limbs and Joints'. It contained camphor and opium. Spilsbury's Antiscorbutic Drops claimed to treat scurvy, but contained antimony. In the late eighteenth and early nineteenth centuries, Dr Sibly's Reanimating Solar Tincture was advertised for the Restoration of Life in cases of sudden death. His advertisement read as follows:

> 'In all circumstances of suicide, or sudden death, whether by blows, fits, falls, suffocation, strangulation, drowning, apoplexy, thunder and lightning, assassination, duelling etc. immediate recourse should be had to this medicine, which will not fail to restore life, providing organs and juices are in a fit disposition for it, which they undoubtedly are much oftener than is imagined.'

Changing pattern of prescribing in the twentieth century

During the first half of the twentieth century, liquid mixtures continued to be the predominant type of preparation given to patients. Analysis of Armitage Dispensing Chemist's Prescription Register for 1938–1940 shows that of the 2,500 prescriptions dispensed in a year from 1938–9, 55 per cent were mixtures, 2 per cent were linctuses, 18 per cent were tablets, 2 per cent were capsules.[14] In the early part of the twentieth century one of the daily tasks in a pharmacy was to make up bulk stock of mixtures in 2-litre Winchester bottles ready for the prescriptions coming in from patients who had seen the local doctors during the course of the day. Typical mixtures were ammonia and ipecacuanha mixture for coughs, aromatic chalk with opium mixture for stomach complaints, and kaolin and morphine mixture for diarrhoea.

By the 1970s, individual pharmacies had largely ceased to make up their own stock of medicines and the liquid medicines supplied on prescription were all commercially manufactured. The *Drug Tariff* is the list of medicines which can be prescribed by doctors on the NHS. Counting all the different strengths of products separately, in 2010 the *Drug Tariff* listed 884 tablets, 220 capsules, but only 90 categorised as mixtures or oral solutions. From the analysis of GP prescribed medicines, we reported in the preface of this book, about 75 per cent are now solid dose forms such as tablet and capsules.

But the preference for tablets and capsules does not mean that there is no need for liquid medicines to be taken by mouth. Difficulty in swallowing is called 'dysphagia'. It probably affects between 16 and 22 per cent of adults aged over 50.[15] Many patients in hospital and care homes also have feeding problems and around 20–50 per cent of patients with head injuries, stroke or suffering from Parkinson's disease are very likely to suffer problems with swallowing. Liquid medicines provide an alternative to solid tablets or capsules for these patients. Several of the drugs for mental health disorders such as depression and schizophrenia are available as oral solutions. Some examples are imipramine oral solution used for treatment of depression, and chlorpromazine oral solution used for schizophrenia and mania.

Many children, particularly infants, find it easier to take an oral solution rather than a tablet. Some of the antihistamine drugs for treatment of allergies such as hay fever are available as oral solutions: cetirizine and loratadine are two examples. As mentioned in Chapter 11, these are now sweetened with an artificial sweetener rather than sucrose, because the older generation of sucrose-sweetened products was associated with an increase in tooth decay in children.

Some medicines are available as suspensions of the active drug in a flavoured liquid vehicle. Paracetamol is available as both a suspension and a solution for mild to moderate pain and fever in children. Sugar-free versions of both the suspension and the solution are available.

The Edinburgh pathologist and professor in the institutes of medicine, John Hughes Bennett (1812–1875), introduced cod liver oil to the English-speaking medical community. He had spent some years in Germany and seen its use in the treatment of rickets, rheumatism, and gout. However, the disagreeable taste of cod liver oil was a problem. Alfred B. Scott came to New York City in 1873 and with his partner Samuel Bowne began work to develop a more palatable preparation.

They established the firm of Scott and Bowne, and began marketing an emulsion of the oil as Scott's Emulsion. Emulsions are dispersions of minute droplets of oil in a water phase. In the 1920s, it was realised that cod liver oil was an excellent source of vitamins A and D and in the 1970s, the health benefits of omega-3 fatty acids contained in cod liver oil were discovered. Scott's Emulsion is now sold by Glaxo Smith Klein as the original and as an orange-flavoured version.

Other examples of emulsions still in use are liquid paraffin emulsion and liquid paraffin emulsion with magnesium hydroxide, which are on sale as a laxative to treat constipation.

Cough medicines

Many liquid medicines such as cough and cold remedies are now sold as over-the-counter (OTC) remedies and are not prescribed. Cough due to a respiratory tract infection is very common, particularly during the winter, and there are many commercial remedies sold to treat this condition. Cough suppressant drugs such as codeine or dextromethorphan are often combined in these products with soothing substances such as syrup or glycerol. Codeine is problematic as it causes constipation and may cause patients to become addicted to it; products containing dextromethorphan have fewer side effects. Some products contain antihistamine drugs such as diphenhydramine which have the side effect of causing sleepiness. There is controversy about the effectiveness of many of these OTC remedies.

Cochran is a global independent network of medical professionals which gathers and summarises the best evidence from research to help everyone make informed choices about treatments. In 2012, a Cochran review was published on OTC medications for acute cough in children and adults, which concluded there was no good evidence for use of OTC medications in acute cough.[16] In another Cochran review, published in 2018, it determined that honey relieved symptoms to a greater extent than diphenhydramine products, but was similar to the dextromethorphan products.[17] There is a strong case for parents to consider using honey as a first line choice to treat coughs in their children.

SOLID DOSAGE FORMS

General introduction

Solid dosage forms offer several advantages over other forms of oral medication. The first is that they present the active ingredient in a concentrated form, thus facilitating transport and administration. By contrast, liquid dosage forms usually contain a large proportion of water which needs a larger container, thereby increasing transport and storage costs. Furthermore, patient convenience is reduced with consequences for compliance – the ability of the patient to stick to the dosage scheme designed to achieve the desired clinical effect.

Many active ingredients break down in the presence of water, that is they undergo hydrolysis, and this is avoided if they are presented in a solid dosage form where water is largely absent. Thus, the solid dosage form is intrinsically more stable and has a longer shelf life.

However, liquid dosage forms are sometimes necessary, since the young and the old patient may have difficulties in swallowing a solid dosage form, but even here, a solid dosage form can bring advantages. A good example is an antibiotic medicine frequently used to treat upper respiratory tract infections in the young. Many antibiotics are unstable in the presence of water, so they are often formulated as a powder or granules containing the active ingredient plus sweetener, flavour and other excipients, all in a dry state. When this is dispensed by the pharmacist, water is added to give a liquid preparation of short but known shelf life. Since antibiotics are usually only given for short periods, this short life is not a problem. Another example is aspirin which also undergoes hydrolysis. If a liquid preparation is called for, aspirin is formulated as a soluble or dispersible tablet, which is then mixed with water immediately before taking it.

Some idea of the changing relative popularity among dosage forms can be gained from consideration of the number of monographs for a given dosage form in successive editions of *The British Pharmacopoeia*, and these data are presented for the period 1864 to 2018 in Table 12.1.

The pill was the most common dosage form in the nineteenth century but dwindled to zero by the middle of the twentieth century. In contrast the number of monographs for the capsule and the tablets markedly increased, particularly the latter. Out of a total of monographs of about

Table 12.1: Monographs relating to solid dosage forms in successive editions of *The British Pharmacopoeia*, 1864 to 2018.

Edition	Powders	Pills	Tablets	Capsules	Total
1864	8	17	0	0	25
1885	15	21	1	0	37
1898	16	20	1	0	37
1914	17	18	1	0	36
1932	8	7	1	0	16
1948	7	5	49	0	61
1953	7	0	63	5	75
1958	3	0	119	10	132
1963	2	0	174	16	192
1968	2	0	226	30	258
1973	1	0	251	42	294
1980	5	0	255	50	310
1988	2	0	274	57	333
1993	1	0	263	52	316
1998	4	0	297	60	361
2003	7	0	336	57	400
2008	6	0	351	77	434
2013	4	0	404	91	499
2018	4	0	456	110	570

1300 in the 2018 edition, there are 456 for tablets, making it the most popular dosage form by a considerable margin. The data in Table 12.1 must be treated with caution, since they give the impression that the tablet was hardly used before 1948. In fact, tablet usage was widespread as early as 1880, as will be discussed later. What delayed its entry into pharmacopoeias until 1948 was the absence of agreed standards for tablet preparations until that date, and without these, an entry was impossible. As we saw from the information given in the preface, by 2015 nearly three-quarters of all GP prescriptions were for tablets or capsules.

Powders and cachets

The powder is the simplest dosage form, being an intimate mixture of the active ingredient(s) and if necessary, a diluent such as lactose (milk sugar).

Powders have been used medicinally for many hundreds of years. One of the most ancient formulae for powders, dating back to about 500 BCE was *hiera picra* or 'sacred bitters'. This contained aloes and was used as a laxative. Other old formulae include Powder of Ipecacuanha and Opium, or Dover's powder introduced by the English physician Thomas Dover in the early eighteenth century, and Aromatic Powder of Chalk, which became known as Dr James's Fever Powder, and which allegedly was devised by Sir Walter Raleigh. Another very popular powder in the early years of the eighteenth century was Seidlitz Powder, patented by Thomas Savory in 1815, and named after the village of Seidlitz, then in Bohemia and now called Sedlec in the Czech Republic. Seidlitz Powders came as two components. One of these was sodium bicarbonate, traditionally wrapped in a blue paper, and a mixture of tartaric acid, potassium tartrate and sodium tartrate, traditionally wrapped in white paper. The contents of the two papers were separately dissolved in water, and the two solutions mixed. Effervescence occurred, giving 'a cooling, agreeable draught', which acted as a mild laxative. After the validity of Savory's patent was rejected, Seidlitz Powders were made by a number of pharmaceutical manufacturers. There was a monograph for Effervescent Tartrated Soda Powders (an equivalent product) in the 1898 edition of *The British Pharmacopoeia*.

For individual powders, the minimum weight is usually about 100mg. In the traditional method of preparation, each dose is individually wrapped in a piece of paper, folded in a carefully defined way. Powders were taken either by mixing with water, or by being ingested in the dry state, followed by a draught of water. Powders have a major advantage over other solid preparations in that the content of active ingredient in each can easily be varied, so that unusual doses of the active ingredient can be obtained. This is in contrast to tablets, which are only economical to make in large quantities of the same product. A major disadvantage of powders is that unpleasant tastes cannot be masked, and this was the main justification for using cachets.

Cachets

A cachet is defined in the *Concise Oxford English Dictionary* as 'a flat capsule containing a dose of unpleasant-tasting medicine'. The word is derived from the French verb 'cacher' meaning 'to hide'. The originator of the cachet in 1853 appears to have been a pharmacist from Lyon, France named M. A. Guilliermond.[18] He made his cachets from a bread paste (cachets de pain). Prior to this, one method of administering powders with a noxious taste was to sprinkle them on to bread, so Guilliermond's choice of an unleavened bread paste for his cachets is a logical progression.

Guilliermond's invention was further developed some years later in 1873 by Stanislas Limousin (1831–1887), a Parisian pharmacist. His invention was a perforated board that would accommodate several sizes of cachet, a powder measure, a powder funnel and a wooden 'presser and wetter' to speed the extemporaneous filling of cachets by pharmacists.[19]

Cachets are now made from a gelatinised starch paste. When moistened, cachets become soft and can be swallowed, so they break down only after the taste buds in the mouth have been by-passed.

The cachet consists of two parts, and there are two types of cachet which differ in the way these parts are joined together. In the flanged or wet-seal variety (similar to those invented by Guilliermond and Limousin), the flanges are moistened after filling so that the two halves stick together. In the dry-seal type, the two halves fit tightly together and no moisture is involved. A typical example of a machine is shown in Picture 14.

An advantage of cachets is that the largest size can contain well over a gram of powdered contents, which is considerably more than the largest acceptable tablet. This is because they are softened before ingestion, and so can be more readily swallowed, unlike the rigid tablet or capsule.

Filling cachets can be a slow and laborious process, so their use is now very limited. One of their last uses was in the treatment of tuberculosis with 4-aminosalicylic acid, which has a very unpleasant taste and needs to be given in doses of several grams daily. This active ingredient is now provided in sachets, each of which contains 4g of 4-aminosalicylic acid presented as gastro-resistant granules, which are sprinkled on to food.

Pills

The Concise Oxford English Dictionary defines 'pill' as 'a ball or disc of solid medicine for swallowing whole'. The word is derived from the Latin *'pilula'*, the diminutive of *'pila'*, a ball.

The pill is an extremely ancient dosage form, though it is now completely superseded by the tablet or capsule. However, the word 'pill' is still in widespread use, albeit incorrectly, as a shorthand term for any sort of solid oral dosage form. Millions of women of childbearing age are said to be 'on the pill': they are actually 'on the tablet', though the latter term is never used. There is an old saying 'there is a pill for every ill', and if that were ever true, it certainly is not true today. In a recent radio discussion on the medicinal use of cannabis, the terms pill, tablet and capsule were used interchangeably by the participants over a period of about ten minutes.

The earliest reference to a pill appears in the Ebers Papyrus (about 1550 BCE). This is the main source of our knowledge of ancient Egyptian medicine. The preparation is described as 'malachite ground fine, added to a cake of bread, made into three pills and swallowed with sweet beer'.

Pills were later included in many formularies and pharmacopoeias such as *The Augsburg Pharmacopoeia* of 1564 and *The Pharmacopoeia Londinensis* of 1618. The 1864 edition of *The British Pharmacopoeia* contained seventeen monographs for pills, many of which were used to treat bowel irregularities.

By the early part of the nineteenth century, the pill had become the most commonly used oral solid dosage form. Pills were made by a process known as massing. All the solid components were mixed together and a viscous aqueous paste added that contained adhesive ingredients such as acacia or tragacanth. The mixing process continued until a very stiff mass was obtained. This was then rolled into a cylindrical shape, ideally of uniform diameter, which was then divided into parts of equal length. This was facilitated by rolling out the cylinder on a pill tile on to which graduations were printed. A pill tile is shown in Picture 8. Alternatively, the cylinder was rolled on a 'pill machine' made of a hard wooden block fitted with equally spaced brass corrugations at one end. The cylinder was placed on these corrugations, and then a wooden part with matching brass corrugations was pressed down on the cylinder, cutting it into equal segments. A pill machine is shown in Picture 9.

The segments were rolled into a spherical shape, which when dried, formed very hard masses. For aesthetic reasons, pills were sometimes covered with silver or gold foil. Because of the hardness of the pill itself, exacerbated by the foil coating, some could pass through the gastrointestinal tract virtually unchanged to be excreted in the faeces. In view of the toxic nature of some of the active ingredients and excipients e.g. lead and opium pills and phosphorus pills, the latter using the toxic liquid carbon disulfide as a dispersant, this was probably just as well.

Pill preparation was a slow and expensive process which required considerable manipulative skill, and pill-making was considered an important part of the pharmacist's training. There was considerable public demand for pills, and it is not surprising that when the first tablets were introduced, they were described as 'compressed pills'.

In addition to being made by individual pharmacists, pills were being produced on an industrial scale by the mid-1880s by a number of manufacturers. Among these was the firm founded by Thomas Beecham. He was born in 1820 near Witney, about 10 miles west of Oxford, the son of an agricultural labourer. When he became a shepherd at a farm near Banbury, he noticed which plants and herbs kept his flock healthy and therefore might be useful to treat human disease. He gained a reputation for curing illness by herbal medicines. His method of manufacture was to grind the hard vegetable material into a powder, and by adding water, make a dough-like mass. He acquired a pill machine and made pills by the traditional method described earlier. As Beecham was employed to buy and sell sheep at local markets, he was able to combine this work with selling his pills. He then decided that he would do better to move from the poorer agricultural areas of England to the more prosperous industrial areas of Lancashire where there was a high demand for medicines, because occupational diseases were so rife. After a short stay in Liverpool, he moved to Wigan in 1847 and then to St Helen's in 1859. Rising demand for his products obliged him to acquire several simple pieces of equipment to speed up production, though he was still using the traditional manufacturing method.

It was at this time that the slogan that made his product famous was coined – 'Beecham's pills, worth a guinea a box'. The impressive claims for the product included 'For a weak stomach, impaired digestion, and all disorders of the liver they act like "MAGIC" and a few doses will be found to work wonders upon the most important organs in the human machine.' Beecham faced stiff competition from other manufacturers, but ultimately succeeded. His pills contained aloes, ginger and soap, and unlike some of their competitors, actually worked as a laxative. Beecham insisted on high standards of quality, and also used bold marketing techniques to keep the name Beecham in the forefront of the public mind. The firm opened a new factory in St Helen's in 1887, and by 1890 was making about 250 million pills per year for sale at home and overseas. He was using a mechanised method of the traditional technique of pill making. Production of Beecham's Pills ceased in 1998.

A comprehensive account of the development of the Beecham organization is given by Corley.[20]

Tablets

On 8 December 1843, a British Patent, number 9977, entitled 'Shaping Pills, Lozenges and Black Lead by Pressure in Dies' was granted. The most important part of this title is 'pressure in dies', which distinguishes products of this type from all others. The grantee was William Brockedon, who in the subsequent British census of 1851 lived in Devonshire Street (now Boswell Street), Bloomsbury, London, and who described himself as 'Artist and Historical Painter', an unexpected description of the inventor of the most popular dosage form now known as the tablet.

Brockedon is an interesting figure, who amply justifies the dictionary definition of the term 'polymath' as 'a person of much or varied learning'. Though his original training was that of a clockmaker, he was a good enough scientist to be elected a Fellow of the Royal Society, a good enough artist to exhibit on many occasions at the Royal Academy, a distinguished travel writer and illustrator, specialising in Italy and the Alps, a founder member of the Royal Geographical Society, and an inventor in a variety of fields.

William Brockedon was born in Totnes, UK in 1787. His initial training was as a watch and clockmaker, firstly by his father and later in London. He returned to Totnes in about 1802 to take charge of the family business because of his father's ill health and subsequent death. Around this time, his skills as an artist were recognised and he was sponsored to commence his studies at the Royal Academy in 1809, where he exhibited regularly. He began by painting a series of large-scale works of a religious nature, but then turned his attention to illustrations of geographical topics, especially Alpine passes. His work circulated as engravings or illustrations in books rather than at exhibitions. In some of these works he wrote the text himself, in others he provided the illustrations for another author's words.

In contrast to his paintings on religious or geographical themes, William Brockedon was also a portraitist of distinction. As an intended inheritance for his son Philip North Brockedon, he completed two volumes of portraits, each accompanied by an autographed letter from the subject. The collection, unofficially entitled *'Philip's Book of his Father's Friends'* provides a measure of Brockedon's interests and friendships. There are over 100 drawings of leading figures in the arts and sciences, including Sir Walter Scott (1830), Michael Faraday (1831), Thomas Telford (1834) and Sir Charles Wheatstone (1837). The last portraits in the series were produced in 1849. Sadly, the son for which the collection was intended died later in the same year. These illustrations are now in the National Portrait Gallery in London, and provide a valuable resource for those interested in the social and scientific life of the first half of the nineteenth century. Many of Brockedon's subjects merit an entry in *Wikipedia*, and these entries are frequently illustrated by Brockedon's drawings. A photograph of a portrait of William Brockedon is shown in Figure 12.1.

In about 1840, Brockedon's interests changed. He became an inventor, and his work as an artist and writer took on minor roles. Of his literary works catalogued by the British Library, only three are dated post 1840, apart from obviously posthumous re-issues. Brockedon's artistic output also ceased. Only his drawing of pencil sketches of his friends continued into the 1840s.

Of the eleven British patents granted to Brockedon, only three pre-date 1840. The last patent he received was in 1851, when Brockedon's

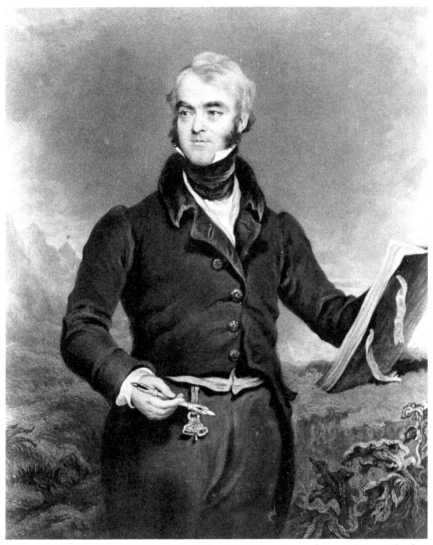

Figure 12.1: Portrait of William Brockedon. (*Wellcome image from a photograph of an engraving*)

health had begun to fail (he died in 1854). These inventions were for a wide variety of topics, but probably one of his most productive areas was a series of inventions involving rubber. Patent grants covered the use of rubber as a substitute for cork as stoppers for bottles and in the covering of roofs and protecting valves used in the propulsion of vehicles by atmospheric pressure. This last was presumably related to work by

Isambard Kingdom Brunel in his extension of the Great Western Railway west of Exeter for which Brunel proposed to use atmospheric propulsion. It is hardly coincidental that Brockedon's son Philip worked for Brunel, though there is no evidence that Brunel used Brockedon's invention. In 1846, Brockedon became a partner in the firm of Charles Macintosh & Co, makers of the eponymous waterproof clothing and who sold rubber stoppers made by Brockedon's process.

In his work leading to the award of British Patent 9977, Brockedon did not set out to invent a medicinal dosage form. Rather it was a reaction to a shortage in the supply of high quality graphite for the production of pencil 'leads', a matter of obvious concern to an artist like Brockedon. For several centuries, the source of graphite for British artists was a deposit of very pure graphite at Seathwaite Fell in Cumbria, UK, and a well-known pencil factory had been established in the nearby town of Keswick. By the nineteenth century, this supply had virtually run out. Brockedon would have been aware that in fashioning pencil leads, much graphite powder was generated, and Brockedon's studies were directed at reducing this waste. It seems likely that an anonymous person suggested to Brockedon that his invention might have medicinal applications.

An interesting feature of British Patent 9977 was Brockedon's suggestion that an improved product could be obtained if a partial vacuum was applied during the compression process. However, he stated that this was not necessary for the small amounts of solid needed to produce medicinal products. Modern research into tablet manufacture has shown that Brockedon's suggestion of production *in vacuo* is valid in medicinal tablet manufacture, though it is not economically worthwhile to do so. It explains the well-known tablet fault of capping, in which the tablet can split horizontally, by showing that it is caused by air being trapped within the porous structure of the tablet.

The validity of Brockedon's patent was challenged by Wolff and Son, another well-known firm of pencil manufacturers, who also used compression to make pencil leads. They too had found it necessary to expel air from the graphite powder prior to compression. However, Wolff used heat to remove the air whereas Brockedon preferred to withdraw the air by means of a pump. So no contravention was committed by either party.

Brockedon enjoyed some success in pencil manufacture, becoming associated with Messrs Reeves and Sons. Reeves exhibited 'a range of specimens of black lead from all parts of the world, and in various stages of preparation by Mr Brockedon's patent process' at the Great Exhibition in 1851. At the close of the exhibition in October 1851, Brockedon was awarded a prize in the mining, quarrying, metallurgical operations and mineral products category for 'Cumberland lead, condenser and blocks'. There is no evidence that an association of the name Brockedon with pencil making lasted for long after his death. In contrast, Wolff and Son continued their success as pencil manufacturers, producing 'Wolff's Royal Sovereign British Pencils' that are still available.

The apparatus described in British Patent 9977 is very simple and is illustrated in Figure 12.2. Compression takes place in a die between two punches. The die consists of a metal block, usually circular, through which a cylindrical hole has been drilled, and which is situated above a base plate that bears a cylinder that is an excellent fit into the die. The baseplate constitutes the lower punch. The upper punch is also cylindrical, and it too is a close fit into the die.

A weighed quantity of powder is poured into the die, and the upper punch is placed on top of it. According to the patent specification, the

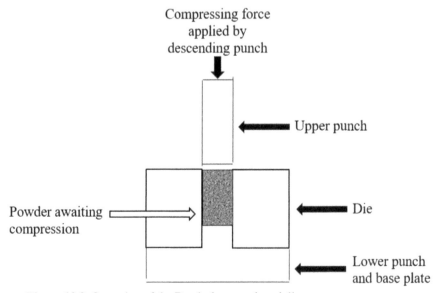

Figure 12.2: Operation of the Brockedon punch and die.

compression force is applied by means of a fly press, which is a simple mechanical press fitted with a fly-wheel to maintain momentum, or 'other convenient means'. It is likely that, initially at least, the press was used to compress the relatively large quantities needed for pencil leads, but for medicinal products, other means were used to apply the compressing force. Most examples of upper punches that have survived from Brockedon's time show signs of damage after repeated blows from a mallet or hammer.[21] Examples of Brockedon's punches and dies are shown in Picture 10.

Brockedon realised that every compressed medicinal product should have the same weight and hence contain the same amount of active ingredient. He also realised that weighing out these quantities would be a tedious and time-consuming task. Therefore, he invented a dosing apparatus, and this also forms part of British Patent 9977. Essentially it consists of two concentric tubes, the outer tube projecting beyond the inner, the end of which is blocked to form a piston. The apparatus is plunged into a bed of the powder contents, and picks up enough to fill the space between the tip of the outer tube and the face of the piston in the inner tube. The apparatus is removed from the powder bed, positioned over the die of the press, and the piston then descends, expelling the powder into the die. It is uncertain if this device was ever used to produce medicinal products, but it is remarkably similar to devices used many years later on machines to fill hard shell capsules.

The pill was undoubtedly the most frequently used oral solid dosage form when William Brockedon was granted his patent in 1843, and it was perhaps inevitable that when this novel form of solid medicine was introduced, Brockedon described it as a compressed pill. The term 'compressed pill' was still being used in publicity material published forty years later.

Brockedon's invention has been described as the mechanisation of pharmaceutical production. However, as originally described, Brockedon's patent does not use a 'machine'. Furthermore output would be extremely limited, due to the fact that the apparatus had to be dismantled after every compression to enable the product to be removed from the die. So this claim is something of an exaggeration.

Brockedon lost no time in announcing his invention to the pharmacy profession. It was reported in *The Pharmaceutical Journal* of May 1844, only a few months after the patent was granted.[22]

'Brockedon's patent process

   We have received a specimen of bicarbonate of potash compressed
in the form of a pill by a process invented by Mr Brockedon, and
for which he has taken out a patent. We understand the process
is applicable to the compression of a number of other substances
into a sold mass without the intervention of gum or other adhesive
material. Mr Brockedon has promised to favour us with a detailed
account of this process for publication in an early number'.

There is no evidence that *The Pharmaceutical Journal* ever published the
promised 'detailed account'.

Brockedon frequently advertised his product in the national press. *The
Times* of 12 September 1844 contained an advertisement which read as
follows:

'HEARTBURN, &c. Certain and immediate relief, in the hours of
business, by night or on a journey, is given by the pure alkaline
preparations of BI-CARBONATE of SODA and POTASS
compressed into pills by Brockedon's patent process. They furnish
an ever-ready and instant remedy to those powerful diseases
of the digestive organs, heartburn, sick headache, indigestion,
& c. produced by acidity. Sold wholesale by Barclay and Sons,
Farringdon--St; and by every chymist (*sic*) and druggist in the
United Kingdom. Price 1s per box or in family boxes half-a- crown'.

This advertisement and others like it appeared regularly in the national
and regional press for several years. Use of the word 'pills' should be
noted, as should the claim for nationwide availability only a few months
after the process had been patented. It is worth pointing out that these
preparations were not cheap. If allowance is made for inflation, a shilling
and a half crown are approximately equivalent to about £3 and £7.50
respectively in current values.

Brockedon's product was certainly well known, since advertisements
contained such phrases as 'Brockedon's, the original. Take no other',
and 'Brockedon', the purest remedy for indigestion'. It would appear
that the use of the name Brockedon as a noun indicated that Brockedon's

Picture 1: Cuneiform medical clay tablet BCE. (*Wellcome Images*)

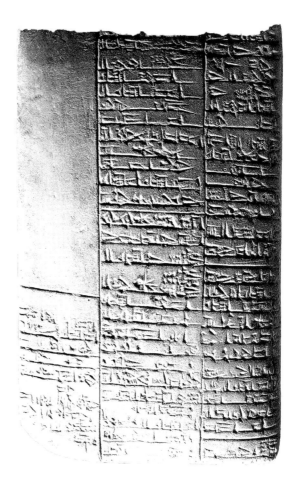

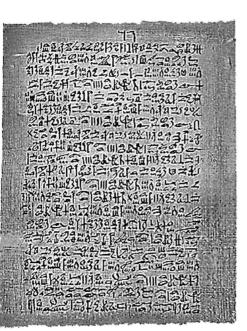

Picture 2: Section of the Ebers Papyrus from National Library of Medicine in Egypt from 1550 BCE, with an asthma remedy to be prepared as a mixture of herbs heated on a brick so that the sufferer could inhale the fumes. (*Wellcome Images*)

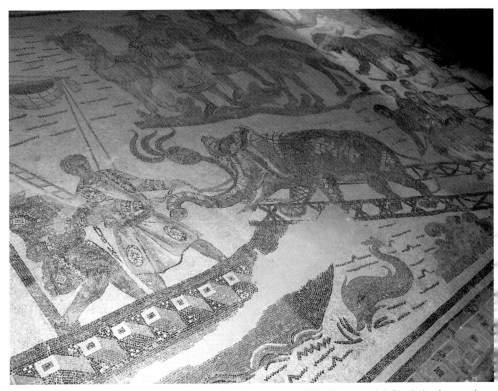

Picture 3: Roman mosaic from the third to fourth century CE Villa Romana del Casale in the province of Enna in Sicily, showing animals being loaded onto a ship in North Africa to go to Rome. (© *Author photograph*)

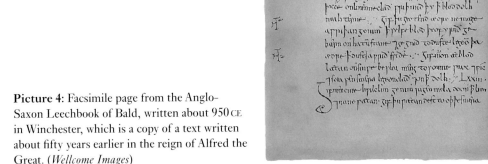

Picture 4: Facsimile page from the Anglo-Saxon Leechbook of Bald, written about 950 CE in Winchester, which is a copy of a text written about fifty years earlier in the reign of Alfred the Great. (*Wellcome Images*)

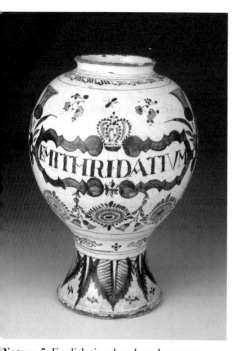

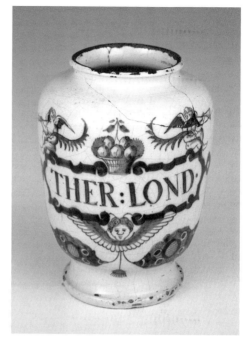

Picture 5: English tin-glazed earthenware drug jar dated 1700–1720 labelled E. MITHRIDATUM – Electuarium Mithridatium. White glaze with bluish tinge and design in blue. (*Royal Pharmaceutical Society Museum image reference LDRPS:KCY1*)

Picture 6: English ceramic, tin-glazed earthenware drug jar dated 1700–1725 labelled THER. LOND – Theriaca Londinensis or London Treacle. (*Royal Pharmaceutical Society Museum image reference LDRPS:KCM1*)

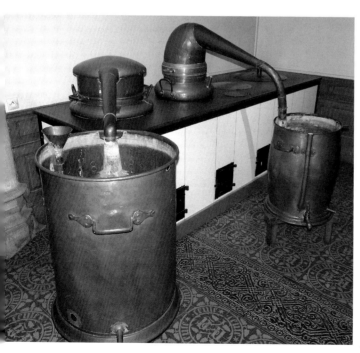

Picture 7: Two distillation alembic stills from the laboratory in the Hospices de Beaune Museum, Beaune, France, founded in 1443. (© *Author photograph*)

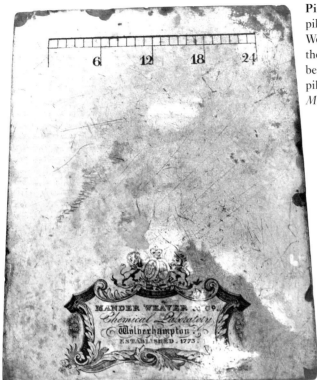

Picture 8: Late eighteenth-century pill tile made by Mander Weaver, Wolverhampton. Used for rolling the pill mass into a long 'pipe' before dividing it into individual pills. (*Royal Pharmaceutical Society Museum image reference ATB2*)

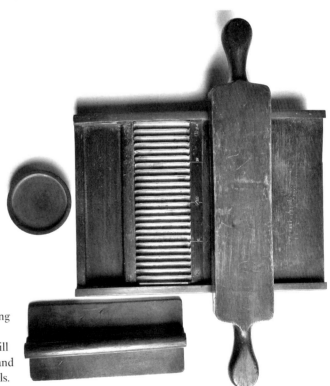

Picture 9: Hand pill-making equipment, twentieth century. For dividing the pill mass into individual pills, and rolling them into round pills. (© *Author photograph*)

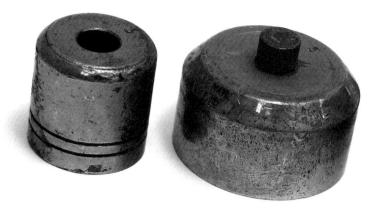

Picture 10: Punch and die set as patented by William Brockedon in 1843 to produce single tablets. Set shown was manufactured by S. Maw, Son and Thompson 1870–1900. (*Royal Pharmaceutical Society Museum image reference ATA3*)

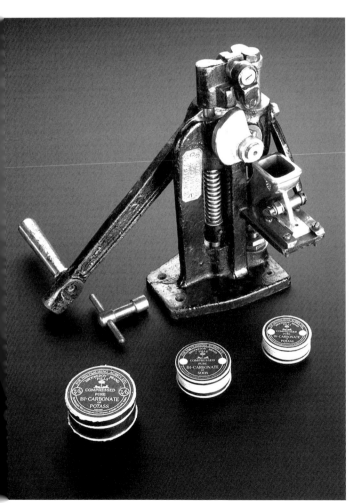

Picture 11: Hand-operated single punch tablet-making machine made by J.W. Pindar and Company 1901–1920 for use by a community pharmacist. (*Wellcome Images*)

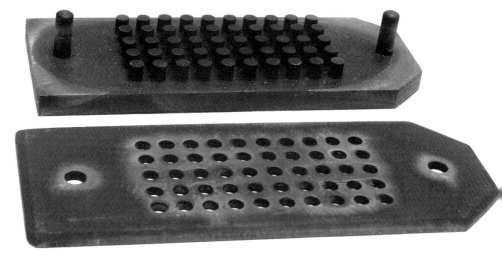

Picture 12: Rubber tablet triturate mould. Manufactured by Whitall Tatum Company, late 1800s or early 1900s. (*Royal Pharmaceutical Society image reference ATA1*)

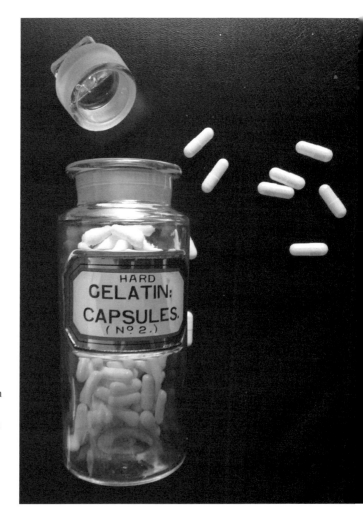

Picture 13: Empty gelatin capsules, as patented by James Murdoch in Britain in 1847. Capsules were filled by the pharmacist or by a pharmaceutical manufacturer. (© *Author photograph*)

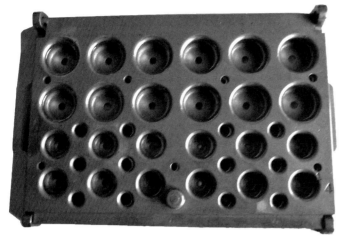

Picture 14: Wet-seal cachet machine from early 1900s. Used to fill the lower halves of the cachet with powder fill, then moistening the rims of the upper and lower halves and bringing the two halves together to seal. (© *Author photograph*)

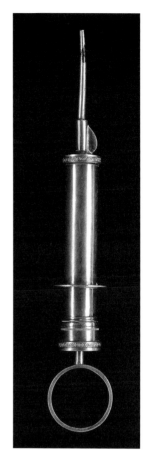

Picture 15: Anel ophthalmic syringe from the seventeenth century. Dominique Anel (1679–1730). (*Wellcome Images*)

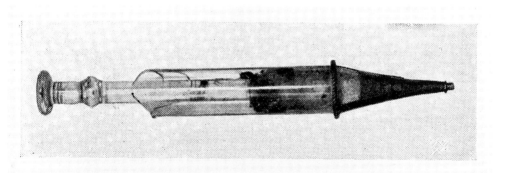

ORIGINAL HYPODERMIC SYRINGE OF

DR. ALEXANDER WOOD

THE FIRST USED IN GREAT BRITAIN

Picture 16: Dr Alexander Wood's hypodermic syringe of 1853, the first used in Great Britain. (*Wellcome Images*)

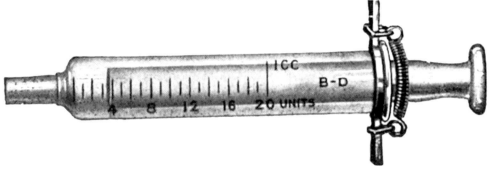

Picture 17: Becton Dickinson insulin syringe introduced in 1924. (*Image courtesy of Becton Dickinson*)

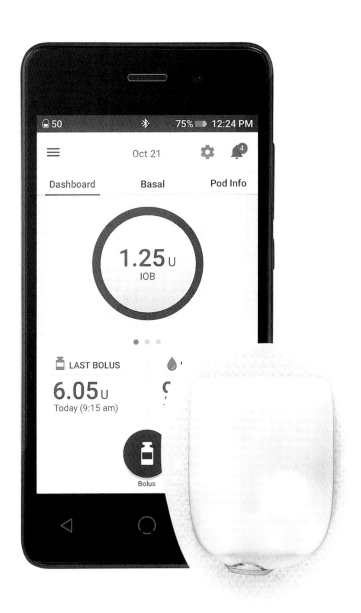

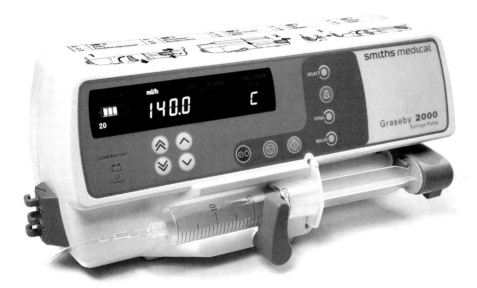

Picture 19: Smiths Medical Graseby® 2000 syringe infusion pump. (*Image used with permission of Smiths Medical*)

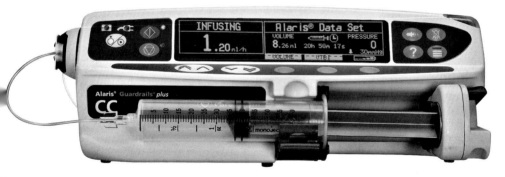

Picture 20: Becton Dickinson Alaris CC Plus syringe pump. (*Image courtesy of Becton Dickinson*)

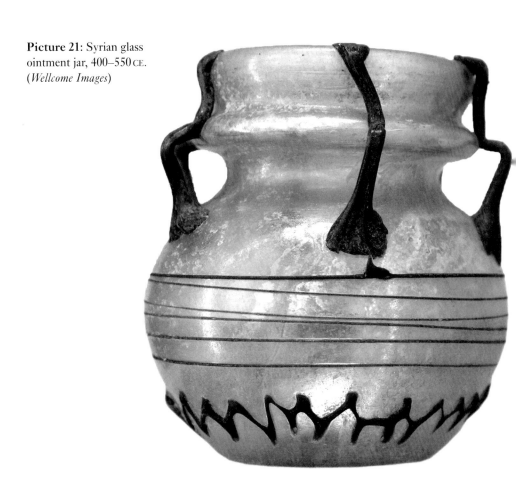

Picture 21: Syrian glass ointment jar, 400–550 CE. (*Wellcome Images*)

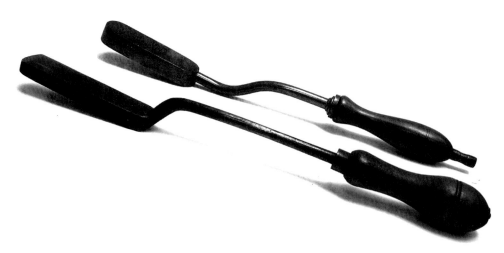

Picture 22: Plaster irons, 1800s or early 1900s. These were used to spread plaster mass onto sheepskin, calico, linen or silk. One shown was gas-heated, the other was heated over a flame. (*Royal Pharmaceutical Society Museum image references APC1/D and APC1/L*)

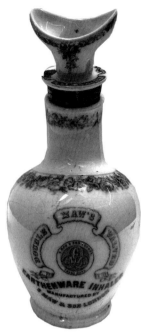

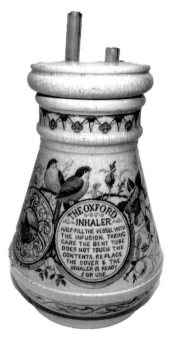

Picture 23: S. Maw and Sons ceramic double-valved vapour inhaler devised by Dr Nelson in 1861. (*Royal Pharmaceutical Society Museum image reference GIA12*)

Picture 24: Oxford ceramic creamware vapour inhaler, c.1880. (*Royal Pharmaceutical Society Museum image reference GIA22*)

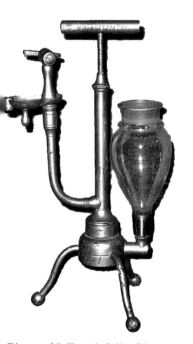

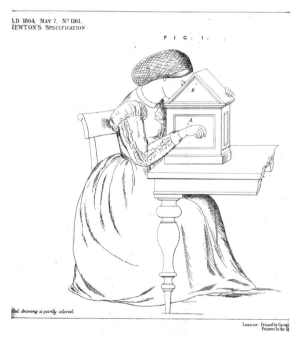

Picture 25: French Salès-Giron Pulvisateur vapour spray inhaler device of 1858. (*With permission from www.inhalatorium*)

Picture 26: Alfred Newton's dry powder inhalation device of 1864. (*With permission from www.inhalatorium*)

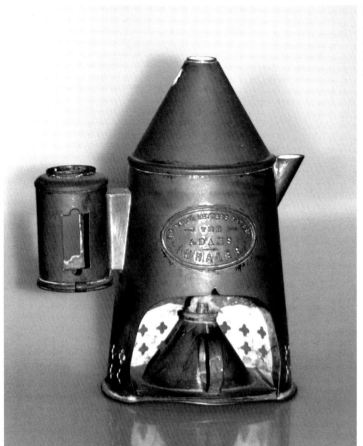

Picture 27: Dr John Adams' spray nebuliser inhalation device of 1868. (*With permission from www.inhalatorium*)

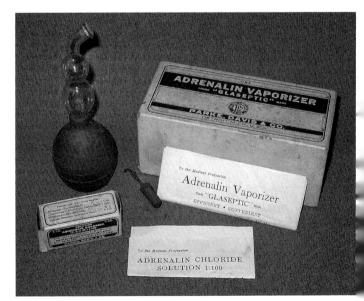

Picture 28: Parke Davis Glaseptic Nebuliser, 1907. (*With permission from www. inhalatorium*)

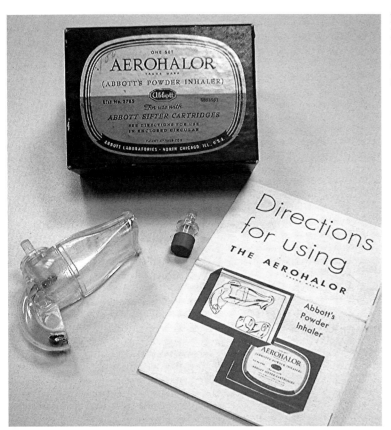

Picture 29: Abbot Laboratories powder Aerohaler, 1948. (*With permission from www.inhalatorium*)

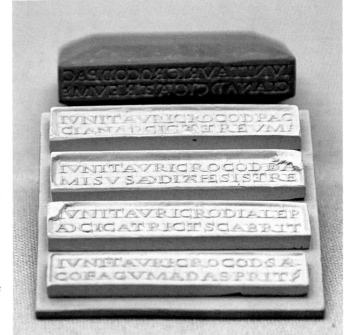

Picture 30: Roman collyrium stamp inscribed with names of four remedies prepared with saffron by Junius Taurus from a prescription of Pacius. Dated between 1 and 299 CE. Used for marking sticks of eye ointment before they harden. From Lorraine, France. (*Wellcome Images*)

Picture 31: Single dose Levofloxacin antibiotic eye drops. (*Wellcome Images*)

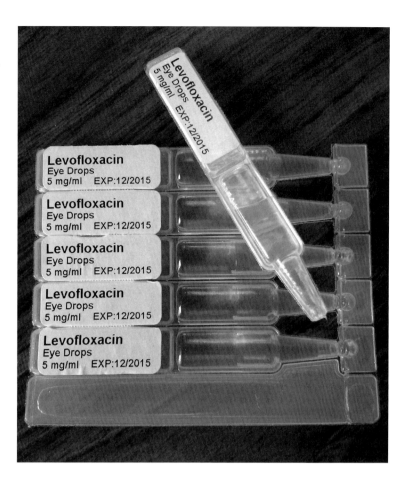

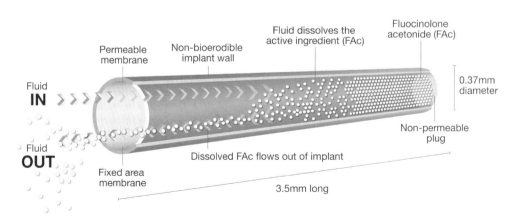

Picture 32: Diagram of Iluvien fluocinolone acetonide intravitreal implant. This is an implant injected into the eye and used for the treatment of diabetic macular oedema. It releases the drug over three years. (© *Alimera Sciences Limited*)

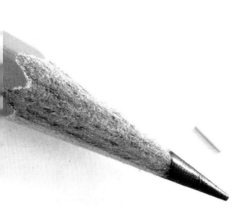

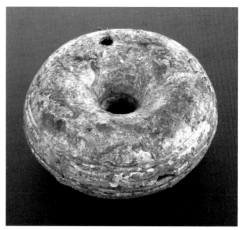

Picture 33: Photograph of Iluvien implant to show its size compared to a pencil tip. (© *Alimera Sciences Limited*)

Picture 34: Roman bronze pessary ring in two halves used to treat uterine prolapse. Dated 200 BCE–400 CE. (*Wellcome Images*)

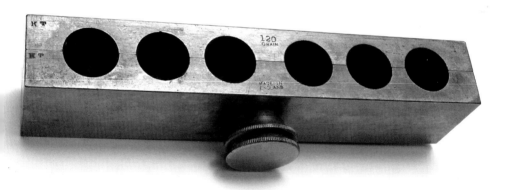

Picture 35: Nickel-plated brass pessary mould to produce six pessaries. Marked 120 grain (7.2 grams) which is the pessary size. (*Royal Pharmaceutical Society Museum image reference APA2*)

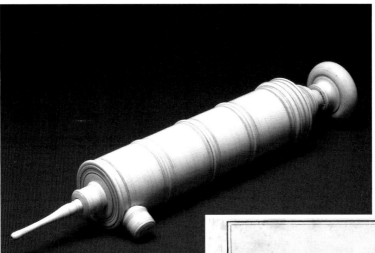

Picture 36: French ivory enema syringe, dated 1701–1800. (*Wellcome Images*)

Picture 37: Black and white etching, entitled 'Apotekeren / l'Apothicaire', designed by Jacques Antoine Arlaud, dated around 1730. It depicts a young, thin and bespectacled apothecary, kneeling in profile to the right, his eyes staring and lips pursed as he prepares to administer a huge clyster (enema) to an unseen lady – only her discarded shoe is visible next to a steaming jug. (*Royal Pharmaceutical Society Museum image reference PZ143*)

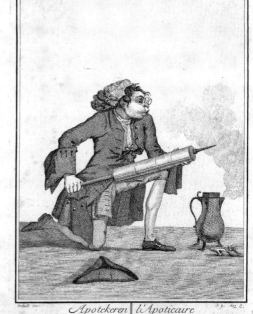

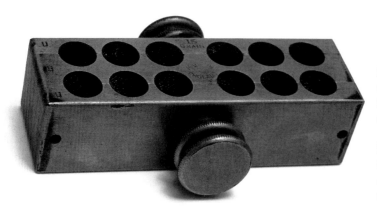

Picture 38: Metal suppository mould to produce twelve suppositories. Marked 15 grain (900 mg), which is the suppository size. (*Royal Pharmaceutical Society Museum image reference ASE3/I*)

name was becoming an eponym, the use of which was specific to a form of medicine mainly used for the treatment of indigestion, and that the public did not need to be told if it was a compressed pill nor what was in it. There are other examples of the name of the original inventor being used as nouns to define a product. Hoover is perhaps the best known, having become a generic name for vacuum cleaners, irrespective of the manufacturer and also as a verb describing the process of gathering up.

Brockedon's compressed pills continued to sell well, so much so that in 1871, Francis Newbery & Sons thought it worthwhile to acquire the right and title to manufacture compressed pills according to Brockedon's process, though they did not actually acquire the patent rights. By this time, Brockedon had been dead for about seventeen years. 'Brockedon's Patent Pills' appeared in their catalogue of 1874. They were exported to many countries, including the US and Germany. So popular were English compressed medicines in Germany that German manufacturers were alleged to stick English labels on to their own products.

In about 1888, Newbery & Sons sold their rights to the Brockedon process to Messrs Burroughs Wellcome & Co.

Brockedon marketed his compressed pills on the basis of their purity i.e. they contained only the active ingredient. Potassium chlorate and the bicarbonates of potassium and sodium seem to have been the most popular. The strategy of emphasising purity was to contrast his product with pills prepared by traditional methods. To quote from Patent 9977:

'It is well known that in making pills, and also medicated lozenges, as heretofore practised, the proper materials are mixed with a suitable liquid into a state of stiff paste, which is divided and shaped and allowed to dry, and it is well known that in some cases the gum and other materials, used as adhesive matter for keeping pills and lozenges in form, when the same are mixed by means of fluids, interfere with and prejudice the desired action of the matters employed in making up or preparing pills and lozenges, and these gums and adhesive matters are rendered necessary by the use of fluids for getting the matters into a condition to be shaped.'

In modern parlance, the excipients present in pills could reduce or even abolish the bioavailability of the active ingredient.

This theme of purity is also apparent in the announcement in *The Pharmaceutical Journal* ('compression of substances into a solid mass without the introduction of gums') and in the advertisement in *The Times* ('pure alkaline preparation') quoted earlier. There is an important limitation to this strategy, because there are very few medicinal substances capable of being compressed into a satisfactory product without the addition of other substances i.e. most need the presence of excipients. For example, a diluent is needed if the dose of active ingredient is less than about 50mg. A lubricant is almost invariably required to prevent the compressed mass sticking to the punch faces and the die. In patent 9977, the apparatus is being dismantled after every compression to eject the product, and so in theory at least, the apparatus could be cleaned, but in any continuous production, a build-up of powder on the punch faces and in the die cavity will bring the press to a halt. For a wider application of compression to the production of solid dosage forms, a different approach was needed.

There is little evidence that making compressed medicines progressed much in Great Britain after the introduction of Brockedon's compressed pills and their marketing by Francis Newbery. It was in the 1860s that significant development of compressed medicines occurred in the US, and enormous strides in their production took place over the next thirty years. Thus, compressed medicines take their place among British inventions which were developed into successful commercial products in the United States. Television, antibiotics and the jet-propelled airliner are other examples that come readily to mind. Indeed, it could be claimed that the entire pharmaceutical industry is an American 'invention' of that period. Many American companies that were formed in the latter years of the nineteenth century are still in existence today, though a considerable degree of amalgamation has taken place.

The question must be asked why this happened in the US rather than elsewhere? It may be due to a lack of entrepreneurial spirit in Britain, a greater availability of finance in a country with enormous material resources and a growing population with a corresponding growing need for medicines. However, there was a factor peculiar to the US in the early 1860s and that was the American Civil War (1861–5). This has been described as the first industrial war i.e. the first major conflict since the Industrial Revolution, and it generated an enormous demand for manufactured items including medicinal products.

The first American name to appear in the development of compressed medicines was Jacob Dunton. He was born around 1830 in Philadelphia, graduated from the Philadelphia College of Pharmacy in 1855, and set up a pharmaceutical wholesale business in Market Street, Philadelphia. He was granted US Patent Number 174790 on 14 March 1876. The introduction to the patent refers to an improved machine for making pills, and so it must be assumed that Dunton was familiar with Brockedon's apparatus. Note that Dunton refers to his product as a pill. There is no indication that the compression force is applied by any other means than by hitting the top of the upper punch with a hammer. Dunton's machine was entirely concerned with making medicinal products, whereas Brockedon's invention was primarily concerned with compressing graphite for pencil manufacture, with medicines something of an afterthought. The most intriguing aspects of Dunton's patent is its date, over thirty-two years after Brockedon had been awarded his patent for what is fundamentally a very similar device, and after the introduction of other presses which were significant advances on Brockedon's invention.

There is evidence that Dunton's interest in compressed pills began well before 1876. It is known that Dunton provided pills for the US Government at the time of the Civil War, but there is no evidence that any of these were compressed pills. What appears more certain is that Dunton was selling 'compressed lenticular (i.e. lens shaped) pills' in 1867. However, more definite information is available. In 1879, Dunton was involved in litigation after his patent was published, perhaps not surprisingly in view of the apparent lack of novelty in his invention. The dispute was with Bennett L. Smedley, another Philadelphia manufacturer, and it is in the record of the court that Dunton's early activities in the field become apparent. [23] Evidence was produced showing that as early as 1864, he had commissioned an engineer to produce a machine similar to that described in the patent. Dunton himself claimed that he had first put his compressed pills on the market in 1869, and between 1864 and 1869, he had made several thousand pills, though he did not sell them. He said that most of these pills had been made on machines that were modifications of that described in the patent. The pressing force was applied by means of a screw, thereby eliminating the hammer blow. He also fitted an eccentric so that the pill could be ejected without dismantling the press. Neither of these developments form part of Patent 174790. By 1869, Dunton stated that he had made over 300 varieties of compressed pill, and by 1876, he had made between two and three million pills, none of which had been made on machines identical to that described in the patent.

Replacing an inconsistent hammer blow with a screw drive constituted a major advance in the reproducibility of the product, especially in its physical strength and ease of disintegration. All other factors being equal, tablet properties depend on their porosity, which in turn is governed by the degree of consolidation that occurs during compression. Turning the screw by the same amount for each tablet would thus provide a consistent porosity, assuming a constant fill weight. Using an eccentric to bring about ejection was a further advance, since it reduced the amount of manual work needed to produce each tablet, and this in turn greatly increased productivity.

Dunton had obviously decided not to file a patent for his original press, and it is not known why he did this, nor why he changed his mind in 1876. It is known that secrecy prevailed in the industrial production of medicines at that time, rather than reliance on patents to protect intellectual property, so Dunton may have been following this practice.[24]

From the early 1870s, there were many developments in press design, which form a bridge between the simple devices patented by Brockedon and Dunton to the presses in use at the present time. Many of these took place in the city of Philadelphia, which was becoming the centre of pharmaceutical production. Particularly noteworthy is the contribution made by the firm of John Wyeth & Brother. John and Frank Wyeth had opened a drug store on Walnut Street, Philadelphia, not far from Dunton's wholesale premises on Market Street, but they later moved into the manufacture of pharmaceutical products. John Wyeth & Brother became part of the American Home Products Company in 1932, and it is now part of the Pfizer organisation.

Though there is very little published material from this period, it is surely significant that as early as 1877, Silas Mainville Burroughs (1846–1895), who graduated from the Philadelphia College of Pharmacy in that year, was able to amass sufficient material to be able to present a thesis entitled '*Compression of Medicinal Powders*'. Burroughs later became the agent in London for John Wyeth & Brother, and later founded Burroughs and Co to import American medicines into the UK. Henry Wellcome (1853–1936) joined the company in 1880, which then became Burroughs, Wellcome and Co. Their company became a major influence in the pharmaceutical field, particularly in the area of compressed products.

The Dunton tablet press showed little advance over the Brockedon press invented at least twenty years earlier, and basically similar presses continued to be introduced. In 1875, for example, and thus pre-dating the Dunton patent, Joseph P. Remington of Philadelphia, then Professor of Pharmacy at the Philadelphia College of Pharmacy, described a simple machine which differed very little from Brockedon's press, force being applied by striking the top of the upper punch with a mallet. All presses like this needed to be at least partially dismantled after each compression to enable the 'pill' to be removed then reassembled, so a slow rate of production was unavoidable. The use of a hammer or mallet to bring about compression was one of the first features of the early presses to be abandoned. As stated above, it was part of Dunton's patent that Dunton himself had already discarded. It was recognised that variation in the way the hammer was wielded led to a proportional variation in the applied force.

Two major developments in press design date from 1874. The first of these was a press with one die and one set of punches, patented by T. J. Young of Philadelphia (US Patent 156398). The upper punch was raised and lowered by means of a cam in the centre of the drive shaft, which could be rotated by a pulley and belt arrangement, and the lower punch was raised by a cam on the drive shaft and lowered by a weight. During compression, the lower punch was stationary, but after compression, it was raised to eject the compressed product from the die. Then the machine was stopped by means of a brake, the product removed, the die refilled and the machine back into gear by actuating another lever. Young improved his machine in 1877 (US Patent 189005) and assigned his patent to Henry Bower. A machine matching this description and dating from the 1870s was apparently still operating in 1913 at John Wyeth & Brother in Philadelphia.

The output of a press can be increased by boring each die so that it contains several parallel individual die cavities. Matching multi-tipped punches are provided, so that each stroke of the press makes several products rather than just one. Another method of increasing output is to have more than one die in the press, and this is the basis of the second major advance in press design in 1874 patented by Joseph A. McFerran, also of Philadelphia (US Patent 152666, entitled 'Improvement in pill machines'). This was described as an automatic compressed pill machine. The key feature of this machine was a rotating disc in which there were eight dies arranged in a circle. There was an automatic feed, upper and lower punches and a brush for removing the 'pills' after compression. The whole apparatus was actuated by a driveshaft, so mechanisation was at least theoretically possible. This is undoubtedly the first published description of a rotary press, and is the basis of most commercial presses operating currently.

It is believed that a similar rotary press had been invented in 1872 by Henry Bower. It must be assumed that Bower's device worked satisfactorily, as it was adopted by John Wyeth & Brother. Further improvements were patented by Jabez H. Gill in 1879 and 1881. The first of these was assigned to Bower and the second to John Wyeth & Brother. There was obviously some connection between Bower and Wyeth. The climate of secrecy surrounding medicine manufacture in Philadelphia has already been alluded to in relation to Dunton's patent, and Wyeth undoubtedly relied on secrecy rather than patents to protect its early machines from imitation. Thus, details of Bower's and Gill's inventions are unclear. However, it is apparent that by the late 1870s, Wyeth were making large numbers of compressed pills. These products were being exported in sufficient quantities to justify Wyeth appointing Silas Burroughs as its European representative in 1878. The scale of production by Wyeth only became public knowledge in 1889, when their premises in Philadelphia were destroyed by fire. John Wyeth stated that, 'The precious formulas were saved. The heaviest separate loss is on the pill presses. The pill pressing process is our own, we control it entirely.' Another member of the Wyeth family stated that at that time, the company had about 25 machines, each of which could make 7,200 units per hour[24].

The presses described above are capable of efficient large-scale production, but this could not be achieved whilst only manual power was available. However, presses which involved some form of rotary motion, whether of the die table or in the means of applying the compressing force, would lend themselves to some form of mechanical drive. The question was what the source of the motive power might be.

An article in *The Pharmaceutical Journal* in 1911 refers to large quantities of tablets being manufactured by 'steam-driven machinery'.[25] To modern users of tablet presses, the suggestion that these machines are driven by steam appears incongruous. However, it must be remembered that the first rotary presses were invented before the widespread availability of a reliable electricity supply. At that time, virtually all machinery was driven by steam power. The normal arrangement was for steam to be generated in a boiler of sufficient capacity to supply the whole factory. The boiler was usually situated in a separate building, which often had a tall chimney, giving a landscape made familiar by L. S. Lowry in his paintings of the textile-producing areas of Lancashire. The steam drove an engine, the output of which was transmitted by a system of gears to rotating shafts, usually suspended from the ceilings of each level of the factory. From these shafts, motion was transmitted by driving belts to the individual pieces of machinery.

In the last years of the nineteenth century, development of the press continued, partly in the USA, but also in Britain and Germany. An indication of the progress that had been made can be gained from a report in 1903 in *The Pharmaceutical Journal* of a press made by the British firm of Allen and Hanbury (now part of Glaxo Smith Kline).[26] Apparently, Allen and Hanbury had visited a pharmaceutical machinery exhibition in Philadelphia in 1876, and had brought back to Britain what was probably the first 'modern' tablet press in the country. They later began building machines to their own design that were capable of making 1,000 items per minute. It is striking how many features of the Allen and Hanbury press are used in the modern rotary press. Early developments in tablet presses have been comprehensively surveyed by Kebler[23] and Foote.[27]

Viewed externally, a modern tablet press looks nothing like the Allen and Hanbury machine, but the underlying layout is essentially the same.

A useful comparison is provided by the TPR700 range of tablet presses from Bosch Packaging Technology. Depending on the model, there are between 49 and 81 dies and sets of punches, and maximum output is between 528,000 and 1,008,000 tablets per hour, compressed at a force of up to 100kN. The press is driven by an integral electric motor, and the machine is enclosed in metal and glass panels for safety reasons, and to cut down noise and possibilities of cross-contamination from neighbouring presses making a different product.

Use of the word 'tablet' with reference to compressed medicines

Languages can be considered analogous to living organisms in that the meaning of words evolves over time. Obsolete uses of a word gradually become defunct, and new uses are introduced. The word 'tablet' is no exception. Even in the last few years, a completely new meaning of 'tablet' has emerged, referring to a small, usually rectangular, hand-held computer.

The online *Oxford English Dictionary* gives nineteen different usages of the word 'tablet', one of which is 'A small flat or compressed piece of a solid substance, originally of rectangular form. Spec: a measured quantity of a medicine or drug, compressed into a small disc or lozenge and designed to be swallowed whole; a pill'. This is followed by a series of references to the use of the word in that context, the earliest of which dates from c. 1425.

According to the *Shorter Oxford English Dictionary* (2008) 'tablet' can also be used as a verb, as in 'make a (medicine, drug etc.) into a tablet'. The derivation of the word is stated to be Middle English, via Old French tablete from the Proto-Romanic. It is the diminutive of the Latin tabula meaning a table, so 'tablet' literally means 'little table'.

Samuel Johnson gave the following definition of 'tablet' in his *Dictionary of the English Language*, the first edition of which was published in 1755: 'A medicine in a square form'. Dr Johnson's description of a tablet being square was to acquire significance more than a century later.

Presumably the word 'tablet' was originally chosen as the name for a form of medicine because of its rectangular shape. The term is widely used in other Northern European languages such as German (Tablette). The word used in Southern European languages e.g. comprimé (French) and comprimido (Spanish) is more descriptive of how the medicine is actually made, being derived from the Latin verb comprimere (to compress).

It is therefore clear that the term 'tablet' to describe a form of medicine was in use for centuries before the tablet as we currently know it was invented. The earliest citations of the term 'tablet' probably refer to what later became known as tablet triturates and lozenges.

The pill was undoubtedly the most frequently used oral solid dosage form when William Brockedon was granted Patent Number 9977 in December 1843, and it was perhaps inevitable that when this novel form of solid medicine was introduced, Brockedon described it as a compressed pill. Irrespective of the name that Brockedon actually used for his new dosage form, it was called a pill when it was reported in *The Pharmaceutical Journal* of May 1844, only a few months after the patent was granted, and in widely published advertisements. It retained this description for some time.

Everyday use of the term 'tablet' in relation to compressed medicines probably dates from 1878 and was coined by Burroughs Wellcome, though independent definite information is lacking.

Use of the term' tablet' was commonplace by the 1880s, (although John Wyeth & Brother, then the largest manufacturer of compressed medicines, was still referring to its products as 'pills' as late as 1889),[24] so acceptance of the word 'tablet' to describe a compressed dosage form must have spread remarkably quickly. The first appearance of the word 'tablet' in the index of the *The Pharmaceutical Journal* was made in 1881, and refers to an article published on 20 August that year entitled '*Pharmaceutical Notes*' by Robert F. Fairhome.[28] This in turn was taken from the *American Journal of Pharmacy*, also of August 1881, and states the advantages that tablets or 'compressed granules for hypodermic use' offer in terms of convenience, accuracy and labelling.

The first indexed entry of the word 'tablet' in *The Chemist & Druggist* appeared a few months later, and refers to two letters published in that journal. The first of these appeared in the 15 November issue, and was from M. Rogerson & Son of Bradford.[29] It bemoans the lack of enterprise among British tablet manufacturers in allowing American competitors to gain a dominant provision in the supply of compressed medicines in this country.

A vigorous response came in the issue of 12 December 1881 from F. Newbery & Son, who at that time owned the rights to prepare medicines by Brockedon's method and who claimed that the demand for such products was increasing.[30]

> 'Sir. We have observed the letter of your correspondent Messrs M. Rogerson & Son in your last issue, and would point out that the idea of compressing pills or tablets, by whatever name they may be called, was originated by the late Professor Brockedon …'

It is worth noting that in this letter, 'compressed pills' and 'tablets' seem to be regarded as synonyms referring to the same item ('by whatever name they may be called').

An extended range of tablets was certainly available in Britain in 1883. The first edition of *The Extra Pharmacopoeia*, published in that year has a section entitled 'Tablets Compressed' and lists twelve preparations. There is, of course, no indication as to whether these tablets were made in Britain or obtained from elsewhere, but they must have had wide availability and usage to justify listing in a book of reference such as *The Extra Pharmacopoeia*.

In the 1885 edition of *The British Pharmacopoeia*, there is a monograph entitled 'Tablets of Nitroglycerin', and this surely indicates that 'tablet' was by now the accepted name for such products. The monograph does not suggest that they were made by compression, and were probably moulded tablets or lozenges. This preparation is not among those listed under 'Tablets Compressed' in *The Extra Pharmacopoeia*, but is included in that publication under 'Lozenges'.

In 1878, Silas Burroughs, an American, came to Britain as the agent for the medicinal products of John Wyeth & Brother, which were, of course, made in the US. By that time, tablets had become a widely accepted form of medication on both sides of the Atlantic, but Burroughs realised that there was hardly any pharmaceutical manufacturing in Great Britain, and this absence presented a considerable business opportunity. He invited Henry Wellcome to become his business partner, the partnership being established in 1880 in London, and the first manufacturing site was set up in Wandsworth in South West London in 1883. The business expanded quickly, as indicated by the Wellcome price list of 1896, which included 354 different varieties of tablet, 255 of which were for oral use.

To assist the marketing of these, Henry Wellcome registered the trademark *Tabloid* in 1884, and this became one of the most renowned trademarks in any commercial sphere. In fact, the name Tabloid was applied not just to tablets but to a major part of the whole range of the company's products including Tabloid first aid kits, Tabloid photographic developer and even Tabloid tea. The fact that Burroughs Wellcome invented the name Tabloid, so clearly derived from 'tablet', shows that by 1884, the term 'tablet' was in common usage. Therefore, Burroughs Wellcome required a new word to distinguish their products from those made by other companies.

Burroughs Wellcome vigorously defended its intellectual property rights to the word Tabloid, and it was only after a series of prolonged legal actions that Tabloid was recognised as being the exclusive property of Burroughs Wellcome in 1903.[31]. Soon after its introduction, Tabloid was soon in everyday use, particularly in relation to compressed medicines. Rather than being just a registered name, Tabloid became virtually a synonym for the word 'tablet', irrespective of the identity of the actual manufacturer of that tablet. This confusion occurred not just among the general public, but also among prescribers, and it is unlikely that Burroughs Wellcome did much to discourage its use in this sense. A good example of the irritation that confusion between Tabloid and tablet could cause can be gauged from a letter that appeared in *The Pharmaceutical Journal* of 9 February 1895. Just prior to this, T. Lauder Brunton, a lecturer in pharmacology and therapeutics at St Bartholomew's Hospital, London, had published an article in the *British Medical Journal* of 2 February 1895, in which he extolled the advantages of tabloids. He suggested that it would be useful 'to have something of that sort in the Pharmacopoeia'. The 1898 edition of *The British Pharmacopoeia* was then being compiled.

There is no suggestion in this article that Brunton was aware that Tabloid was a trademark.

This article generated an irate response from a pharmacist writing to *The Pharmaceutical Journal* under the nom-de-plume of 'Galen', who had obviously seen the original article in the *British Medical Journal*, [32] and who took Brunton to task. Was he aware

> 'that the word "tabloid" is a registered trademark of a firm of Americans, who can claim neither originality nor superior excellence for the manufacture of medicines compressed into this form? The way in which prescribers are led by the nose by the advertisements of monopolists, who assume to themselves the right to influence the mode of medical prescribing is intolerable.'

He then recounted an incident when he received in his pharmacy a prescription for 'Tabloids' of a drug needed urgently. He had then wasted much time before discovering that Burroughs Wellcome did not make this product and so it could not be a Tabloid. He then had to supply another manufacturer's tablets.

In recent years, a new usage of 'tabloid' has arisen in relation to newspapers with a compact format. Originally so-called tabloid newspapers were aimed at a mass market, as distinct from the 'broadsheets', but this distinction has become progressively blurred. It is ironic that the term flourishes in respect to newspapers when the Tabloid brand name and that of its originators are no longer in being, the latter losing their identity when they were taken over by Glaxo PLC in 1995.

In addition to successfully defending its intellectual property rights to the word 'Tabloid', Burroughs Wellcome also attempted to claim that the word tablet was part of its intellectual property. In a letter published in *The Chemist & Druggist* of 1892 they made the following statement:[33]

> The word 'Tablets' was first applied by us to the class of drugs (compressed medicines) at the commencement of our business in 1878. This form of medication had hitherto been known in this country as 'compressed pills'. We registered the word 'Tablets' in this connection as a trade-mark and therefore regard it as our rightful

property, also because we introduced the word here, and because it is in our opinion non-descriptive and therefore eligible for use as a trade-mark. We still employ it on some of our goods. A 'Tablet' has never been described or considered as a substance having a round or oval surface, but rather having a flat or squared surface. In the compressed form of medication, the surface is rounded or curved. Some firms have, we presume inadvertently, used the word 'Tablets' in connection with compressed drugs. To certain of these firms, we have explained that we claimed the exclusive employment of the word in this connection and have received replies from them that they would make no further use of that word.

In all twelve firms were named.

It is of interest that Burroughs Wellcome were drawing a distinction between square and round tablets. They obviously had in mind the definition in Johnson's dictionary that a tablet is a 'medicine in a square form'. Presumably, therefore, any medicine that is not in a square form is not a tablet in the generic sense. Hence registering the word as a trademark for round tablets is permissible.

It is not surprising that such a claim elicited a vigorous response from some of their competitors.

Obviously, Burroughs Wellcome were making determined efforts to keep the name 'tablet' for solid medicines which did not have a square shape as their exclusive intellectual property. What is peculiar about these arguments is that they were being made as late as 1892. As described earlier, the first edition of *The Extra Pharmacopoeia,* published in 1883, listed twelve preparations which were presumably in common use at that time, describing them as 'compressed tablets' of 'lenticular shape', i.e. they were made by compression and they were round in cross-section. This list appears to demolish Burroughs Wellcome's claims. The use of the word 'tablet' in the title of a monograph in the 1885 edition of *The British Pharmacopoeia* would cause further damage to Burroughs Wellcome's claims for exclusivity, since it is highly unlikely that the publishers would knowingly use 'tablet' in such a situation if it was the intellectual property of one company. If Burroughs Wellcome felt they had a case, surely, they should have made it in 1883 or 1885 rather than several years later. After 1892, no further reference has been found to this dispute, so it is likely that Burroughs Wellcome decided to concentrate on protecting the word 'Tabloid'.

The attempt by Burroughs Wellcome & Co to protect the title 'tablet' long after the term had appeared in *The British Pharmacopoeia* was not unique. As late as 1896, Messrs Allen and Hanbury were trying to protect 'tabellae' as their exclusive property when this word had been used in the title of a monograph in the 1885 edition of the pharmacopoeia. Up to the 1953 edition, the main title of monographs in the pharmacopoeia were in Latin, e.g. *Tabellae Glycerylis Trinitratis*.

Reactions by the pharmaceutical profession to the increased use of the tablet

By the 1880s, the tablet was a frequently used form of medication, and a wide range of active ingredients were available as tablets. The advantages of the tablet were already obvious to the medical and pharmaceutical professions and also to the general public, some of these advantages being accuracy of dosage, stability and convenience of administration. However, there was one other factor which led to the increased use of the tablet, and that was that tablets could be produced in relatively large quantities by means of an industrial process. Prior to this, virtually all medicines were produced either by the prescriber or the dispenser for a specific patient, but no longer. Medicines could be made by machines at a relatively small number of locations rather than in thousands of individual dispensaries, the distribution of such medicines being facilitated by improved transport networks. This is typical of changes brought about in virtually all manufactured items.

With hindsight, the introduction of relatively cheap, machine-made items would be regarded by the majority of the population as 'progress'. But for parts of the population at that time, they were nothing short of disastrous. Small businesses, which in many cases had existed for generations, found they could not compete with much cheaper, mass-produced goods transported economically by rail from distant factories, and so ceased trading. Some workers found that there was no demand for their skills, often obtained after a long period of training, and so had to seek alternative employment elsewhere. With the coming of railways, small towns situated along major highways virtually lost their complete livelihoods, since this depended on the horse-drawn transport of passengers and goods. Hence such trades depending on the horse, such as ostlers and blacksmiths, became redundant, as did the employees of coaching inns which had lost their 'passing trade'.

As the Industrial Revolution did not impinge on the manufacture of medicines until the middle of the nineteenth century, it is not surprising that, as the US had become the major innovating force by that time, the important modernising influences came from there. Pharmaceutical manufacturing in the modern sense was initiated there, and spread rapidly to other parts of the world, especially Europe.

It is therefore understandable that considerable unease was felt throughout the pharmaceutical profession on the possible redundancy of their traditional craft skills, acquired during a lengthy and probably expensive period of apprenticeship.

For a period of about twenty years at the end of the nineteenth century, there was considerable discussion about the role that tablets might play in the professional lives of pharmacists. There was an element of xenophobia in addition to concern over the possible loss of professional skills. A good early example is the letter by Rogerson and Son cited earlier, which interestingly forms the very first indexed entry of the word 'tablet' in *The Chemist & Druggist*. Rogerson was perturbed by the seeming lack of enterprise by British manufacturers.[29]

A typical contribution to the debate on the perceived reduction in the importance of traditional pharmaceutical skills appeared in *The Pharmaceutical Journal* of September 1891. Entitled 'Compressed tablets', it appeared under the nom-de-plume of 'Apprentice'.[34] The article opens by citing a communication that 'Apprentice' had recently received in which it was advocated that: 'It would be a vast improvement if all drugs were to be prescribed and dispensed in the form of compressed pellets.'

'Apprentice' begged to differ, giving several reasons, some professional and some commercial. He alludes to the facilitation tablets offer to adulteration of ingredients, stating that there have been several incidents of this. He suggested it was 'better by far to keep a stock of "the good old pill", which has been and always will be, co-existent with the healing art itself'.

He also suggested that if the use of tablets became universal, how long would it be before 'every grocer and oil man' would be selling them at 1½d per dozen whereas a pharmacist would be able to sell twelve doses of a liquid medicine for at least a shilling.

'It would simply be handing over to the unqualified dealer that last sheet anchor of the pharmacist's profession – dispensing.'

He concludes:

'How in the world is a poor apprentice to pass his Minor (i.e. his examinations) nowadays, when dispensing only too frequently consists of filling a bottle with some quack medicine in disguise, which medicinal men are inveigled into prescribing by specious advertisements and crafty commercial travellers, whose sole purpose in life seems to be to worry the physician on whom he calls to test his precious samples; when galenical preparations are to be bought at a lower price than the raw ingredients; when infusions, tinctures and the like are made by adding seven litres of water to somebody's 'liquors'; and now, when by the look of matters, the required three years' dispensing experience is to mean nothing more than writing labels and wrapping up bottles of somebody else's 'tablets?'

Disgruntled pharmacists such as 'Apprentice' might have received encouragement from an article reproduced in *The Pharmaceutical Journal* in January 1895, and originating in *Alumni Report*. The article was entitled '*The Passing of the Tablet Fad.*'[35]

The opening sentences of the article are intriguing: 'Unquestionably one of the greatest evils from which legitimate pharmacy and medicine suffer is the indiscriminate use of compressed tablets. Beginning in a small way, they have gradually increased in use until now they threaten to overthrow all other forms of preparations.'

The use of the words 'evil', 'threaten to overthrow' and the suggestion that tablets have no place in 'legitimate pharmacy' is strong language indeed, as is the use of the term 'tablet faddist' later in the piece. The article is particularly scathing on the use of tablets for drugs of vegetable origin, stating that the heat involved in the tablet manufacturing process must cause reduction in the amount of active principles.

It concludes: 'We believe that tablets have had their day, or rather have reached the zenith of popularity, and like every other form of drug preparation that has preceded them, will pass away, at least in part, to make room for something else.'

The 'fad' theme is continued in a leading article in *The Pharmaceutical Journal* in 1896, entitled '*The Tendency of Tablet Medication*'. It quotes extensively from US sources and refers to an article (presumably American in origin) in which a medical writer expresses the opinion 'that the addition of a class of compressed tablets and tablet triturates to the *USP* [*United States Pharmacopeia*] would regulate what is at present a somewhat irregular but widespread and popular method of medication and one that has real advantages and merits'.[36]

The Pharmaceutical Journal then quotes with approval, a vigorous response which appeared in *The American Journal of Pharmacy*. This denies that the tablet is an improvement.

> 'Whilst the tablet may be a boon to the lazy physician, it is also a boon for the quack. The sugar coated pill fad, it is pointed out, has been followed in the US by the elixir craze and this in turn by the gelatine coated pill, the tablet and synthetic remedies which may be administered in any of the forms mentioned'.

Bearing in mind that this article was written in 1896, when there were numerous tablets on the market, and monographs on tablets were included in several pharmacopoeias, it does seem rather dated.

The debate was really about whether or not factory-made medicines were in competition with the professional skills of the pharmacist. Two good examples are found in the discussion which followed the presentation of a paper by Parry and Estcourt entitled: '*Compressed drugs. Accuracy of dosage in tablets.*'[37] The chairman of the meeting said that it was often remarked that the chemist was becoming a mere retailer of tabloids (*sic*) and patent medicines. He went on:

> 'As long as, however, a doctor prescribed medicine in a compressed form, the chemist must be prepared to supply it. The physician

himself ought to be the best judge as to the desirability of ordering medicines in this form, but it devolved upon the chemist to see that when so ordered, it was what it represented to be.'

Further discussion at the same meeting emphasised the 'de-skilling' involved in producing factory-made tablets. It was felt that 'pellets' were prepared by 'quite inexperienced persons, sometimes even by girls, instead of, as they should be, by properly qualified pharmacists.'

Other contributions to the discussion adopted a more pragmatic approach. The crux of their argument was that, like it or not, the tablet was playing an increasingly important role in medicine. Both prescribers and pharmacists ignored the tablet at their peril.

Some writers did not accept that the use of tablets should affect professional attitudes, provided the pharmacist made the tablets himself, and they encouraged pharmacists to do so. For example, an article in *The Pharmaceutical Journal* pointed out that: 'although tablets are manufactured in large quantities by steam-driven machinery, the tablet also belongs legitimately to dispensing, and no one should consider himself a competent dispenser if he has not learnt how to prepare them properly in small quantities.'[25]

In an address to the Philadelphia College of Pharmacy, and originally published in *The American Journal of Pharmacy* and reprinted in *The Pharmaceutical Journal*, McFerran[38] stated that:

'compressed tablets are very frequently used. Enterprising manufacturers will not only furnish them directly to physicians but also to druggists … the whole boundless domain of physic is embraced by their all-embracing love. Nor will the doctor stop his ears to the seductive arguments of the travelling salesman. The manufacturer sees the opening of trade, the retail druggist tries to ignore it but it is useless. Doctors want compressed goods and if they cannot get them from the retail druggist, they will get them where they can – it is useless to say they are not used or they cannot be made by the retail druggist. They are used and the retail druggist can furnish them in better conditions than the manufacturer. It is urged by many druggists that they can buy tablets at a lower price than they can make them, but this is not so for goods of better quality.'

He continues:

> 'If you understand the principles of pharmacy, you can soon learn
> how to make compressed tablets and knowing how, you will become
> better druggists. A retail druggist can make his own tablets and
> furnish physicians who desire to think for themselves any tablet they
> wish to prescribe without buying 100 to dispense a prescription for
> ten.'

The address given by McFerran goes on to provide guidance on
manufacturing aspects, including setting up and maintaining the tablet
press, and gives hints on specific preparations. McFerran's article was
immediately followed by a scathing editorial in which strong views were
expressed on the provision of factory-made medicines.[39]

> 'McFerran regards the work of physicians in selecting remedies and
> that of the druggist preparing them as being equal professional
> duties involving personal responsibility. We do not suppose any
> are likely to disagree. But we live in progressive times. The use of
> factory-made medicines as a circumstance by the insidious influence
> of which physicians are too often led to forget the great purpose of
> their profession and druggists, eager for trade, are induced to lower
> themselves to the position of mere vendors of ready-made medicines.
> This cannot be conducive to the interests of the professions. When
> the physician prescribes factory-made medicines, he deprives his
> patients of the advantages they should derive from the pharmacist's
> skill in preparing them. If the pharmacist obtains these medicines
> as well as extracts, tinctures etc. from manufacturing firms, supplies
> them under his own name and still calls his place a pharmacy, he is
> neglecting his special duty, sacrificing his professional position, and
> damaging his individual interest.'

Clearly *The Pharmaceutical Journal* is of the opinion that the professional
status of the pharmacist would be compromised by the use of medicinal
preparations that the pharmacist did not personally make, a point of view
it was to hold throughout most of the 1890s.

A few weeks later, *The Pharmaceutical Journal* repeated its opinion in another editorial, prompted by a letter it had received from a Mr Ball. This gentleman had averred that the paper presented by McFerran was 'undoubtedly intended as a trade puff for tablet machines made in Philadelphia'. Though McFerran's presentation might not have been entirely a trade puff, Ball was quite correct in his statement that McFerran sold tablet machines, some of which were of his own design, but in the report of McFerran's paper, no mention is made of this. Yet McFerran must have been aware that one of the great advantages of the tablet was that of mass production, and so his suggestion quoted above of making a batch of only ten tablets is at best disingenuous.

Leaving aside contentious questions about 'quality', it was all very well to encourage pharmacists to make their own tablets, but where was the individual pharmacist to obtain the necessary knowledge and equipment? It is unlikely that the pharmacist's education would have included much about tablets, and he almost certainly would not be familiar with the practical aspects of tablet manufacture and the use of a tablet press. The first edition of Little and Mitchell's text book on tablet-making was not published until 1949, and pharmaceutics textbooks published as late as the 1950s provided little useful information on tablets and their preparation.

This dilemma is well illustrated by a letter in *The Pharmaceutical Journal* of 1895 from Mr W. A. Wall, writing from Rome.[40] He states that he wanted 'a machine that will enable me to dispense 2–3 dozen tablets as quickly as the same number of powders'.

He received a prompt reply in the same journal from Mr F. Foster.[41]

'There is not any machine that will do this. In all the automatic feeding or measuring machines, the powders must have certain preparation as they will not flow evenly and tablets will vary in weight. In all other machines in which the tablets are made from separately weighed powders (this was essentially Brockedon's process), the time required to compress the powders is much greater than is required to fold the powders in papers.'

In other words, Foster had grasped the point that tablet manufacture only makes sense with a relatively large batch size: that is by mass production.

In an anonymous article in *The Pharmaceutical Journal* in 1895 entitled *'Chapters in Practical Pharmacy: the Preparation of Compressed Tablets'*, the author states that the reason pharmacists are reluctant to make their own tablets 'is the difficulty of obtaining suitable apparatus at a moderate cost for making them on a small scale. These difficulties are now non-existent, and British pharmacists should consider it incumbent on them to be able to prepare compressed tablets as required.'

The production of relatively unsophisticated tablet presses was for pharmacists who wished to manufacture small quantities of tablets themselves rather than obtain them from elsewhere.

In an article in *The Pharmaceutical Journal* in 1897, Gibbs states that:

'the extemporaneous manufacture of perfectly compressed tablets is placed within the power of dispensers ... the more the modern pharmacist fits himself to meet all demands on his skill, without having to resort to manufacturers and wholesalers, the greater will be his reward and the higher the esteem in which he is held by the public.'[42]

A good example of a small tablet press suitable for a dispensing pharmacist is that made by J. W. Pindar & Co., a small engineering company in South East London, who specialised in making pharmaceutical equipment. This is in the reserve collection of the Science Museum in London. It was apparently purchased by a Mr J. Phillips for his pharmacy in Bournemouth, and was obtained by the Wellcome Collection when that business closed in 1970, after which it was acquired by the Science Museum. It consists of one die and one set of punches, the upper punch, lower punch and the feed shoe being interconnected to enable continuous production. It is hand-operated using a lever and its 'footprint' on the dispensing bench is about 25cm square. It is shown in Picture 11.

Pharmaceutical education and training

Despite the fulminations of the professional bodies against the tablet, and the urging by some correspondents that all pharmacists should be capable of preparing tablets, it must have been obvious by the early years of the twentieth century to most pharmacists that much of the medicine they dispensed had been prepared by the pharmaceutical industry. The trend would increase as advances in medicinal chemistry produced new active ingredients that had a preventative or curative effect on an ever-increasing range of diseases. The intellectual rights to these substances would reside with their inventors, who would either prepare dosage forms containing them, or permit their production by an industrial third party.

The preparation of medicines at individual pharmacies then became limited to liquid preparations or to solid medicines with an unusual combination of active ingredients or with unusual doses of active ingredient. Most exceptions like this would usually be packed into hard shell capsules. Traditional solid dosage forms whose production could not be easily mechanised, such as the pill, went into rapid decline. Thus, the 'ordinary' pharmacist was dispensing products about which he knew little, but his education included training in the preparation of products that were rapidly becoming obsolete.

It is surprising how long it took for pharmaceutical education to reflect what was actually happening in current pharmaceutical practice. Two examples illustrate this: pill preparation was last tested in the pharmaceutics practical examination of the University of London in 1954, and tuition in pill preparation continued at schools of pharmacy until about 1960.

A few major hospitals retained facilities to make their own tablets, but these became progressively fewer as the workers who had retained the necessary skills retired and were not replaced. An example of this is University College Hospital, London, which continued to produce tablets until 1976. The pharmacy at the University Hospital in The Hague, The Netherlands still produced a few tablets as late as 1979, but ceased soon afterwards.

Tablet preparation and formulation

The first tablets to appear in *The British Pharmacopoeia* in 1885 were those containing *glyceryl trinitrate*, but the monograph does not mention the word 'compression', and it is likely that these tablets were lozenges or moulded tablets. The lozenge was made by adding water to the solid ingredients, mixing to form a stiff mass, rolling this out into a sheet and cutting out the required shapes. The preparation was intended to dissolve in the mouth, releasing the active ingredient which was absorbed through the buccal membranes. The moulded tablet was also made into a stiff paste, which was then pressed into cavities in (usually) a rubber block. A tablet mould made by Whitall Tatum Company is shown in Picture 12.

As previously described, Brockedon marketed his 'compressed pills' on the basis of their purity to contrast them with the conventional pill, which usually contained several other ingredients that might interfere with the efficacy of the preparation.

To be made into satisfactory tablets, a substance must have three essential properties.

1. Particles must flow readily and reproducibly into the die of the press, otherwise a non-uniform tablet weight will be obtained with a consequent variation of the content of active ingredient.
2. Particles must form a coherent structure when subjected to a compressing force and retain that structure when the force is removed.
3. Once formed, the tablet must be capable of being removed from the press without particles sticking to the die and punches.

Very few substances possess all of these three qualities without some pre-treatment or the addition of other materials, and some possess none of them. This limitation became more apparent as more complex and faster tablet presses were introduced, and tablets were being made from an ever-widening range of active ingredients. The use of excipients in the tableting process, pioneered in the US, became universal.

As far as can be ascertained, Jacob Dunton was the first person to obtain a patent relating to the preparation and formulation of materials that are to be made into tablets (US Patent 168240, dated 28 September 1875). This patent, entitled 'Improvement in the manufacture of tablets', thus predates the patent for his simple press. He observed that if the materials to be compressed contained moisture e.g. from the atmosphere, then in some cases cohesion was impaired. He also noted that cohesive forces between particles were often exceeded by the adherence between particles and the die and punches of the press. In other words, particles stuck to the machine and reduced the quality of the tablets, and in extreme cases, the tablet could be ripped apart when the punches separated after compression.

His invention consisted firstly of drying the material to be compressed, and secondly lubricating the die or the material. To quote from the patent:

> 'In carrying out my invention, the powdered materials are first dried, preferably at a temperature of 90° Fahrenheit so as to deprive them of the natural moisture absorbed from the air, which would have a tendency to decompose them or interfere with the compression or stability of compression.
>
> The materials are now in proper condition for compression and the cohesion of particles. In order to compress, however, some substances which leave a portion of themselves adhering to the mold after compression, which adherence prevents the formation and withdrawal of a successive pill of the same material in a perfect or merchantable condition, it becomes necessary to get rid of the adherence, and also to prepare the mold before another pill can be made.
>
> [...] a small portion of a liquid may be added to the powder (1 per cent being in some cases sufficient), which under pressure will ooze out at the surface of the pill, and act as a lubricant, so as to allow the pill to be removed from the mold without leaving any particles adhering to the mold, and leaving the latter in fit condition for the next pill. In lubricating the mold a portion of paraffin, oil of cacao, butter of cocoa, or other equivalent material may be used.'

The continuing relevance of this invention to modern tablet-making is immense. In adding a lubricant to the material to be compressed, Dunton is going away from Brockedon's 'purity' selling point, but he is introducing the concept of excipients on which current tablet formulation depends. As Brockedon was principally concerned with tableting graphite for pencil production, he would not have needed to add another lubricant, as graphite itself has lubricant properties. But it is surprising that he could make a range of medicinal tablets without using some additional form of lubrication.

The oils used by Dunton are no longer employed in the production of medicinal tablets. By far the most commonly used lubricant is magnesium stearate, but the insoluble and indeed water-repellent nature of this can cause problems for the formulator, as will be discussed later.

With regard to flow properties, these did not cause difficulties to the earliest tablet-makers, as the dies in their presses were filled by hand. In a modern tablet press, each die must be reproducibly filled in a fraction of a second.

There are three techniques that can be used. The traditional one is called wet granulation, in which the active ingredient and any diluent are mixed together and formed into coarser aggregates by the addition of a solution or dispersion of an adhesive. This was often a starch paste in water, but now synthetic polymers such as povidone are preferred. The disadvantage of wet granulation is that water has been introduced into the formulation, and must now be removed by drying, with an expenditure of time and thermal energy. The second approach is to use an excipient known as a glidant, colloidal silica being the most common. Its function is to smooth out irregularities on the particle surfaces. The third approach is to use a diluent that has good flow and compressive properties. This acts as a carrier for the active ingredient. The process is known as direct compression and has obvious advantages. Its main limitation is that it can only be used with highly active ingredients where the diluent is then the major component in the formulation. If it were to be used with lower potency ingredients, the resultant tablet would be too large for it to be conveniently swallowed.

For tablets to be used medicinally, other factors must be considered beside those involved in compression. The tablet will contain an active substance, and its medicinal properties must not be compromised. Also, the physical properties of the tablet, such as its size and shape should not deter the user from taking it. Factors such as appearance, size, shape and taste must be taken into consideration at the outset.

The weight of a tablet is primarily governed by the dose of active ingredient contained within it. The tablet must not be so large that it presents difficulties in swallowing it; neither must it be so small that the user finds it difficult to handle or detect in the mouth prior to swallowing. Tablets rarely weigh less than about 50mg, and hence, if the dose of active ingredient is much less than this, the formulation must be bulked up with a diluent. This may thus be the major component by weight of the formulation, and it is the properties of the diluent rather than those of the active ingredient that will dominate the compression properties of the formulation.

The most common tablet diluent is α-lactose monohydrate. This is readily available, being a by-product of the cheese-making industry. It is much less hygroscopic than other possible carbohydrate diluents such as sucrose. If a diluent is to be present, it is mixed with the active ingredient prior to any pre-treatment such as granulation.

As regards the upper limit of tablet weight, there are few commercial tablets that are intended to be swallowed intact that weigh more than 700–800mg.

The majority of tablets are circular in cross-section, with a height-diameter ratio of about two to three, and have convex faces. This has been the case since the earliest tablets of Brockedon and Dunton. Non-circular tablets can also be produced using suitably shaped punches and dies, and tablets often bear identification marks or break lines engraved on their surfaces by means of embossed punches.

Tablets are frequently coated, this being an attempt to mask unpleasant flavours. The earliest method of tablet coating was sugar coating, a technique originally developed in the confectionery industry. The process took place in a revolving pan, usually made from copper, and the coating was built up gradually by adding small quantities of a sucrose syrup before removing the solvent by a stream of warm air. The process was laborious and highly skilled, and approximately doubled the weight of the tablet. Tablet disintegration was also impaired. Because of these problems, sugar coating was only used when necessary, and is rarely encountered today.

In the 1960s, the process of film coating was introduced. In this a polymeric solution or suspension is sprayed on to the tablets. The polymers are usually cellulose derivatives such as hypromellose, and the coating often contains titanium dioxide as an opacifier and perhaps an acceptable colouring agent such as iron oxide. The process is rapid, and the increase in tablet weight is minimal, as the thickness of the coating layer is only a few micrometres. Identification markings engraved on the tablet surface remain visible. Because of the ease of the process, most medicinal tablets are now film-coated.

The tablet represents a paradox. Compression results in aggregates of low porosity, yet most tablets are intended to be swallowed whole, then disintegrate rapidly so that the active ingredient can dissolve in the gastrointestinal fluids. The addition of another excipient, termed the disintegrant, is often added to bring this about. The need for disintegrants in some tablet formulations has been known for many years. This is shown by an article in *The Chemist and Druggist* of 4 October 1890, describing advances in tablet disintegration made by Messrs Burroughs Wellcome and Co in their 'Tabloids', and Messrs Allen and Hanbury in their 'Tabellae'.[43]

This article was followed by a series of letters from both companies extolling the superior disintegration properties of their products. It is likely that both companies used starch as their disintegration aid, though neither disclosed this. Until comparatively recently, various types of starch were almost invariably used, but synthetic materials known as 'super disintegrants' such as crospovidone and sodium starch glycolate are now more common.

All tablets are made by a compression process, but by the use of appropriate excipients, the tablet has been developed into a variety of different dosage forms. The tablet has a versatility that is not matched by other dosage forms. Of the total of 456 tablet monographs in the 2018 edition of *The British Pharmacopoeia*, no fewer than 109 (almost 24 per cent) are for some form of modified method of use by the patient or method of release of the active ingredient. Details are shown in Table 12.2.

The 'conventional' tablet is taken by mouth, swallowed and it disintegrates in the gastrointestinal tract. This releases the active ingredient which dissolves in the aqueous contents of the gut, is then absorbed into the circulatory system, and carried by the blood to its target. Rapid disintegration is usually aimed for, so that it does not become the rate-controlling step in the absorptive process.

The part of the gastrointestinal tract where tablet disintegration actually takes place is not usually important, so long as it is not delayed until the tablet reaches the large intestine, since after this point, absorption of substances other than water is significantly reduced. However, in some

Table 12.2: Tablet monographs of the 2018 *British Pharmacopoeia* involving modified method of use by the patient or method of release.

Description of tablet	*Definition*	*Number in* The British Pharmacopoeia, *2018*
Buccal	Tablets dissolve slowly in the mouth, often sticking to the gum	1
Chewable	Tablets chewed and the fragments swallowed	14
Dispersible	Tablets break up in cold water. Not all the ingredients dissolve	12
Effervescent	Tablets effervesce in water, giving a solution or dispersion	6
Gastro-resistant	Tablets have an acid-resistant coating. They pass unchanged through the stomach but disintegrate in the small intestine	15
Orodispersible	Tablets break up in the mouth, giving a dispersion	5
Oromucosal	Tablets which release the active ingredient when held in the buccal cavity	2
Prolonged-release	Tablets release the active ingredient slowly after they have been swallowed	38
Soluble	Tablets dissolve completely when added to cold water	9
Sublingual	Tablets dissolve when held under the tongue	4
Vaginal	Tablets administered via the vagina	3

circumstances, disintegration of the tablet in the stomach should be avoided, particularly with active ingredients which irritate the gastric mucosa. This is achieved by coating the tablet with polymers that are insoluble in the strongly acidic medium of the stomach, but soluble in the less acidic surroundings of the small intestine. An example is cellacefate (cellulose acetate phthalate). This process was formerly called enteric coating, but the currently used term is 'conferring gastric resistance'.

The gastro-resistant tablet is one which does not disintegrate in the stomach, but does so when it reaches the small intestine. A more common modification of the tablet is the prolonged-release tablet, when the active ingredient is gradually released along the length of the small intestine and perhaps the stomach. Formerly used terms for this behaviour were slow release and controlled release. Prolonged-release is usually achieved by coating, but an alternative method is to disperse the active ingredient in a non-dissolving matrix from which it is leached out by the gut fluids.

Other varieties of tablet are designed to dissolve or disperse before ingestion. A requirement of soluble tablets is that all ingredients must be completely and rapidly soluble in water, and this can be a challenge to the formulator. In particular the tablet lubricant can present difficulties. The most commonly used lubricant, and probably the most effective, is magnesium stearate, which is not only virtually insoluble in water, but is also water-repellent. Soluble lubricants sometimes used are sodium stearyl fumarate and high molecular weight macrogols. Difficulties in finding a satisfactory lubricant is probably why dispersible tablets are more common. These give a dispersion rather than a complete solution, but if rapid disintegration in cold water is required it is often achieved using an effervescent mixture as the dispersing agent. This usually consists of a bicarbonate or carbonate with a solid organic acid such as citric acid. When this mixture comes into water, carbon dioxide is generated, which disrupts the tablet structure. The oro-dispersible tablet is a variation of this type of formulation, when the tablet is ingested intact and dispersion takes place in the mouth.

Some tablets are designed to be taken intact, and either dissolve or disperse relatively slowly in the mouth. Such tablets are usually intended to deliver the active ingredient to the mucous membranes of the mouth. Since slow disintegration is required, they do not contain any disintegrating agent, since if the tablet broke up in the mouth, almost certainly fragments of the tablet would be swallowed, and hence the active ingredient would not be available at the intended site of action. Lozenges, sublingual tablets and buccal tablets come into this category.

Chewable tablets are taken intact, but are then broken up by chewing, after which the fragments are swallowed.

A wide variety of tablets are now available, brought about by careful selection of excipients. In contrast to the secrecy which prevailed in the pharmaceutical industry in its early days and for many years following, information on the composition of the tablet is now available to the consumer, usually by means of a leaflet contained in the pack. In the four tablet preparations used regularly by one of the authors of this chapter, the number of excipients is three, four, ten and fourteen. The modern tablet is therefore a multicomponent mixture, each component being present to carry out a specific function.

Capsules

The word 'capsule' is in common use in a variety of fields, ranging from anatomy (for example, the lens of the eye is enclosed in a capsule) to space flight. In the area of medicines, the *Oxford English Dictionary* defines 'capsule' as a 'small soluble case of gelatin enclosing a dose of medicine, and is swallowed whole'. The word is ultimately derived from the Latin 'capsula' meaning a small box or case. There are two types of capsule used in pharmaceuticals: soft shell capsules and hard shell capsules.

Soft shell capsules

The original patent for a pharmaceutical capsule was granted to two Frenchmen, I. G. A. Dublanc and F. A. B. Mothes (French patent 5648, granted on 25 March 1834). Therefore, the capsule predates the compressed pill or tablet. Mothes was the actual inventor, but as he was a student at the time, he had to be associated with a more senior figure. Therefore Dublanc, a qualified pharmacist, became co-grantee. The spur to the invention was an epidemic of venereal disease sweeping Europe as a result of the social upheavals caused by the Napoleonic wars. At that time, the oleoresin of copaiba was believed to be the most efficacious treatment available, but this substance had an extremely unpleasant taste that was difficult to mask.

The method as originally devised by Mothes was very slow and laborious. A mould was formed by tying a small piece of leather to the end of a slender metal funnel. Mercury was poured down the funnel into the leather to make it firm, and this was then dipped into a solution of gelatin. The mould was removed from the gelatin, dried, the mercury removed, and then the film of gelatin surrounding the mould was carefully detached from the leather, thus forming the capsule. This was then filled with the oleoresin and sealed with a drop of gelatin solution. Very soon, moulds made from mercury-filled leather pouches were replaced by moulds made from brass and later iron. The invention proved extremely popular as it appeared to meet an urgent social need, and Mothes prepared capsules filled with other oily liquids, as well as supplying fellow pharmacists with empty capsule shells.

Essentially, manufacture of capsules of this type continued to use variations of the original method, albeit mechanised to a certain extent. Other patents were granted describing improvements in Mothes' original method, indicative of the popularity of the dosage form. Extemporaneous production by individual pharmacists rapidly declined as industrial-scale manufacturers offered an ever-widening range of products and also contract manufacturing facilities to other pharmaceutical companies, a progression similar to that involving the tablet. A major development was the incorporation of glycerol into the shell in amounts ranging from 20 to 40 per cent. This acts as a plasticiser, and gave rise to the name 'soft gelatin capsule', later contracted into 'softgel' which is in use today.

An important step forward was taken in 1933, with the invention of the rotary die process by Robert Pauli Scherer, an American of German birth. This gave a product with a greater uniformity and accuracy of fill, and is now the usual method of production. Two continuous gelatin ribbons are brought together by a pair of revolving cylinders, into the surface of which are cut depressions which will form the capsule. A range of capsule shapes can be obtained. As the two ribbons converge, a precisely measured volume of liquid is injected between them. Sealing between the two ribbons now takes place, and the capsule is cut out from the gelatin ribbons by the slightly raised rims of the revolving dies.

The earliest soft capsules in *The British Pharmacopoeia* all contained oily fluids, such as oil-soluble vitamins and also organic fluids such as carbon tetrachloride which was used as an anthelmintic. Use of such materials fell into abeyance, but a new development saw the introduction of a non-oily or hydrophilic fill for the soft capsule. The basis of this is to use low molecular weight polyethylene glycols (PEGs). These are water miscible but do not react with the shell, especially if the fill also includes glycerol. As both shell and fill contain glycerol, no migration takes place between shell and fill, and so the plasticity of the shell remains constant.

PEG-based fills have considerably widened the usefulness of the soft capsule, since non-oily active ingredients can be dispersed in them.

Hard shell capsules

As the name implies, hard shell capsules do not contain a plasticiser and so have a more rigid structure. They were invented by a Parisian pharmacist, J. C. Lehuby, who was granted a patent on 20 October 1846 for '*mes enveloppes médicamenteuses*' (French Patent 4435). These capsules had two components, both cylindrical with slightly different diameters and hemispherical ends. The parts fitted tightly together, one inside the other. Unlike soft capsules, which immediately became popular, take-up of the hard shell capsule was slow to develop. There are two possible reasons for this. The first is that many medicinal substances were of vegetable origin and were frequently in liquid or semi-solid form. The second was that the two parts of the capsule had to fit tightly together so the contents did not leak. Moulds of high accuracy were needed.

The first successful manufacturer of hard shell capsules was a Detroit pharmacist, F. A. Hubel. He was able to produce relatively low-cost moulds by using iron wire or rod set in wooden blocks. In 1874, Hubel started manufacturing capsules using two sets of mould pins, one of slightly greater diameter than the other. The pins were dipped into a gelatin solution and were withdrawn covered with a gelatin film. The films were allowed to dry then removed from the pins. The capsule thereafter quickly achieved popularity when in 1875, the whole of Hubel's output was sold to Parke Davis and Company, also from Detroit, who employed aggressive sales methods. Hubel improved his manufacturing procedures, and when he retired in 1900, his firm was producing a million capsule shells per day.

Later Parke Davis, in conjunction with the Arthur Colton Company, introduced a new type of apparatus in which the two halves of the capsule were produced separately though on the same machine. The significance of this was that the body and the cap could be made in different colours, a major advance in product identification. The capsule manufacturing part of Parke Davies evolved into a company called Capsugel, now part of the Pfizer Corporation.

A second US company, Eli Lilly of Indianapolis became involved in hard shell capsule manufacture in 1895. A distinguishing feature of their product was that they were self-sealing which prevented the two halves separating after they had been filled. This was achieved by interlocking projections on the body and the cap.

Medicinal hard shell capsules are usually filled with a mixture of active ingredient plus diluent in powder form, though techniques for a liquid or semi-solid fill are available. This can be advantageous if a powder fill has poor flow properties, as it can be dispersed into a semi-solid and pumped accurately into the capsule shell. In contrast to soft shell capsules, when the capsule and fill are produced at the same time, empty hard shell capsules are often sold by one manufacturer for filling by another, so a range of standard-sized shells is needed. See Picture 13.

By the time capsules became popular, the individual pharmacist had become used to 'factory-made medicines'. Although empty shells could be purchased, few pharmacists were prepared to fill these to make a batch of product in their own dispensary. Therefore since there was no question of pharmacists producing their own capsule shells, capsule-filling machinery 'that could fit on a dispensary bench' was never invented. It meant there was not the controversy that arose with the introduction of tablets.

It is striking how the tablet, the soft shell capsule and the hard shell capsule were all European inventions, but their commercial development into useful medicines took place in the US.

Some active ingredients, such as paracetamol, are available as both tablets and hard shell capsules. It was thought that the active ingredient was released more quickly from capsules, since the disintegration time for these was governed by the time it took for the capsule shell to be disrupted –usually about five minutes. After this, the active ingredient is released as a disperse powder. Using modern disintegrating agents such as crospovidone, tablet disintegration can take place just as rapidly, even if the tablet is film-coated.

A further attraction of the hard shell capsule is its shape, which many people find easier to swallow than a round tablet. Tablets can be made in the same shape by use of appropriate dies and punches. Tablets of this shape are often called 'caplets'.

A comprehensive history of the development of both types of gelatin capsule has been given by Jones.[44]

Chapter 13

Products Given by Injection

Theories of the function of the heart and circulation of the blood

Blood-letting was widely practised from the time of Hippocrates through to the nineteenth century. In Hippocrates' treatise '*On the nature of man*', it states that living matter is composed of four components – blood, phlegm, yellow bile and black bile. Illness was regarded as an imbalance between these four humours, and one way in which this could be restored was purging and blood-letting.

But injections and transfusions had to wait until there was an understanding of the function of the heart and the circulation.[1] According to the views of Galen, which held sway for centuries after his time, blood simply ebbed and flowed through the veins with some blood passing through pores in the septum of the heart between the two chambers, the right and left ventricle. Galen held that there were several types of spirits (pneuma). Digested food was sent to the liver where it formed blood. The blood which reached the right ventricle was transported to the lungs where impurities were removed and the blood that reached the brain found animal spirit, which was then distributed in the body *via* nerves.

The Arab physician Ala' al-Din ibn al-Hazm, better known as Ibn al-Nafis (1210–1288) was born in a village near Damascus.[2] He studied medicine at the Great Nuri Hospital in Damascus. In 1236, he moved to Egypt and became chief of physicians and private physician to the ruler Sultan Al-Zahir Baybars al-Bunduqdari. He was a prolific writer on medical and theological topics. In one of his manuscripts, the *Sharh Tasrih al-Qanun*, he was the first to describe the circulation of blood through the lungs (pulmonary circulation). Ibn al-Nafis' works were translated into Latin in Venice by Andreas Alpago of Belluno, a physician working in Damascus in 1547.

Miguel Serveto, better known as Michael Servetus (1511–1533), was born in Aragon in Spain.[3] In 1526, he attended the University of Toulon where he studied law. He entered into the service of a Dominican friar, Juan de Quintana, who became the confessor to Charles V. Servetus travelled widely as part of the imperial court. He published his first book *On the Errors of the Trinity* in 1531 and in 1536, travelled to Paris to study medicine. However, after controversy about his views and a dispute with the Dean of Medicine, he left and completed his studies in Montpellier. He started to practise medicine in Vienne, as physician to the archbishop. Whilst there he published another religious text *Christianismi Restitutio* (the Restoration of Christianity). The text included an attack on the conventional views of the church on baptism and the Holy Trinity. He was convicted of heresy and sentenced to be burned with his books. He escaped to Geneva, but was recaptured, tried again, condemned to death and burnt alive. His theological book *Christianismi Restitutio* contained a description of the pulmonary circulation of blood, where he stated that blood mingled with air in the lungs and that the change in blood colour occurred in the lungs. Although most copies of the *Restitutio* were destroyed, some survived and it has been argued that Servetus' views on circulation influenced some of his contemporaries such as Juan Valverde de Amusco and Realdo Columbus, and became known through their works.

William Harvey (1578–1657) was born in Folkestone in Kent. His early education was at the King's School in Canterbury, then at Gonville and Caius College in Cambridge. He graduated with a BA in Arts at Caius in 1597. He travelled through France and Germany, then studied medicine at the University of Padua from 1599 to 1602. On his return to England he was awarded a Doctor of Medicine at Cambridge. He began practice in London from 1604 and worked at St Bartholomew's Hospital there for most of the rest of his life, being physician in charge from 1609. He had a lucrative private practice and was Physician Extraordinary to King James I, and from 1625 to King Charles I. From 1632 he was Physician in Ordinary to King Charles I, and accompanied him on his hunting expeditions. This gave Harvey access to deer carcases which he could dissect. In 1628, he published his book *Exercitatio de Motu Cordis et Sanguinis in Animalibus* (Anatomical

Account of the Motion of the Heart and Blood in Animals) in Frankfurt, which held an annual book fair. This revolutionary book, based on many experiments in animals and observation of dissections, was the first complete account of the action of the heart and the circulation of the blood.[4] Inevitably his theory was met with scepticism and took some years to become the established wisdom.

The first intravenous injections

Harvey's book stimulated research into injections and infusions. The first experiments into intravenous injection were reportedly carried out by a German huntsman Georg von Wahrendorff in 1642 who injected wine into his hunting dogs, through chicken bones.

Christopher Wren (1632–1723) was born in East-Knoyle in Wiltshire.[5] He was the only son of Dr Christopher Wren, the Dean of Windsor, who had been educated at Oxford University. In 1650, Wren obtained a BA degree at Wadham College, Oxford, then an MA in 1653. He was elected a Fellow of All Souls in the same year. In 1657, he was chosen as Professor of Astronomy at Gresham College in London, and in 1660 became Professor of Astronomy at Oxford, where he also obtained the degree of Doctor of Civil Law in 1661.

During his time in Oxford in the 1650s, Wren was part of a group of distinguished scientists who formed the Oxford Experimental Philosophy Club. The other group members included Robert Boyle, the iatrochemist physician Thomas Willis, and Robert Hooke. In 1656, Wren carried out experiments on intravenous injection. Wren wrote to Sir William Petty in Ireland with a brief account:

> 'The most considerable experiment I have made of late is this: I injected wine and ale into the mass of blood in a living dog, by a vein, in good quantities, till he became extremely drunk; but soon after voided it by urine. It will be too long to tell you the effects of opium, scammony and other things which I have tried in this way. I am in further pursuit of the experiment, which I take to be of great concernment, and what will give great light to the theory and practice of physic.'

Robert Boyle's account of the same experiments gives more detail, describing Wren opening a superficial vein in the dog's back leg and 'putting into them slender Syringes or Quills, fastened to Bladders (in the manner of Clyster Pipes) containing the Matter to be injected.' Wren continued with biological and other scientific research, and in 1680 was elected as president of the Royal Society. He is best known for his work as an architect for the Royal Hospital Chelsea, and for the rebuilding of fifty-two churches in the City of London after the Great Fire of London in 1666, including St Paul's Cathedral, on Ludgate Hill, completed in 1710.

Johann Daniel Major (1634–1693) studied philosophy at Wittenburg, then medicine at Leipzig, finally becoming a Doctor of Medicine in Padua in 1660. He became the professor of theoretical medicine, chemistry and botany at the Christian-Albrechts University in Kiel in 1665. In 1664, he published, in Leipzig, his book *Prodromus inventae a se chirugiae infusoriae,* in which he described the use of therapeutic injections.[6] Rather than the goose quills from feathers which had been used by Wren, Major used silver pipes for injection. He believed that illness could arise from corrupted blood and that it could be cured by injecting a healing medicament, or by making a blood transfusion from a healthy person into a sick person.

Johann Sigismund Elsholtz (1623–1688) was born in Frankfurt. Before travelling to Holland and France, he studied medicine in Wittenberg and Königsberg. He also practised medicine in Padua. When he returned to Germany he became the state physician in Berlin to Friedrich Wilhelm Hohenzollern, the Elector of Brandenburg and Duke of Prussia, otherwise known as the Great Elector. In his book, *Clysmatica Nova,* which was first published in 1665, he described his experiments on intravenous injections. A translation of the text into English by Ethel Gladstone of the University of California Library was published in 1933.[7,8] In 1661, he opened the artery on the arm of a drowned woman and was able to inject warm water into it using a syringe. In two later experiments on a dog, he first injected opium and then crocus metallorum (impure oxysulphide of antimony used as an emetic). The dog recovered from the dose of opium. After vomiting, the dog died the next day after the injection of the dose of crocus metallorum. Elsholtz was also able to carry out experiments on three soldiers from the Elector's bodyguard. Elsholtz also quotes from experiments on transfusion of blood carried out by Richard Lower in Oxford and by Junius in France. At the end of his book, Elsholtz exhorts physicians 'to become interested in the safe remedies which can be applied in this new way, to be eager to get profits of this discovery whenever the occasion presents itself.' Elsholtz was the first to use a syringe for intravenous injections.

Syringe Design

There are two components needed for injections: the syringe itself, and the needle. Early syringes had been used since the time of Hippocrates in the form of animal bladders attached to pipes or quills from feathers. They were used to irrigate wounds or to give clysters (enemas).

Hero of Alexandria, who is reported to have lived in the reign of Ptolemy VIII in about 100 BCE, is credited with the invention of the syringe, as a tube with a piston with an attached fine tube.[10] This could be used to draw off pus from a wound or to inject a liquid.

Abū al-Qāsim Khalaf ibn-'Abbās al-Zahrāwī al-Ansari (936–1013 CE), popularly known as Albucasis, was an Arab Muslim physician, surgeon and chemist who lived in Cordoba in Spain. He is considered as the greatest surgeon of the Middle Ages, and has been described as the father of surgery. Later copies of works by Albucasis show metal cannulas for extraction of worms from the ear. For irrigation of the bladder, he used a syringe with a plunger made from silver or ivory, combined with a pipe put into the urethra. In anatomy, the urethra is a tube that connects the urinary bladder to the apparatus for the removal of urine from the body – in males, this is the penis. In the seventeenth century bone and silver urethral syringes became popular.

Dominique Anel (1679–ca. 1730) was a French surgeon who invented a syringe for treating patients with infections and obstructions of the tear duct in the eye. He published his results in 1713.[10] His syringes were made of a silver alloy, with the barrels engraved and having three rings to allow an easier grip. The piston rods were made of solid metal with a round knob at one end and the plungers were made of waxed linen over a cylindrical frame. The cannula attachments were pipes which were screwed onto a mount at the bottom of the barrel. Anel syringes to a similar but more modern design continued to be available until the 1960s for use by ophthalmic surgeons. It is likely that the design of Anel's syringe influenced the development of the hypodermic syringe. An Anel syringe is shown in Picture 15.

In 1839, two American physicians, Isaac Taylor and James Washington used a method to inject morphine subcutaneously by making an incision in the skin with a lancet and inserting the nozzle of an Anel syringe and injecting the morphine solution. They did not claim their method as being original – they had obtained the idea from a French publication.

Francis Rynd (1801–1861) was a surgeon at the Meath Hospital in Dublin. In 1845, he described in an article in the *Dublin Medical Press* how he had treated a patient with acute facial pain due to neuralgia by injecting a solution of morphine acetate in creosote into the facial nerves using a special device. This was a trocar – a metal tube (cannula) into which was fitted a rod with a sharp tip. The trocar was made to spring back into the device and the solution was poured in and allowed to gravitate to the nerve tissue. Rynd reported on the success of his treatment: 'In the space of a minute all pain (except that caused by the operation, which was slight) had ceased, and she slept better that night than she had for months.' Rynd's hollow cannula could be thought of as the predecessor to the hollow needle used with a hypodermic syringe.

In 1853, Dr Charles-Gabriel Pravaz (1791–1853) from the Veterinary College in Lyon, France, described (just before he died) the use of a special syringe with a screw mechanism which allowed the dose to be standardised.[11]

An aneurysm is a weak spot on a blood vessel wall that causes an outward bulging, similar to a bubble or balloon. Pravaz used his syringe with a hollow needle to inject mercury perchloride into aneurysms in a sheep and two goats to treat them by blocking the blood vessel by coagulating the blood.

Alexander Wood (1817–1884) was a Scottish physician who, in 1855, used a syringe he obtained from a surgical instrument maker, Mr Ferguson of Giltspur Street, London.[12] This syringe was designed for injecting perchloride of iron (ferric chloride) solution into naevi (skin lesions such as moles, birthmarks, or beauty marks) to remove them.

It occurred to Wood that it could be used for treating neuralgia pain. He injected his patients at the site of their pain with Battley's Sedative Solution (an opium solution). This was found to be very effective as a painkiller and he published his findings in the *Edinburgh Medical and Surgical Quarterly Journal*. Wood continued to develop the syringe with the help of instrument makers, adding graduations to the glass barrel of the syringe. He described the hollow needle as 'having an aperture near the point like the sting of a wasp'. His syringes were advertised as 'Dr Alexander Wood's narcotic injection syringes' and were sold as narcotic injection syringes by Archibald Young, the Queen's Cutler in Edinburgh. Wood maintained that the injections only had a local effect, and that the drug was not available more generally in the body. This was even though he had observed a patient sleeping for twelve hours after an injection of the opium solution. Wood's syringe is shown in Picture 16.

Charles Hunter (1835–1878) was the house surgeon at St George's Hospital in London and also the surgeon to the Royal Pimlico Dispensary. In the 1860s, he improved Wood's syringe design by adding a locking mechanism, which prevented the needle becoming loose when the plunger was pushed, and by using a pointed needle with a lateral opening. In his first trials, he followed Wood by injecting opium into the area of the body where the pain was located. However, in one of his patients where this area had become infected, he injected elsewhere and realised that the drug was distributed and worked across the body. In 1865, he published a book with his findings on the injection of morphine, atropine and quinine in patients.[13] He coined the term 'hypodermic' to convey that the drug was being injected beneath the true skin or dermis. Wood challenged Hunter's idea that the injected drug could work across the body. In 1867, the Medical and Chirugical Society of London appointed a committee to consider the controversy and concluded that Hunter was correct.

In 1856, when in Edinburgh, Dr Fordyce Bake was presented with a syringe made by Ferguson, the London surgical instrument maker. He took it to the US where the US firm George Tiemann and Co in New York started manufacturing them.[14] A number of other US manufacturers followed suit, making syringes from a variety of materials – glass, silver, and celluloid. Celluloid was the first plastic, invented in about 1860 when it was made from nitrocellulose and camphor.

Karl Schneider, the instrument maker for H. Wulfing Luer of Paris invented an all-glass syringe in 1896. This was patented in the US and the rights sold to Becton Dickinson & Company in 1898. Luer syringes continued to be developed, with better and smoother grinding to give a longer lasting tight fit. In the 1920s, Luer syringes were produced with alkali-free glass, which had better resistance to medicaments and to sterilisation. One issue with the Luer all-glass syringe was the need to have an easy method to attach and remove the needle to the syringe. In about 1925, Colonel F.S. Dickinson of Becton Dickinson & Company designed the Luer-Lok syringe. This had an inside thread which engaged with the needle, so that the needle could be fixed with a half turn.

In 1906 the German company Dewitt and Herz of Berlin invented the Record syringe which had a metal plunger and a glass barrel ground to a good fit. Record syringes were very popular in Europe.

The Becton Dickinson insulin syringe which was introduced in 1924 is illustrated in Picture 17.

Needle design

Early syringe needles were made of carbon steel, but these had issues in that they rusted and could break. Harry Brearley (1871–1948), a metallurgist, was asked to lead a research project for two of the Sheffield steel manufacturers at Brown Firth Laboratories. He experimented by varying the levels of carbon and chromium. The new chromium steels were much more resistant to acid attack. In 1915, Brearley left Brown Firth, but his successor Dr W.H. Hatfield continued the work and in 1924 developed 18/8 stainless steel which included nickel as well as chromium. Needles were made from this new stainless steel from the 1920s. In the US, manufacturers used a stainless steel V2A made by the Krupp Works in Germany during and after the First World War. Different gauges and lengths of needle were used for different purposes. Needles could also be sharpened for re-use.

Injection solutions

In the 1879 book, *Manual of Hypodermic Medication*, Roberts Bartholomew gave details of how to prepare injections, by grinding the drug in a mortar, then adding the water, then passing through a filter paper in a funnel. The solution was then stored in stoppered glass vials. However, the medical profession complained that the solutions were often contaminated with fungal growth. In 1870, the *New York Medical Record* recommended boiling hypodermic solutions then storing them in stoppered bottles. Others investigated the use of preservatives such as phenol or chloroform water. Another solution to the issue of contamination was to package a powder which was then dissolved in water in the syringe. Another answer to the problem was devised by an American pharmacist L. Wolff who prepared hypodermic tablets made with a tablet press. The tablets contained the active ingredient and sodium chloride (salt) as the other main ingredient.

In 1883, an editorial in the *Philadelphia Medical Times* drew attention to the need for injections to be sterile. The article pointed out that:

'In view of the inoculation experiments of Koch, Pasteur and many others, it is evident that unless the little instrument is rendered aseptic before use, abscesses are likely to occur. It is believed that the solution administered is the most frequent cause of superficial abscesses. A microscopic examination of the solution will generally show the presence of microorganisms which are sufficient to explain the result.'

The editorial went on to describe one of the first sterilisation techniques: sterilising vials with boiling potassium permanganate solution, then rinsing them and filling with the medicament solution and bringing it to a high temperature, then corking them. In France in 1890, a report by Schilmmel-Busch documented numerous cases of infection due to non-sterile solutions and injections, and in 1893 in a treatise on surgery, he reported the development of microorganisms in distilled water and injection solutions. In 1895, the French *Codex Medicamentarius* published a method of sterilisation in a supplement to the *Codex*. The method used was to prepare the injections or infusions with boiled and filtered water and then to heat the injection for fifteen minutes at 100°C, before filling it into a stoppered vial. This method is not sufficient to destroy spores and it was superseded by the use of autoclaves.

Charles Chamberland (1851–1908) was the French microbiologist who worked with Pasteur and Roux; he helped develop the germ theory of disease. In 1884, he developed a bacterial filtering apparatus known as the Chamberland filter or the Chamberland-Pasteur filter. This was an unglazed porcelain filter candle, which had pores smaller than bacteria, so making it possible to remove them from the solution. Chamberland also led a research project that resulted in about 1880 in the invention of the autoclave for sterilising using pressurised steam.

The French pharmacist Stanislas Limousin (1831–1887) was a prolific inventor. We have encountered him earlier in Chapter 12 in relation to the development of cachets. In 1886, he invented the glass ampoule, which when sterilised at 200°C could then be filled with an injection solution.

Despite these advances, many official standards did not keep up with these developments. The 1914 *British Pharmacopoeia* did not have any requirements for sterilisation of any of the injections it included and it was not until its 1932 edition of the *British Pharmacopoeia* that the requirements were stated. In contrast, in 1916, the *United States Pharmacopeia* (USP) published its first chapter on sterilisation in USP Volume IX. Several methods were described: dry heat in an oven for containers, autoclaving for solutions, sterile filtering for solutions and a process called Tyndallisation. This last process is named after the scientist John Tyndall (1820–1893) and consisted of heating containers at 80°C for one hour for three successive days. Tyndallisation is now discredited as a process.

Disposable syringes

The Second World War created the need for packaging for injections which could be carried easily into battlefield areas and used quickly on the spot. Examples were the Syrette and the Ampin. The morphine Syrette consisted of a sealed, flexible metal tube with an attached needle containing 30mg morphine acetate in 1.5ml of solution. The needle punctured the skin and the metal tube was squeezed to inject the drug. The Ampin was a glass ampoule with an attached needle, where the solution was allowed to flow into the tissue without application of pressure.

Charles Rothauser (1914–1997) was the Australian inventor of the plastic disposable hypodermic syringe at his Adelaide factory. Penicillin was being used to treat infections, but it tended to block up glass syringes, so an alternative was needed. Rothauser first developed a polyethylene syringe in 1949, but it was difficult to sterilise because polyethylene melts when subjected to the required temperature for sterilisation. In 1951, he improved on this original design to produce injection-moulded syringes made of polypropylene which could be heat sterilised. Millions of syringes were made for the Australian and export markets.

The use of vials of an injection needs a separate syringe to be used. Prefilled syringes, although more expensive, have become popular and offer convenience to the healthcare staff and the patient.[15] Most biological medicines must be injected and many of them are provided in prefilled syringes. Syringes consist of the barrel, piston, plunger rod, needle, and tip cap/needle shield. These can be made of a variety of materials. Syringe barrels are made from glass or plastic of several types: cyclic olefin polymer, cyclic olefin copolymer, polypropylene and polycarbonate.

Some of the new injectable biological medicines can be used by the patient with auto-injection devices, and these are much more convenient than conventional syringes; patients prefer them for some chronic conditions like diabetes, migraine and multiple sclerosis. For other conditions such as rheumatoid arthritis, the patients are likely to have limited dexterity due to swelling of the hands, so would find use of a syringe difficult. An example of an auto-injection device is the Humira Pen developed by the US company AbbVie for use with its drug adalimumab for treatment of rheumatoid arthritis and Crohn's disease.[16] This has one-touch activation to give a subcutaneous injection. The needle is not seen during the injection.

One area in which auto-injectors are used is in the emergency management of anaphylactic reactions to food, such as nuts, particularly in children. Anaphylaxis is a serious allergic reaction that comes on quickly and may cause death. It typically causes one or more of the following symptoms: itchy rash, throat or tongue swelling, shortness of breath, vomiting, light-headedness, and low blood pressure. Patients need to carry an emergency epinephrine (adrenaline) auto-injector with them and be trained in its use. The first EpiPen manufactured by Mylan was approved in the US in 1987 and also marketed elsewhere. Other epinephrine auto-injectors are now available.

Intramuscular injections

An intramuscular injection is the injection of a drug substance directly into muscle. Muscles have larger and more blood vessels than subcutaneous tissue and injections usually have faster rates of absorption than subcutaneous injections. Injections are commonly given in the upper arm for small volumes or in the buttock for larger volumes. A large range of drugs are given by this route: antibiotics, steroids, antipsychotic and anti-schizophrenia drugs, vitamin B_{12}, painkillers, and interferon.

Infusion solutions

Cholera first appeared in Britain in 1831, when the disease spread across Europe, killing many thousands. We know now that the disease is caused by an infection in the small intestine from the bacterium *Vibrio cholerae*. The classic symptom is large amounts of watery diarrhoea lasting a few days. Diarrhoea can be so severe that it leads within hours to severe dehydration and electrolyte imbalance. In 1854, John Snow showed that cholera was transmitted by drinking water contaminated with sewage from patients who already had the disease. In 1831, doctors were invited to submit reports on possible treatments to the Central Board of Health in London.[17] One report was from a young general practitioner from Leith, near Edinburgh: Dr Thomas Aitchison Latta (*ca.* 1790–1833). That year, three reports had been submitted to the *Lancet* by Dr William O'Shaughnessy on the problem of what he called 'blue cholera'. He ascribed this to 'stagnation of the venous system and rapid cessation of arterialisation of the blood'. He had the idea of injecting into the veins, substances 'most capable of restoring it the arterial qualities'. In a further report, O'Shaughnessy found that the blood in cholera patients 'had lost a lot of its water and of its saline ingredients' and he now recommended introducing into a vein 'the normal salts of the blood'. Latta immediately took up O'Shaughnessy's suggestion and sent in a case report on his treatment of an elderly female patient to the Central Board of Health which was then printed in the *Lancet*.[18] He punctured a basilic vein (in the forearm) with a lancet then inserted a tube into it, injecting six pints of a solution of sodium chloride and sodium bicarbonate. The patient improved but died the next day. Latta reported on a number of his cases – both successes and failures.

Sydney Ringer (1835–1910) trained in medicine at University College Hospital, London and worked there all his professional life. As well as his clinical work in the hospital, he had a physiology laboratory. With the aid of a series of co-workers, between 1875 and 1895, Ringer published more than thirty papers devoted to the actions of inorganic salts on living tissues. He was trying to find a solution which would keep an animal heart beating outside the body. By accident his technician prepared one solution with London tap water rather than distilled water, and this enabled the heart to beat longer. When he replaced the tap water with distilled water, the heart became weaker and stopped. The fluid he devised containing calcium was called Ringer's Solution, and it became one of the solutions most commonly used to rehydrate patients and support the circulation.

In 1879, Kronecker and Sander in Germany carried out clinical studies and recommended the use of saline injections in cases of life-threatening haemorrhages. Schwarz confirmed this recommendation in a further study in 1881 and recommended a minimum volume of 500ml to be injected. In the same year, Bischoff in Basel used this solution in a case of haemorrhage in childbirth. In 1882, in England, Jennings used saline infusions in cases of serious haemorrhage in childbirth. In addition to this use in women in childbirth, infusion solutions were also used for other haemorrhages and bleeds, wounds, typhoid fever, and tuberculosis.

In the twentieth century, work was carried out to develop suitable containers for large volume infusions. Early glass bottles had problems because of the alkalinity of the glass. In 1931, Baxter Laboratories in the US produced the first glass bottle with a rubber stopper (the Vacoliter) which could be pierced with a needle to allow it to be used as a transfusion. The bottle was used with a rubber tube with two needles, one to pierce the stopper of the bottle, the other to insert in the vein of the patient – this is called the 'giving set'.

In 1971, Baxter Laboratories launched a PVC infusion bag instead of a bottle, and a PVC giving set to connect the bag to the vein of the patient.

This was transparent, light, and was impossible to contaminate with air. However, some problems remained, particularly those of the drug being adsorbed onto the surface of the plastic, altering the concentration of the drug being given to the patient. Other manufacturers followed, using other polymers for construction of the bags, such as ethylvinylacetate, and multi-layer ones made from polyethylene, polyamide and polypropylene.

Many drugs are added to infusion solutions for administration to patients. Examples are antibiotics and chemotherapy drugs for cancer patients. These have to be shown to be compatible with the other components of the liquid infusion.

Pumps and patch pumps

After the discovery of insulin by Banting and Best, the first injection into a patient was in January 1922 to 14-year-old Leonard Thompson at the Toronto General Hospital in Canada. The subcutaneous injection using a syringe became the main treatment for Type 1 diabetics. In 1964, the idea of continuous delivery of insulin emerged from the work of Arnold Kadish, a private physician working in Beverly Hills, California.[19,20] His device was a pump, together with equipment for sensing the blood glucose levels. It had an on-off switch that controlled the pump when the blood glucose level was outside the normal ranges. The size of Kadish's device was similar to a small microwave and the patient needed to have it strapped to his back, so it was impracticable. In 1974, Slama and colleagues in Paris tested an intravenous insulin pump, but this had disadvantages because of the risks of infection and blood clots. Professor John Pickup from King's College, London carried out pioneering work in the late 1970s as a research fellow at Guy's Hospital, London, where he developed a simple, portable pump for continuous subcutaneous insulin infusion.

Other groups were also working in this area. Dean Kamen in the US, who is also the inventor of the Segway (the two-wheeled, self-balancing personal transporter) and a peritoneal dialysis system, developed the AutoSyringe wearable drug infusion pump, which was initially used for chemotherapy and for treating newborn children, and was later adapted for insulin treatment. It was marketed in 1978 and was popularly known as 'The Big Blue Brick' because of the similarity of its size to a house-brick. Other insulin pumps were developed in the 1980s, such as the Nordisk Infuser developed by a team from the National Institute for Medical Research at Mill Hill and Guy's Hospital. These early devices had problems with reliability, with syringe and tubing blockages, and infections at the injection site. These issues caused clinical problems for the patients and their carers.

In the 1990s, design of insulin pumps improved, with longer-life batteries, additional safety measures, much smaller pumps and plastic catheter infusion sets which minimise infections. They can be programmed to deliver different insulin needs at different times of the day based on the carbohydrate intake of the patient. Until 2000, the main pump manufacturers were Medtronic Mini-Med, which dominated the US market, and Roche's Disetronic Medical Systems, which dominated the market outside the US. Animas, which is part of Johnson and Johnson, launched its first pump in 2001. Sooil and Nipro now manufacture pumps for Dana Diabecare and Amigo pumps respectively.

A newer type of pump is the patch pump – a very small pod which fixes to the skin which contains the pump and a reservoir for insulin. Patch pumps involve no tubing, readily adhere to the body, are small, lightweight, and completely or partially disposable, and are capable of being worn under clothing. The Omnipod sold by Insulet and shown in the illustration in Picture 18, consists of the pod which is controlled by a Personal Diabetes Manager, an electronic device which controls the pod wirelessly. The Omnipod is waterproof and can be worn in the shower and even when swimming. It is filled with insulin and will last for about three days. The patient takes a measurement of blood glucose using a glucose meter on a finger prick sample of blood and inputs this into the Personal Diabetes Manager. Together with information on the next meal, the Diabetes Manager calculates the required insulin dosage. The Diabetes Manager stores the data on insulin deliveries and blood glucose values.

Syringe drivers

Continuous subcutaneous infusion is widely used for palliative pain care of patients in hospitals and hospices, using a variety of painkiller medicines such as morphine, diamorphine (heroin), alfentanil, fentanyl, tramadol and dihydrocodeine. It is also used to control intractable nausea and vomiting with medicines such as cyclizine and metoclopramide, or for medicines used in psychiatry such as clonazepam and haloperidol.

Basil Martin Wright (1912–2001) was born in Dulwich.[21] He went to Winchester School, read Physiology at Trinity College Cambridge, then studied medicine at St Bartholomew's Hospital, qualifying in 1938. In 1942, he joined the Royal Army Medical Corps and initially worked as a pathologist, before setting up the laboratory service in Sierra Leone for British forces in North Africa. After the end of the Second World War, he was recruited by the Medical Research Council. Although he worked as a pathologist, he was an accomplished inventor, and in 1956 invented the Peak Flow Meter to measure lung function. In 1957 he moved to the National Institute for Medical Research to continue to work on medical instruments. Here he developed a device for measuring breath alcohol levels: the breathalyser used by UK police forces. In 1970, he moved to the Clinical Research Centre at Northwick Park Hospital. He was asked by a paediatrician, Bernadette Modell, to produce a device which could be used to treat thalassaemia. Thalassaemia is a group of inherited conditions that affects haemoglobin in the blood. People with the condition produce either too little or no haemoglobin (which is used by red blood cells to carry oxygen around the body). Infants with the disease often died within the first year of life due to anaemia. The treatment was blood transfusion, but this could result in iron building up in the body. A new medicinal drug treatment was being used, desferrioxamine, which prevented the build-up of iron by helping it to be excreted. Richard Propper at the Children's Medical Centre in Boston, Massachusetts had shown that a continuous subcutaneous infusion was the most practical way to administer the drug. Wright worked with Pye Dynamics to develop a syringe driver – a portable battery-operated device to deliver the drug by continuous subcutaneous infusion. The clinical trial of the new device in treating thalassaemic children was successful and Pye put it into production. After this initial success, Wright thought that the device might have a role in treating pain in terminal cancer patients, who could not take painkillers orally. In 1979, an article was published in the *British Medical Journal* on a trial of its use. The UK hospice movement enthusiastically took it up. Pye Dynamics became Graseby Medical, then Smith's Industries.

The current version of the Graseby 2000 syringe driver (which is shown in Picture 19), is one of the range which is sold by Smiths-Medical; it was developed in 2005 by the Chinese company Z D Medical which was acquired by Smiths-Medical in 2008. This can deliver medication as a continuous infusion at a rate between 0.1ml per hour and 1200ml per hour depending on the syringe size

Another syringe pump which is also illustrated in Picture 20 is the Becton Dickinson Alaris CC Plus intravenous pump which is programmable for up to 3,000 drug treatment protocols.

Needle-free injections[22]

Fears of hypodermic needles are very common in adults and even more so in children. This affects the uptake of immunization. In one Canadian study, two-thirds of children had needle fear. The use of needle-free injections can overcome these fears, and a number of different systems have been developed. They use a variety of forces such as shock waves or gas pressure to propel drugs through the skin, offering painless and highly efficient drug delivery.

One group of patients who benefit from the availability of needle-free injectors is the diabetics, since they have to self-administer multiple injections each day. A needle-free device to provide insulin injections to patients is available to NHS patients in the UK: the Insujet (European Pharma Group). This uses jet injection technology where the insulin is drawn into the nozzle, then a spring pressurises it through a small orifice and creates a high-speed insulin jet which penetrates the skin.

Some vaccinations have also been developed which can be delivered through needle-free devices.

Depot injections

Long-acting injections, sometimes known as depot injections, are meant to be injected intramuscularly and the effect will usually last for several weeks.

One of the earliest depot injections was Depo-Provera, a long-lasting injection of the steroid medroxyprogesterone acetate.[23] It was originally used for a variety of purposes including treatment of cancers of the uterus and kidney. In the early 1960s, it had been shown that it was an effective contraceptive and was used by thousands of women across the world. It is now given as a subcutaneous or deep intramuscular injection every twelve weeks for this purpose.

The first generation long-acting injectable medicines were developed in the 1960s to improve the long-term treatment of patients with schizophrenia. Reviews of how well schizophrenic patients take their oral tablets have shown that 40–60 per cent are either partially or completely non-adherent, and they will then be at risk of relapse and may need to be readmitted to hospital.[24] About 5–10 per cent of patients with schizophrenia think about suicide. The depot injections will last at least a week. The medicinal chemical compounds are esters formed from the alcohol group of the drug and a long-chain fatty acid. This ester is then dissolved in an oil. Some examples of the first generation long-acting injectable drugs are flupenthixol decanoate, fluphenazine decanoate, and haloperidol decanoate. The newer second generation long-acting injections date from about 2000 and include paliperidone palmitate, aripiprazole and olanzepine embonate.

Chapter 14

Products Delivered on or Through the Skin

As mentioned in Chapter 1, the first written records of the use of medicines are from ancient Mesopotamia from the surviving clay cuneiform tablets written in Sumerian, Akkadian, Hittite and other languages. The *materia medica* comprised of trees and plant materials, grains such as barley and flour, animal products and mineral materials. These were dissolved in a variety of liquids or mixed with animal products such as sheep fat and lard, which would now be called the 'vehicle' for the preparation. The medicinal preparations applied to the skin included salves to be rubbed on the body or applied on a bandage or poultice.

An example of a skin preparation is given by Geller in his translation of a medical tablet from Nippur, dating approximately from the eighteenth century BCE: 'If a man is covered in red spots, you blend malt-flour in pressed oil in equal measures, you apply and he will get better.'

Egyptian medicine

Egyptian medicine also used a variety of medicinal substances and dosage forms. The Ebers papyrus, the main source for our knowledge of ancient Egyptian medicine, dates to the reign of Amenophis in about 1536 BCE. Its text describes dermatitis, pustules, scurf, scabies, sores, ulcers, moles, tumours, bites and stings. Amongst the *materia medica* used were antimony, calamine, sulphur, red lead, balsam, onions, honey and sea salt. Ghalioungui's translation gives us some insight into the types of medicine used:[2]

Ebers 104: Ointment to cure skin disease – mix acacia leaves, resin, mineral, liquid of laundryman, red natron, honey, and oil/fat into a mass and apply.

Ebers 109: Another skin ointment – cook together roasted barley dough, roasted grass, roasted emmer seeds [ancient variety of wheat], mineral, milk from a woman who has given birth to a boy, fresh behen oil [behen is the description of various herbs and plants of the genera *Limonium, Centaurea, Silene*], and oil/fat, then apply to the skin for a week.

Ebers 113: A remedy to eliminate skin disease – mix ox bile, lower Egyptian salt, honey, and water into a mass and apply.

The preparations used in Egyptian medicine included creams composed of animal fat, oil and beeswax mixed with water or alcohol; liniments for application to unbroken skin, which could be bandaged in place; lotions consisting of wine with oil applied to the skin; ointments consisting of vegetable oils or animal fats with honey; pastes consisting of finely powdered ingredients mixed with honey, acacia or carob; poultices applied warm to the skin consisting of statue clay or similar material; and solutions of soluble ingredients. The Ebers papyrus mentions the use of a plaster for treating burns. One of the poultices containing thirty-five ingredients was used for treating weakness of the male member.

The most popular ingredient in all of the preparations was honey. A standard treatment for wounds is mentioned in the Edwin Smith papyrus, named after the dealer who bought it in 1862, and which is the oldest known surgical treatise on treatment of injuries. This treatise, dated about 1600 BCE, mentions a mixture of grease, honey, and lint/fibre.

The Egyptian physicians who used honey would have based their treatment on an empirical knowledge of its efficacy. It is now known that the therapeutic value of honey is related to its high sugar content, hydrogen peroxide, and its low pH. Honey also contains a range of antibacterial compounds derived from the various plants from which the bees have collected the pollen. Dr Jennifer Hawkins, in her PhD thesis at the School of Pharmacy and Pharmaceutical Sciences at Cardiff University, has shown that many commercial honey samples contain antibacterial compounds that have activity against methicillin-resistant *Staphylococcus aureus* (MRSA), *Escherichia coli* and *Pseudomonas aeruginosa.*[3] Other studies have shown that it is active against *Salmonella shigella*, and *Vibrio cholera*. When applied to a wound, honey absorbs water from surrounding swollen tissue, cleans the wound and protects it from further infection. There have been modern clinical studies showing that honey is an effective treatment for infected wounds, leg and foot ulcers, chilblains, cracked nipples, abscesses, and burns. Honey is effective in cleaning infections in wounds where other treatments, including antibiotics, have been unsuccessful.

The Hippocratic Corpus

This collection of medical texts attributed to Hippocrates, which were written in about 400 BCE and later, includes a catalogue of skin diseases. These diseases included dermatitis, weeping eczema, skin eruptions, purulent wounds, gangrene, burns, boils, buboes, leg inflammation, anthrax, warts, freckles, and urticaria. The remedies include a range of preparations containing vegetable and mineral drugs in oil, lard or tallow vehicles.

The preparations cited in the Hippocratic Corpus included ointments, poultices, medicated plasters, powders and sitz-baths. A sitz-bath or hip bath was one in which the patient sat in water or a solution of medicaments up to their hips. It was used to treat conditions in the lower part of the body, for example, due to haemorrhoids, anal fissures, or pain in the lower limbs.

One particular ingredient widely used by Hippocratic physicians was wine. The Hippocratic treatise *Use of Liquids* includes a chapter on the use of wine to treat wounds, since they claimed that it had a cooling or hard action on a wound. The author of the Hippocratic treatise *Fractures* states that bandages soaked in dark wine should be wrapped round an open fracture. Wine was also to be used after surgery, for example, after the removal of genital warts the wound was washed with wine in which some oak gall had been soaked. The alcohol in wine would have had some antiseptic properties although we have to wait until the fourteenth century for distillation to produce higher concentrations which were much more effective.

Menecrates

Menecrates was a Greek physician who practised during the reigns of the Roman emperors Tiberius and Claudius I and he dedicated to the latter a treatise on drugs. He is credited with the invention of the diachylon plaster made from oil, litharge (lead oxide) and plant juices, which was adopted by Galen. Lead plasters continued to be used until late Victorian times.

Dioscorides

The Greek physician Pedanius Dioscorides of Anazarbus wrote his monumental work *De Materia Medica* in the second half of the first century CE. It included a huge range of over 600 items comprising plants and plant products, animals and animal products, and minerals and inorganic products.[4] His work influenced his better-known successor Galen, and his book continued to be used throughout the Middle Ages. The remedies in his book included treatments for a long list of conditions – birthmarks, freckles, wrinkles, chilblains, wounds, ulcers, chaps and callous lumps, boils, scars, warts, pustules, shingles, snake and scorpion bites, scurf and dandruff. He also included external applications for conditions such as hip disease and leprosy. He recommended an ointment containing *Saussurea lappa*, (costus root) combined with oil to prevent the shivering associated with a fever, to prevent epilepsy, and to treat those who were paralysed. The same herb mixed with water or honey was used to remove freckles.

Within the book are about 2,000 recipes and formulas, including powders, poultices, plasters, caustic powders, decoctions, oils, ointments, cerates, lotions and sitz-baths. Some examples of treatments are (using the numbering system used in *De Materia Medica*):

I, 1. Iris, *Iris germanica*: A treatment for scrofulous swellings and lesions in the neck [now known to be mainly caused by the tuberculosis bacteria] with a plaster made from boiled Iris roots.

I, 15. Nepal cardamom, *Amomum subulatum*: Used combined with basil in a poultice to soften boils and help to treat scorpion bites.

I, 20. Camel's-thorn, *Alhagi maurorum*: Used in a wash to treat spreading ulcers.

I, 32. Castor oil: Used for mange [a skin condition caused by mites], boils, scurf and for unsightly scars.

Galen

Galen of Pergamum (129–216 CE) was a Greek physician living in the Roman Empire. He was a prodigious writer on a variety of subjects. In his book, *De Simplicium Medicamentorum* (On the Powers of Simple Drugs), Galen provided a catalogue of the medicinal materials he used: herbs and plants, earths, mineral substances, and animal products. He listed 440 different plants and 250 other substances and described the effect of these drugs in *De compositione Medicamentorum per locos* (On the Composition of Drugs by Part), providing a 'head to toe' list of recommended treatments.

In *De compositione medicamentorum per genera* (On the Composition of Drugs by Type), he discussed the method of administration of the drugs. There were four books on plasters, two books on multifunctional medicines and one book on emollients, laxatives and painkillers. One of Galen's compositions, his Cerate, is very similar to today's cold cream.

It is all too easy to dismiss, out of hand, many or indeed most of Galen's compositions as irrational and likely to lack efficacy compared to modern dermatological products. However, a recent study by Harrison and his colleagues from the University of Copenhagen indicates that we need to be cautious in making such a sweeping generalisation.[5] They studied the skin penetration of Galen's Olympic Victor's Dark Ointment. This was an opium-based ointment which was applied to the skin of athletes. This ointment comprised Cadmia (zinc carbonate), acacia gum, Stibii (antimony), Croci (saffron), myrrh, Mastic gum resin, Pomphylox (zinc oxide), frankincense, raw opium, aloe vera juice, and beaten egg. In the study, the ointment was applied as a layer to abdominal skin dissected from 8-week-old mice that had been killed for the experiment. The skin was mounted in a diffusion chamber to measure the delivery of morphine from the Olympic Ointment through the skin. The ointment had a thick consistency and formed an elastic layer, which adhered strongly to the skin and so was resistant to peeling. The rate of delivery of morphine through the skin was high and comparable to 25 per cent of the most efficient modern transdermal patches (see later in this chapter). The authors speculate that the saffron contains saponins (soap-like substances), which allowed the morphine to pass more easily through the skin. Galen described this ointment as 'useful for extreme pain, providing relief immediately'.

Picture 21 is of a Syrian ointment jar from 300–450 CE.

Arab physicians

The *Canon of Medicine* written by Avicenna (980–1037) was one of the most widely used books on medicine during the Middle Ages. It was in five parts. Part Two dealt with medicinal simples and mentioned 760 drugs, whilst Part Three was a head to toe review of the pathology of each organ or system. Part Four was a discussion of diseases not associated with any particular body part, and included treatment of wounds, bruises, pustules, and other skin conditions. Avicenna provided good descriptions of anthrax (now known to be an infection caused by *Bacillus anthracis* from contact with infected domestic or wild animals), boils and diseases of the scalp.

Anglo-Saxon medicine

We have already described, in Chapter 5, some of the medical texts which have come down to us from Anglo-Saxon times – the *Leechbook of Bald*, the *Lacnunga* and the *Herbarium of Pseudo-Apuleius*. A variety of medicinal products were used to treat skin conditions and wounds, mainly as ointments and plasters. Some of the remedies included a large magic component, and this may have contributed to their efficacy as a placebo effect, in the same way that a supportive healthcare professional can today. But other remedies can now be shown to have a rational basis.[6]

Plantain, *Plantago lanceolate,* was used in forty-eight remedies in the three books comprising Bald's *Leechbook*. One remedy containing plantain ground with vinegar was for sore feet or swelling from walking. A wound ointment was made with plantain, ground and mixed with old lard. The plants in the *Plantago* species have been found to contain a number of biologically active chemical compounds such as aucubin, catalpol and acteoside. These have emollient and antibacterial properties, so there is a rationale for the use of plantain in wound treatments.[7]

Another wound treatment from the *Leechbook* consisted of hazel lichen, and the lower part of holly rind and githrife (corn cockle) mixed with butter. Lichens are actually a combination of two organisms, a fungus and an alga or a cyanobacterium (a bacterium that is blue-green in colour and gets part of its energy from photosynthesis). One of the most common components in lichens is usnic acid which has been shown to have antimicrobial and anti-inflammatory properties. Other antioxidant and antimicrobially active compounds in some species of lichen include altranorin, lobaric acid, salazinic acid and physodic acid.[8]

A remedy for sunburn given in the *Leechbook* consisted of tender ivy twigs boiled in butter and smeared on the affected area. Ivy, *Hedera helix*, has been shown to have anti-inflammatory properties in a study in mice reported in 2013.[9]

Medieval formularies

One of the first formularies was the 1498 *Nuovo Receptario Composto Dal Famotissimo Chollegio Degli Eximii Doctori Della Arte et Medicina Della Inclita Cipta Di Firenze*. This included a variety of dermatological preparations – 25 plasters, 9 honey products, and 35 ointments. It also included many oils, some of which would have been applied to the skin.

Early pharmacopoeias

The first national pharmacopoeia was the March 1618 *Pharmacopeia Londinensis* (*London Pharmacopoeia*) produced in Latin by the College of Physicians in London. The revised second edition was issued in December 1618. This contained one wound potion, 38 simple oils, 20 compound oils, 54 ointments and 51 plasters and 3 ccrates. A plaster was made by melting the ingredients together, then spreading the preparation on cloth or leather and sticking it or binding it to the affected part. A cerate, which had a consistency intermediate between that of an ointment and a plaster, was a preparation for applying to the skin. It was spread upon cloth without the use of heat, but did not melt when applied to the skin.

The first (unauthorised) translation of this book was by Nicholas Culpeper in 1649 in his *A Physical Directory: A Translation of the London Dispensatory*.[10] The *London Pharmacopoeia* was intended for use by physicians and the apothecaries and did not include any information on the uses to which the various preparations should be put. Culpeper filled the gap with his own personal and often highly idiosyncratic commentary on the usefulness of the medicines included in the *London Pharmacopoeia*, and also those which the College of Physicians had omitted.

Culpeper's chapters in the section *'Of the Use of Oyls'* listed oils to be used as 'Anodines' to ease pain, such as linseed oil, oil of St John's Wort, hen's grease, duck's grease, and oils of camomile, fenugreek, dill, rosemary, earthworms, and turpentine. Culpeper says that these oils can be made into ointments by adding hog's grease, and into plasters by adding wax or rosin. Where there is inflammation as well as pain, Culpeper recommends oil of poppies, roses, violets, or fleawort (probably a plantain *Plantago psyllium* or *P. indica*, whose seeds resemble fleas).

The chapter *'Of Resolving Medicines'* listed preparations which open the pores to evacuate excessive humours by sweating. These included oils of rosemary, oregano, dill, anise, hyssop and turpentine. It also included Oyl of Euphorbium. It is now known that euphorbium contains a compound called resinifratoxin, which is a potent capsaicin. Capsaicins are the main component of hot chilli peppers, and when rubbed on the skin, euphorbium oil has irritant properties.

Culpeper's chapter *'Emollients'* listed preparations 'to soften hard swellings'. The simple emollients included gum ammoniacum, bdellium gum resin, turpentine, rosin, colophony, pitch and the emollient herbs. The oils, ointments and plasters could be made of oil of lilies, camomile, earthworms, or foxes. Culpeper also includes ointment of marshmallows.

Culpeper's chapter *'Of Clensing Medicines'* to draw out pus from wounds included oils and ointments of wormwood, agrimony, betony, myrrh, aloes, turpentine, briony, gentian, hellebore and birthwort (*Aristolochia clematis*).

The chapter *'Of Aglutinative Medicines'* to dry out the moist area in a wound, included mastic, frankincense, myrrh, colophony, Dragon's

Blood, Lemnian earth (gray to yellow or red clay obtained from the Greek island of Lemnos), St John's wort, rosemary flowers, comfrey, marjoram, tragacanth gum, ivy gum, red wine, vervain, yarrow, cobwebs, horsetail and cinquefoil.

The chapter *'Of Cathetericks, Septicks and Causticks'* included drugs and preparations to apply to ulcers to remove dead flesh. The drugs mentioned included verdigris (copper sulfate), copperas (ferrous sulfate), burnt salt, antimony, mercury sublimate (mercuric chloride), and euphorbium. Culpeper lists Unguentum Egypticum as a caustic; this contains verdigris, honey and vinegar.

In the time of Culpeper, all plasters were made by melting the ingredients together in a pottery dish then spreading the mixture on a cloth or on white leather. In the 1800s and early 1900s, plaster spreading irons were used and two are shown in Picture 22.

Later pharmacopoeias

We have described the history of the early pharmacopoeias in *The History of the British Pharmacopoeia: 1864 to 2014*.[11] By reviewing the development of the official UK formulary and quality standards for pharmaceutical products in the *British Pharmacopoeia* during the nineteenth and twentieth centuries, we can see the changes in the type of dermatological products in Table 14.1.

Oils included in the table will have been used both for application to the skin and as components of various products.

In the nineteenth century, the medicated plasters would have been produced by hand-spreading using a heated plaster iron (see illustration) to spread the plaster mass on to leather, linen or calico cut to the shape needed for the area on the body on which the plaster was to be placed.[12] The popular diachylon base made with lead oxide was a common base for plasters and was made by heating litharge (lead oxide) with olive oil to form the lead oleate adhesive. One of the most widely used plasters was belladonna plaster which was made from extract of *Atropa belladonna*, (deadly nightshade), and would have contained the alkaloids atropine and hyoscyamine. It was used to treat rheumatism and neuralgia.

Table 14.1: The changing pattern of use of official skin preparations in the *British Pharmacopoeia.*

Type of Preparation	Edition of the British Pharmacopeia				
	1864	*1885*	*1914*	*1932*	*1948*
Poultices	6	6	—	1	1
Plasters	12	15	9	4	—
Liniments	15	16	15	8	6
Collodions	1	2	2	1	1
Oils	28	35	41	37	36
Oleates		2	2	2	2
Ointments	29	44	54	21	30
Lotions	—	4	2	1	1
Creams	—	—	—	—	1

By the middle of the nineteenth century, commercial plasters were being prepared using a combination of India rubber (latex harvested from the rubber tree) and gums as the adhesive component.[13] But by the end of the century, commercial plasters were being manufactured by machine. The current non-medicated plasters for covering minor wounds use an acrylate adhesive.

The oleates (oleate of mercury and oleate of zinc) were made by reacting oleic acid with mercuric oxide or zinc oxide. They were liquid and could be painted on the affected part of the body. Less messy than a mercurial ointment, oleate of mercury was painted on tissue affected by syphilis, and used for treating ringworm.

The liniments listed in the *British Pharmacopoeia* would have been applied with friction. They included liniment of camphor and liniment of turpentine. Turpentine liniment was used to rub in to treat rheumatic pains and stiffness. It was a rubefacient: it caused redness of the skin by dilating the capillary blood vessels.

Kaolin poultice which contains 52.7 per cent kaolin and 4.5 per cent boric acid, with thymol, methyl salicylate, peppermint oil and glycerol, has been in continuous use from the early twentieth century. It is heated in boiling water and applied to the skin under a patch or dressing to relieve pain and irritation. Although no longer included in the current *British Pharmacopoeia* it is still commercially available.

Modern dermatological preparations

Modern skin preparations are more diverse than their historical ancestors. They include applications (viscous emulsions or solutions), creams (generally oil in water emulsions), gels, lotions, ointments, pastes and dusting powders. The type of preparation can alter the degree of hydration of the skin and also alter the penetration of the medicinal active drug into the skin.

These dermatological preparations are used for treatment of dry, scaly skin conditions, for skin infections, for inflammatory skin conditions such as psoriasis and eczema, for excessive perspiration (hyperhidrosis), pruritis (itching), for acne, for scalp conditions such as alopecia (baldness), as skin cleansers, for wounds and injuries, and for treatment of warts. Salicylic acid ointment, used for treating warts and first mentioned in the 1898 *British Pharmacopoeia*, is still used for the same purpose, and salicylic acid is also the active ingredient in corn plasters, where it works by attacking the horny cells of the corn.

Transdermal patches [14]

For over 100 years, scientists have been studying whether the skin is permeable to different substances.[15] Schwenkenbecker in 1904 suggested that the skin would be permeable to oil-soluble substances but not to water or inorganic materials. An example found in the early 1900s was nitroglycerin absorption through the skin of workers involved in explosive manufacture, which caused them to have a severe headache. In 1948, a nitroglycerin ointment was used to treat Raynaud's disease (reduced blood flow in the fingers and toes causing pain, particularly in cold conditions), and later to treat angina. In the same decade the skin absorption of the oestrogens (female hormones) was discovered when men working in the chemical manufacturing plants producing the hormone stilboestrol discovered that they had enlarged breasts. Dale Wurster and Sherman Kramer from the University of Wisconsin studied the skin absorption of various esters of salicylic acid in the 1960s to see which kinds of chemical compound were absorbed.

Alejandro Zaffaroni (1923–2014) was born in Uruguay and in 1945 moved to New York where he gained his PhD in biochemistry. He worked first at the US National Institute of Health and then at Syntex where he investigated steroid hormones to control skin complaints. He noted that the steroid hormones were penetrating the skin and into the blood circulation. In 1968, he founded the Alza Corporation, the first of a string of biotechnology companies and filed a patent for the use of a rate-controlling membrane to control the delivery of drugs through the skin into the circulation in 1971. In 2001 Johnson and Johnson bought Alza. Janssen-Cilag is a subsidiary of Johnson and Johnson.

Historically the Ebers papyrus in 1550 BCE had mentioned the use of *Hyoscyamus* (the plant which contains hyoscine) to be applied to the skin or taken by mouth for abdominal discomfort. In 1873, Paul Audouit had filed a US patent for a diachylon (lead) plaster containing Theriac Andromachi and extract of Belladonna which were to be applied to the pit of the stomach to prevent sea-sickness.[16]. Belladonna extract contains atropine, hyoscine and hyoscyamine alkaloids. Alza started development of a patch for transdermal delivery of hyoscine for the treatment of motion sickness. The patch had a drug reservoir and a microporous membrane to control the drug release into the skin and was worn behind the ear where the skin was found to be very permeable. The first test was on Alza employees sailing in a yacht in rough water near the Golden Gate Bridge in San Francisco. The employees wearing an inactive placebo patch were sick, the ones with the hyoscine patch were not. The patch was also tested as part of the US Spacelab missions, and in a number of clinical trials. The product was marketed in the US in 1979 as the Transderm Scop patch. A patch is marketed in the UK by Novartis as Scopoderm which releases 1 mg hyoscine over seventy-two hours.

In 1973, the Alza Corporation filed another patent, this time for a rate-controlling membrane adhesive bandage for drugs such as nitroglycerin (which is known as glyceryl trinitrate in the UK). It included the concept that a skin penetration-enhancing substance could be included in the drug reservoir. Several US companies marketed nitroglycerin patches in 1981. In the UK there are currently four commercial glyceryl trinitrate patches, marketed by UCB Pharma, Meda Pharmaceuticals, Merck Sharp and Dohme, and Novartis Pharmaceuticals. The Merck Sharp and Dohme patch, Nitro-Dur, contains the glyceryl trinitrate in the adhesive layer. These products are used to treat angina.

In the 1980s, a gel product containing estradiol was marketed as a female hormone replacement therapy for control of the symptoms of the menopause. Alza filed a patent for an estradiol bandage with a polymer membrane to be applied to the skin with ethanol (alcohol) as a penetration enhancer in 1983. After clinical studies in women showed that it was effective in preventing hot flushes, Alza marketed its patch and other manufacturers followed suit with varying designs. Six manufacturers market estradiol patches in the UK.

Fentanyl had been first synthesised in Belgium by Paul Janssen for his company Janssen Pharmaceutica in 1959. It was developed as a painkiller by screening chemicals similar to pethidine for opium-like activity. In the 1980s, Alza started development of a patch for the treatment of pain containing fentanyl, and filed a US patent in 1986, following which clinical trials started in the late 1980s. They marketed it as the Durogesic patch – now sold in the UK by Janssen-Cilag. There are now a large number of other manufacturers of fentanyl patches.

The average cigarette contains about 10mg nicotine, the addictive component in tobacco, but only about 1–2mg of nicotine is absorbed by inhaling tobacco smoke. However, tobacco smoke contains a very large variety of other substances, many of which cause cancer, such as acetaldehyde, benzene, hydrazine and polycyclic hydrocarbons. Nicotine products are used as a means of reducing smoking and helping to stop smoking.[17] Trials of nicotine patches in the 1980s showed that they reduced the craving for cigarettes in smokers and a number of patches were approved in the early 1990s. Smokers who smoke more than 10 cigarettes per day are given high strength patches for six to eight weeks, followed by a medium strength patch for two weeks and eventually the lowest strength patch for two weeks. Originally the sales of nicotine patches made them a blockbuster product, but sales are now slowing since many cigarette smokers are switching to electronic cigarettes instead.

A number of other patch products have now been marketed. Evra, a contraceptive patch containing ethinyloestradiol (an oestrogen) and norelegestrone (a progestogen) is marketed by Janssen-Cilag. A number of different manufacturers market patches containing rivastigmine for treatment of mild to moderate dementia in Alzheimer's disease and Parkinson's disease. There is an over-the-counter patch containing

5-hydroxytryptophan for boosting brain serotonin levels which claims to be an anti-depressant (serotonin is a brain neurotransmitter).

Microneedles

The outer layer of the epidermis in the skin is the *stratum corneum*, which consists of dead cells. This is the main barrier to absorption of chemicals, so is an important protection for workers exposed to them as part of their work, such as agricultural workers. As we have seen, some drugs have the correct physico-chemical properties that enable them to be absorbed, and so are used in transdermal patch products but the range of them is fairly small. One answer to this issue, which is being developed, is a system that punctures the outer stratum corneum layer and delivers the drug to the epidermis, the 150–200μm thick layer of skin under the *stratum corneum*.[18] Microneedles, which are degradable/dissolvable, can be solid or hollow and can penetrate the epidermis to the depth of 70–200μm. The layer of skin below the epidermis is the dermis and this is the layer with the nerves. So, a microneedle injection is painless. A range of medicines has been investigated using microneedles: vaccines, biopharmaceutical products such as growth hormone and insulin.

Chapter 15

Products Delivered to the Lungs

T he recorded history of inhalation products dates back to their use by the Chinese; some writers have claimed that the oldest accounts of the treatment of asthma date back to the mythical Yellow Emperor of China over 4,000 years ago. The treatment was with inhalation of Ma Huang herb, which is from the *Ephedra* species.

Early history of inhaled medicines

The early Egyptian Ebers papyrus (dated to 1550 BCE) includes a reference to the use of black henbane, *Hyoscyamus niger*, used to treat patients who were struggling to breathe.[1] The plant contains hyoscyamine, hyoscine and atropine alkaloids and it was placed on heated stones and a jar with a hole placed over it; the patient then inhaled the vapour through the mouth using a reed stalk placed into the hole. In the nineteenth century, herbal cigarettes containing *Datura stramonium* for asthma were widely used; they would have contained the same alkaloids. Known as anticholinergic drugs, more modern drugs with the same properties are still used to treat asthma.

Herodotus (484–425 BCE), wrote the first history book; it recorded the clash between the Greek city states and the army of the Persian Empire during the period 550–480 BCE.[2] He also included information on the cultures of the various peoples he describes. One group were the Scythians, an ancient tribe of nomadic Eurasian warriors. Herodotus describes their use of vapour-baths as part of funeral rites:

'[….] they make a booth by fixing in the ground three sticks inclined towards one another, and stretching around them woollen felts, which they arrange as tightly as possible, inside the booth is placed upon the ground into which they put a number of red-hot stones, and then add some hemp-seed. The Scythians, as I said, take some of this hemp-seed and, creeping under the felt coverings, throw it upon the red-hot stones; immediately it smokes, and gives out such a vapour as not Grecian vapour-bath can exceed; the Scythians, delighted, shout for joy, and this vapour serves them instead of a water bath, for they never by any chance wash their bodies with water.'

The Scythians were inhaling tetrahydrocannabinol, the hallucinogenic compound from *Cannabis* (marijuana) plants which was making them 'high' or 'stoned'.

Later, the *Hippocratic Corpus*, the body of works from 450–340 BCE attributed to the physician Hippocrates, included a treatment which consisted of vapours of resins and herbs boiled with vinegar and oil and drawn into the lungs *via* a tube.

Dioscorides (40–90 CE) in Book III of his *De Materia Medica* described the properties of anise stating that when burnt below the nostrils to produce a thick smoke, it stops headaches.[3] Later in Book III he described the properties of galbanum (juice of the giant fennel), which if smelled could revive epileptics and those suffering from dizziness. In Book V he discussed sulphur stating that it is good for asthma (and also treated people affected by lethargic fever) when burned so as to produce smoke.

In the second century CE, Galen described the inhalation of powdered medicinal substances such as myrrh and nutgall (a nut-shaped gall on oak trees) powders. These were inhaled through a bent reed to treat angina.

The Persian physician Rhazes (850–923 CE) advocated the inhalation of arsenic and in his encyclopaedia of medicine, *The Canon of Medicine*, Avicenna (980–1037 CE) recommended inhaling the fumes from arsenic and sulphur.

The Spanish-born Sephardic Jewish physician Moses ben Maimon, otherwise known as Maimonides (1135–1204 CE), was the court physician to the Egyptian Grand Vizier Al Qadi al Fadil, then to Sultan Saladin, after whose death he remained a physician to the royal family. He wrote the first book on asthma entitled *A Treatise on Asthma* in 1190. His recommended treatments included chicken soup, sexual abstention and inhalation of herbs such as *Aloe vera* thrown onto a fire.

A number of physicians investigated possible treatments for consumption (tuberculosis). In 1767, Philip Stern published a booklet in which he recommended using his own proprietary product Dr Stern's Balsamic Ether, which was used by adding twenty drops to half a pint (284ml) of boiling water and asking the patient to hold his mouth over the vessel so as to draw in the vapour.[4] Stern claimed that the antiseptic power of the product would 'preserve the sound part of the lungs, and give an opportunity to nature to regenerate the parts that were already destroyed.' Sir Alexander Crichton published a pamphlet in 1817 entitled *An Account of Some Experiments made with the Vapour of Boiling Tar in the Cure of Pulmonary Consumption*. In 1834 Sir Charles Scudamore, a Scottish physician to the Imperial Russian Court, recommended inhaling the vapour of hot water medicated with iodine and conium (*Conium maculatum* or hemlock).

Asthma Cigarettes[5]

In the eighteenth century, Indian physicians recommended their patients to smoke parts of the *Datura* plant to relieve their asthma. Early in the nineteenth century, in 1802, Dr James Anderson, the Physician General to the East India Company, mentioned this herb to General William Gent of the Madras Army and recommended it from his own personal experience. Gent wrote to an English physician, Dr Sims, stating that there was 'a specific for relieving the paroxysm of asthma and that it was prepared from the roots of the wild purple-flower thorn apple (*Datura ferox*).' Sims enthusiastically took up the use of the herb and recommended it to colleagues and patients. A Hackney surgeon who had run out of supply of *Datura ferox*, substituted *Datura stramonium* (the common thorn apple), which then started to be used by asthma patients.

By the end of the nineteenth century, a number of inhaled remedies were being marketed, designed either to be used in a pipe and inhaled or in the form of cigarettes. The products included Potter's Asthma Cure, Asthmador Cigarettes and Kellogg's Asthma Remedy and all contained stramonium – a source of atropine, hyoscyamine, and scopolamine alkaloids. The celebrated French writer Marcel Proust (1871–1922), author of *In Search of Lost Time*, used asthma cigarettes to relieve his asthma and hay fever. However, there were cases of poisoning following the use of Potter's asthma cigarettes.

Smoking stramonium-containing cigarettes was a recommended treatment for asthma patients until the middle of the twentieth century, with surveys and clinical studies recommending their use.[6] However, by the 1930s, other treatments were available such as adrenaline, theophylline and aminophylline. The sales of these preparations continued until at least the 1980s, but they had declined rapidly as asthmatics were prescribed more effective metered dose aerosols.

The development of inhaler devices[7]

The first description of an inhaler machine was in the 1654 book *Theatri Tabidorum vestibulum seu Exercitationes Dianoeticæ cum Historiis et Experimentis demonstrativis* by the physician Christopher Bennet (1617–1655). The book is about the treatment of consumption (tuberculosis). One of the first popular inhaler machines was devised by John Mudge (1721–1793), a Devon physician who lived in Plymouth. In 1778, he published a book *A Radical and Expeditious Cure for a Recent Catarrhal Cough*, which described his invention. This consisted of a pewter pot which was three-quarter filled with hot water. Air was drawn through the hot water for twenty minutes by the patient breathing in and out of a hollow tube connected to the lid. The air came in *via* the hollow handle and bubbled through the water.

The first pressurised inhaler was invented in France by Jean Salès-Girons (1808–1879). This was presented to the Academy of Science in Paris in 1858 where it won a silver medal. It consisted of a glass reservoir linked to a pump device which forced liquid through a nozzle to atomise it. This is shown in Picture 25.

In 1861, Dr Nelson exhibited a ceramic inhaler to the Royal Medical and Chirurgical Society in London and it was marketed by London pharmacy supplier S. Maw and Sons as the Nelson Inhaler in 1865. It was advertised widely in medical journals such as the *Lancet* and *British Medical Journal*, but also mentioned in domestic handbooks intended for use by the general public; it consisted of a ceramic pot with a mouthpiece tube at the top for inhaling using the mouth and a spout at the side for exhaled breath. The pot was not more than half-filled with nearly boiling water and the steamy vapour could be inhaled. Herbal and other ingredients were placed in the pot and boiling water poured onto them. Nelson inhalers can still be purchased today and are mainly used by singers and performers. An example is shown in Picture 23.

A number of official inhalation solutions were introduced into the 1867 *British Pharmacopoeia* to be used with this type of inhaler. These were hydrocyanic acid, chlorine, coniine (from juice of hemlock), creosote, iodine and fir-wood oil. Most of these now appear quite irrational – for example, hydrocyanic acid (prussic acid) was used for treatment of coughs but is lethal at concentrations above 2,000 parts per million (hydrocyanic acid was used for executions in the gas chambers in a number of US states). Creosote would have contained a mixture of various phenols and cresols which would have been antiseptic, and creosote inhalation was a treatment for phthisis (another name for tuberculosis).

In 1864, Alfred Newton applied for a patent in London for a dry powder inhalation device. This consisted of a large wooden box with an orifice on one side. Inside the box was a mesh and a shaft fitted with feather beaters. A handle was turned to make the feathers beat the powder within the box to create a fine dust, and the patient inhaled the dust through the mesh using the orifice. Newton used potassium chlorate as the active ingredient in his device. A drawing of the Newton inhaler is shown in Picture 26.

The first nebuliser devices were introduced in the 1860s. These produced a fine spray of solution which could be inhaled. One device was patented by Dr Siegle of Stuttgart in 1863, using aspects of earlier designs by Bergson and Reichenheim. This device utilised the principle of a glass steam boiler to produce steam for a jet atomiser where suction was applied to a tube of liquid when a high velocity fluid was passed over it, then forcing the liquid through a nozzle to nebulise it. In 1868, Dr James Adams from Glasgow exhibited a much-improved version with a tubular metal boiler to produce a high-pressure jet of steam. Adams wrote that the design of his improved device had been pirated by Sicgle, who then added insult to injury by selling the device at an inflated price all stamped 'Siegle's Patent' in what Adams described as 'an act of shameless plagiarism and spoliation'.[8] The device is shown in Picture 27.

Another interesting device was the Carbolic Smoke Ball invented by Frederick Roe in 1889. It was an early dry powder inhaler, consisting of a rubber ball fitted with a vulcanite nozzle with a gauze sieve near the end of the nozzle. The ball was filled with a mixture of glycyrrhiza (liquorice), hellebore and carbolic acid (phenol). The patient squeezed the rubber ball, which caused a fine powder to be produced as it passed through the gauze sieve, then inhaled the powder. The company made a number of grandiose claims for their product in newspaper advertising, stating that it cured coughs, cold on the chest, catarrh, bronchitis, loss of voice, sore throat, influenza, hay fever, headache, croup (an infection of the voice box and windpipe), and whooping cough (pertussis). The advertisements offered a £100 reward for anyone who contracted influenza when using the Smoke Ball (an amount which would be equivalent to about £12,600 in 2019). They also claimed that during the last epidemic of influenza, many thousands of carbolic smoke balls were sold as preventives against this disease, and in no ascertained case was the disease contracted by those using the carbolic smoke ball. During the 1889–90 influenza pandemic, over a million people were estimated to have been killed worldwide. The company was sued by Mrs Louisa Elizabeth Carlill who had seen the rather reckless advertisement, bought one of the balls and used it three times daily for nearly two months until she contracted influenza on 17 January 1892. The company lost its case both at the Queen's Bench Division of the High Court and subsequently in the Court of Appeal, in what became a landmark legal judgement, where the judges held that offers made in advertising constituted a binding contract. Ironically Mrs Carlill died in 1942 at the age of 92 – of influenza.

Advances in therapy

At the end of the nineteenth century, extract from the adrenal gland was identified as containing a substance which dilated the bronchi and bronchioles, increasing airflow to the lungs. In 1897, the active substance in the extract was identified as adrenaline (epinephrine). In 1900 Jokichi Takamine working in John Hopkins University in Baltimore improved the procedure for manufacture of adrenaline, patented it and sold the rights to the Parke-Davis Company in Detroit, Michigan. In the same year Solomon Solis-Cohen showed that tablets containing an extract of the adrenal gland would increase the airflow to the lungs. Bullowe and Kaplan from New York reported in 1904 on five cases where they had injected adrenaline to treat asthma.[9] Three years later Parke-Davis Company marketed their Glaseptic Nebulizer. This consisted of one piece of glass with a rubber bulb and tube and glass throat-piece. By pressing on the rubber bulb, liquid was drawn to the top of the inner tube and expelled as a fine spray. They also supplied solutions of adrenaline chloride in ampoules which were snapped open to be used with this nebuliser (see the illustration in Picture 28). The device was portable and could be carried in the pocket or handbag. In 1929, Percy Camps, a GP from Teddington, described treatment of asthma by inhalations of oxygen with adrenaline for every type of patient, which he said stopped attacks. Adrenaline chloride solution became widely available in the 1930s.

In the 1940s, Professor Konzett at the University of Vienna studied some chemicals related to adrenaline. The most promising compound was isoprenaline. It had fewer side effects on the heart and it was marketed in the UK in the 1950s; it became the most widely used inhaled treatment for asthma for about the next twenty years. However, it also stimulated the heart and this led researchers to try to find a drug with a more selective action. In 1968, researchers at Allen and Hanburys (now part of GlaxoSmithKline PLC) developed salbutamol, which was marketed as Ventolin.

The next step by the researchers at Glaxo was to make a derivative of salbutamol which had a longer-lasting action. They produced salmeterol which dilated the bronchioles for over twelve hours. This product was introduced in 1990. Another long-acting drug used in inhalers is formoterol.

In 1950, a study by Reeder and Mackay showed that cortisone solution given by inhalation treated the symptoms of bacterial pneumonia and in 1951, Gelfand showed that inhaled cortisone was effective in treating asthma. Steroid tablets were increasingly given to patients with severe asthma, but the side effects were a problem, for example, causing stunting of growth in children. Other steroids were investigated and in the early 1970s, beclomethasone dipropionate was marketed. Combination inhalers containing a long-acting bronchial dilating drug with a steroid are now a very effective treatment for asthma.

Khellin is the active drug found in the fruits and seeds of the Egyptian plant El khella. The herb khella was used by the local people as a diuretic and antispasmodic drug. In 1938, investigators at the University of Vienna analysed the structure of khellin, and Professor Samaan of the University of Cairo found it was a smooth muscle relaxant. This led to the investigation of chemical derivatives of khellin. Fisons in the UK developed sodium cromoglycate. This was not a bronchodilator; it was used to prevent attacks of asthma. Fisons had to develop a new dry powder inhaler system to deliver the product to the lungs.

Nebulizers[10]

The Sales-Giron, Siegle and Adams nebulizers marketed in the nineteenth century have already been mentioned. In the early twentieth century, hand-held nebulizers came into common use, usually powered by a rubber squeeze bulb to create pressure. In 1930, the Pneumostat, the first electric nebulizer, was made in Germany and marketed by Francis Riddell Ltd in London. This produced a fine mist of solution which was inhaled by the patient using a face mask. It was used with a product called Bronchovydrin, produced by Pharmaca Dr Weil, and subsequently made in the UK in the 1950s by William Martindale Ltd. It contained a mixture of papaverine hydrochloride, methyl atropine nitrate, amethocaine hydrochloride, pituitary lobe extract and adrenaline.

By the late 1940s, a large number of commercial nebulizers were available, and many of these continue to be used. They include small portable jet nebulizers and ultrasonic nebulizers. Manufacturers include Pari, Omron and Beurer. The Phillips Respironics Innospire system is a small portable device that includes a valve which opens when the patient breathes in to allow the medication to be delivered and closes when the patient breathes out. The Phillips I-neb AAD battery powered portable system produces an aerosol by forcing the medication liquid through a fine mesh when the patient breathes in. Nebulizers are used for treatment of patients with asthma, chronic obstructive pulmonary disease (COPD) and cystic fibrosis.

Metered Dose Inhalers[11, 12]

The first metered dose aerosol was developed by Riker Laboratories (now 3M Pharmaceuticals). In spring 1955, 13-year-old Susie Maison was struggling with the glass nebulizer with a rubber squeeze bulb which she used to control her asthma. The glass containers were fragile, often broke and were inconvenient. She asked her father, 'Why can't they put my asthma medicine in a spray-can like they do hairspray?' Her father was Dr George Maison, the president of Riker Laboratories (then part of the Rexall Drug Company). He asked Irvine Porush, head of Riker's pharmaceutical development team, to see if this would be possible. Porush went down the hall to the Rexall laboratories for help from the cosmetic chemists who formulated hairsprays. Equipped with some basic knowledge he ordered aerosol equipment, propellants and other supplies. His first experiments used Coca-Cola bottles, which he knew would withstand a pressure of about 1,300lbs per square inch. At about this time, Emson Research had patented a design for a metering valve, and Dr Maison was able to negotiate a two-year exclusive licence for their use for medicinal aerosols. The Wheaton glass company made multi-dose injection vials, and Riker decided that if these were coated with vinyl plastic, they would be protected against being dropped. Porush was able to use the 10ml Wheaton vial with the Emson metered valve, a plastic mouthpiece to go into the patient's mouth, together with propellants from Du Pont to formulate the new metered dose aerosol. He used two drugs for his trials – isoprenaline and adrenaline. Some animal studies were carried out as part of a check on safety of the isoprenaline and adrenaline aerosols. A clinical trial on the two products was carried out by Dr Karr at the Veterans Administration Hospital at Long Beach, California in June 1955. These trials showed that the products worked in patients. Riker set up a manufacturing facility and filed New Drug applications with the US Food and Drug Administration in January 1956. The two products Medihaler-Iso containing isoprenaline and Medihaler-Epi containing adrenaline were approved in March 1956.[13] These products were also marketed in Europe.

One of the issues found with the early metered dose inhalers was that the patient needed to breathe in at the same time as actuating the inhaler.

Patients needed to be trained to do this, otherwise the product would not work properly. In 1970, Riker produced an aerosol that was actuated when the patient breathed in – this was the Autohaler.

The first beclomethasone dipropionate aerosol, used to prevent asthma attacks, was marketed as Becotide by Allen and Hanbury's (now part of GlaxoSmithKline) in 1972. In 2004, Glaxo marketed the Seretide Evohaler, a combination of the long-acting bronchial dilating medicine salmeterol with the steroid fluticasone propionate. This was the first product with a dose counter to help patients know when their inhaler is near the last dose.

By the 1980s, metered dose inhalation aerosols had become the method of choice for many patients to control their asthma. They were powered by chlorofluorocarbon (CFC) propellants. Since these chemicals were inert, they diffused into the upper atmosphere and it was found that when exposed to sunlight, they were broken down into chlorine radicals, which in turn broke down ozone molecules. The ozone layer in the atmosphere prevents most harmful UVB wavelengths of ultraviolet light (UV light) from passing through the Earth's atmosphere. These wavelengths of UV light cause skin cancer, sunburn and cataracts, which were all projected to increase dramatically as a result of the thinning ozone layer. In 1987, the Montreal Protocol was signed, an international agreement to eliminate the CFC propellants, meaning the pharmaceutical manufacturers had to find new propellants and reformulate their products. The new propellants were the hydrofluoroalkanes (HFAs) and products were gradually reformulated from 1996 onwards to use them. All CFC propellant aerosols were phased out in Europe by 2010.

Dry Powder Inhalers[14, 15]

The first commercially successful dry powder inhaler was the Aerohalor developed by Abbott Laboratories and marketed in 1948. This device contained a steel ball which moved when the patient breathed in and tapped a cartridge which contained the medicine to generate a fine powder. The drugs used in the device were isoprenaline for asthma, and penicillin for lung infections (see Picture 29).

In the early 1960s, Roger Altounyan, himself an asthmatic, worked on sodium cromoglycate at Bengers (later taken over by Fisons). He invented the Spinhaler, an inhaler that delivered powdered drug from a capsule in a cavity connected to an impeller. The capsule was pierced and when the patient inhaled, the impeller rotated and drew powder from the capsule and sent it to the patient to breathe in. The drug was dispersed onto carrier particles of lactose.

Other powder inhalers were also developed and marketed. In 1977, the Rotahaler inhaler for salbutamol was marketed by Glaxo; this was a device with the dose in a single capsule. The first multidose inhalers were marketed – the Serevent Diskhaler by Glaxo and the Pulmicort Turbuhaler by Astra in 1988. The Diskhaler used disks containing four or eight doses of medicament/lactose blend with each dose in a foil blister. When the patient opened the mouthpiece, the foil was pierced and the powder could be inhaled. The current Ventolin Accuhaler by Glaxo is a multi-dose device with sixty doses of the drug/lactose blend in foil blisters which are opened ready for inhalation when actuated; it also includes a counter for the number of doses.

Chapter 16

Products for the Eye

Anatomy of the eye

To help the reader the basic features of the anatomy of the eye are shown in Figure 16.1 and are:

Cornea – the transparent, curved structure at the front of the eye.

Iris – the coloured part of the eye: blue, brown, green, grey etc., which can be seen through the cornea.

Pupil –the black part of the eye in the middle of the iris. It dilates or contracts depending on the amount of light passing through it.

Lens – the transparent disc (with both sides being convex) immediately behind the iris and pupil.

Aqueous humour – the transparent fluid (with consistency similar to water) that circulates behind the cornea and in front of the lens.

Vitreous humour – the material (like transparent jelly) that fills the eyeball between the lens and the retina.

Retina –the light-sensitive layer of nerve cells that line the back of the eyeball.

Macula – the small centre of the retina, responsible for reading vision

Babylonian medicine

Babylonian medicine from 2000 BCE is recorded in the cuneiform clay tablets written in Sumerian, Akkadian, Hittite and other languages. Healing involved a complex relationship between magical incantation and therapeutic recipes. There were incantations to treat cloudy vision, eyes

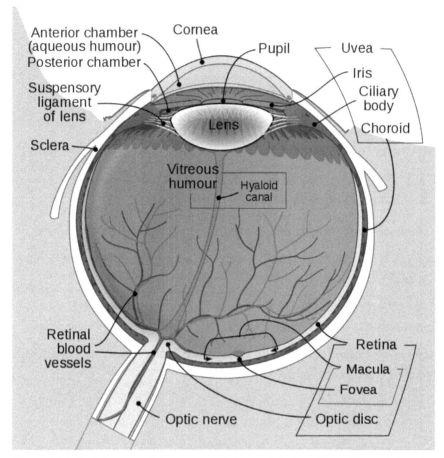

Figure 16.1: Basic features of the anatomy of the eye. (*Authors: Rhcastilhos and Jmarchn. Licensed under the Creative Commons Attribution-Share Alike 3.0 Unported license*)

filled with blood, and filmy eyes. The medicines used in this period were often liquid solutions or semi-solid ointments. The Mesopotamians were the first to use belladonna herb, and they also used alum, tannin from gall-nuts, and other astringents. Verdigris, which is copper acetate, was in common use, probably as a treatment for trachoma. The word 'trachoma' is Greek and means 'roughness'. It is now known to be an infectious eye disease caused by the bacterium *Chlamydia trachomatis*. It starts as an irritation of the conjunctiva (the membrane that covers the front of the eye), and can proceed to scarring and eventually an opaque cornea (the cornea is the transparent front part of the eye shown in Figure 16.1).

Copper salts are known to have a bactericidal action, so the remedy may have been effective.

Egyptian medicine

Egyptian doctors were apparently renowned for their skill in treatment of eye conditions. Herodotus in his *Histories* from the fifth century BCE records that Cyrus, the founder of the first Persian Empire, who reigned from 559 to 530 BCE, sent to Amasis, who was the Pharaoh of the twenty-sixth dynasty in Egypt, to ask for the service of the best eye doctor in Egypt.[1]

The Ebers papyrus which dates to about 1550 BCE is one of the main sources of knowledge about Egyptian medicine. As with Babylonian medicine it contains a mixture of magical incantations and remedies. The papyrus included sixty eye preparations including products to eliminate blood in the eyes, to eradicate blindness, to treat white spots, weeping of the eyes, eye injuries, and to get rid of red inflammation. The drugs used were from plants, minerals and of animal origin.[2]

Some remedies from Ghalioungui's 1987 translation are given below:

E358: Treatment for blindness: Mix colocynth with honey and apply to the outside of the eyes.

E381: Treatment for an eye injury: Apply a mixture of cooked valerian, colocynth and honey to a cloth and bandage over the eyes.

E408: Treatment for eye inflammation: Make a mixture of colocynth, leaves of acacia, green eye-paint, and the milk of a woman who has given birth to a boy into a mass and apply to the eyes.

As can be seen, honey was used as the base for many of the remedies. As mentioned in Chapter 14 on skin products, it is now known that the therapeutic value of honey is related to its high sugar content, hydrogen peroxide, and its low pH. It also contains a range of antibacterial compounds derived from the various plants from which the bees have collected the pollen. Malachite is a copper carbonate/hydroxide mineral. It was a constituent of green eye-paint. It is probable that these constituents would have had an antibacterial effect due to copper leaching out from them into solution.

The rationale for many of the other ingredients is more doubtful. Colocynth, the bitter apple, *Citrullus colocynthis*, for example, contains the chemical cucurbitacin, which is extremely irritating to the mucous membranes and so would irritate the eye. Another remedy (E382) which was for white spots in the eyes was granite, sieved and sprinkled over the eyes, and this must have been very irritant.

Kohl was used as an eye cosmetic for the upper and lower eyelids by both noble women and others in ancient Egypt. It was used as decoration and as a protection against eye diseases. Kohl used stibnite (antimony sulphide) or galena (lead sulphide). Lower eyelids were painted green using kohl made with green malachite. Kohl is still used in the Middle East, North Africa, the Mediterranean and South Asia.

Hippocratic Medicine

The *Hippocratic Corpus* described numerous eye diseases such as ophthalmic catarrh, modification of the pupil diameter, and glaucoma. Glaucoma is a common eye condition caused by fluid building up in the front part of the eye, which increases pressure inside the eye potentially damaging the sight. The treatments recommended in the *Hippocratic Corpus* included drinking wine.

Dioscorides

Pedanius Dioscorides (40–90 CE) recorded many of the uses of herbal and other ingredients in his five-volume book *De Materia Medica*.[3] Examples of his eye treatments include:

Spikenard (oil from *Nardostachys jatamansi*, a flowering plant of the valerian family): This is ground with wine and moulded to provide eye medication for purulent blepharitis [red inflamed edge of the eyelids].

Malabar [leaves from *Justicia adhatoda*, a shrub medicinal plant native to Asia]: Boiled in wine and plastered on the eye to treat inflammation.

Cinnamon: Applied with myrrh to clear away those elements that cast a shadow over the pupils of the eyes (probably meaning cataracts).

Galen and Roman medicine

In Galen's book *De compositione medicamentorum secundum locos* (On the Composition of Drugs by Part), he included about 200 recipes for eye preparations including many named after their originators such as Collyrium of Zoilus, Collyrium of Gaius, Collyrium of Sergius, Collyrium of Antonius Musa, and Collyrium of Asclepiades. For example, the Collyrium of Hermon contained twenty-one ingredients. Most of these preparations were semi-solid, prepared by mixing the active ingredient with honey, gum, a resin or white of an egg. They were made into a form resembling a little loaf. The word 'collyrion' is Latinised Greek and means 'little bread'. Galen used herbal ingredients from plant juices, seeds, fruits, minerals and animal materials. He recorded that the Collyrium of Hero contained mandragora (mandrake) and poppy, and warned that it would send patients to sleep – not surprising since it would have contained atropine, hyoscyamine, hyoscine, and scopine from the mandragora, and morphine from the poppy.

At the end of the second and in the third centuries CE, most eye preparations were in the form of a rectangular hard block or stick. [4,5] Liquid eye preparations had to be prepared just before use as they would degrade if stored for any period. These sticks were carried with the Roman Army on various campaigns. When the soldiers wanted to use them, they were mixed with water, milk, oil or honey. The sticks were usually 60–100mm in length, 30–50mm in width and stamped with the name of the physician who devised the medicine, the name of the medicine, and the disease for which the medicine was to be used. Before they hardened, the sticks were stamped using special stone collyrium stamps. The inscriptions on the stamps were engraved in small Roman letters and read on the stone from right to left, so that when the stick was stamped the text read from left to right. Some hundreds of these collyrium stamps have now been found made from different stones such as soap stone. They have been discovered in archaeological excavations in Spain, Germany, Britain, France and the Netherlands near where the Roman Army legions had set up their camps, and are made from different stones such as soap stone. An example of a Roman collyrium stamp found in France is shown in Picture 30.

Anglo-Saxon medicine

The *Leechbook of Bald* is a medical text probably compiled in the ninth century for Bald. A considerable part of the text is given over to diseases of the eyes, and these were obviously common. The conditions of living in smoky houses with no chimney, and the unsanitary life, would have led to eye infections. The *Leechbook* includes remedies for dimness of vision, pain in the eye, albugo (white spot on the cornea), watering of the eyes, styes, trachoma and infected eyelids. Many of the remedies were derived from earlier Roman authors such as Pliny, Oribasius, and Marcellus (from his book *De Medicamentis*). A couple of examples are:

> For dimness of the eyes: Mix celandine juice or blossoms of celandine and mix with honey, cook in a brass vessel.

> For dimness of the eyes: Mix balsam and virgin honey in equal parts and put in the eyes.

In M.L. Cameron's 1993 book *Anglo-Saxon Medicine*, he speculated that one of the remedies in the *Leechbook* for an eye ointment for styes could be effective in treating the staphylococcal infection of the eyelid, which is the usual cause of a stye. The remedy was a mixture of cropleac (an *Allium* species) and garlic mixed with wine and oxgall and put in a brass vessel for four days, then filtered through a cloth to clarify. In 2015, Harrison and other researchers at the Centre for Biomolecular Sciences at the University of Nottingham investigated this remedy to test its antimicrobial properties.[6] They used either onions or leeks for the 'cropleac'. They found that the remedy killed *Staphylococcus aureus* in biofilms in a laboratory model, and also killed methicillin-resistant *Staphylococcus aureus* (MRSA) in a mouse wound model where the mice were wounded and the wounds infected with the bacteria. The investigators argue that this product was carefully designed using empirical knowledge of the ingredients in the eye-salve, and was based on the experience and training of the Anglo-Saxon practitioners. They conclude that other old remedies may also have untapped potential for providing new antimicrobial therapies.

Arab medicine

Avicenna (980–1037) wrote more than 200 books on medicine and philosophy. His major work, the encyclopaedic *Canon of Medicine*, was completed in 1025. This included discussions of ophthalmic anatomy and disease. He believed that the development of cataracts could be slowed by diet (roasted and fried meat), avoidance of drinking and sexual intercourse, and use of appropriate medication.[7] He recommended the use of fennel juice mixed with honey and wild marjoram for treating the early stages of cataracts. The *Canon* included details of surgery for cataracts by choosing appropriate patients, then using a surgical instrument to push the opacity down with the tip of the instrument until the vision became clear.

Ibn al-Nafis (1213–1288 CE) was born in Damascus. He studied medicine at the Nuri hospital in Damascus. In 1236, he moved to Egypt at the request of the Sultan al-Kamil. Ibn al-Nafis was appointed as the chief physician at al-Naseri hospital which was founded by Saladin. He lived most of his life in Egypt and was a voluminous writer and commentator on the works of Hippocrates, Galen, and Avicenna. His main claim to fame is that he challenged Galen's ideas on the circulation of blood in the body by his belief that blood reached the left ventricle of the heart through the lung. This was three centuries before William Harvey announced his discoveries on circulation. Amongst his books was one entitled *Kitab al-Muhadhdhab fi 'l-Kuhl* (The Perfected Book on Ophthalmology). It was divided into three main sections and comprised about 370 pages. The second section was on the anatomy of the eye, eye diseases and general principles of good health. The third section was on eye remedies.[8] It includes remedies for kohls – powdered mixtures for the eyelids, and collyria – eye ointments or solid eye sticks. One example of a kohl is ash-coloured kohl, which was used to dry up excessive tears, strengthen the vision and for treating trachoma. Its recipe was:

> Stibnite from Isfahan (antimony sulphide)
> Tutty from Kiman (probably impure zinc oxide)
> Scales of copper
> Celandine

All of these were powdered together and applied.

An example of a collyrium remedy for trachoma and other eye conditions was Green Collyrium whose recipe was:

> Ceruse (lead carbonate)
> Acacia gum
> Gum ammoniac (juice of a giant fennel)
> Starch
> Verdigris (copper carbonate or copper acetate)

The gum ammoniac was dissolved in fresh extract of rue and the remaining ingredients ground together with it and dried.

Middle Ages

Many of the ophthalmic preparations continued to be based on herbal medicines using plants such as hamamelis, fennel, rue, saffron and others.[9] Poultices were used for afflictions of the eyelids.

Sixteenth to eighteenth centuries

During this period there were scientific advances in anatomy with Andreas Vesalius's publication of *De humani corporis fabrica* in 1543 and in discoveries on the physiology of the eye. The anatomy of the eye was studied by Professor Johann Zinn of the University of Göttingen and he published his book *Descriptio Anatomica Oculi Humani* in 1765, which gave the first detailed description of its anatomy. Samuel Sömmerring of the University of Mainz in his book *Icones Oculi Humani* described the macula in the retina at the back of the eye – the oval-shaped pigmented area near the centre of the retina, now known to be responsible for colour vision. The Maltese-born Joseph Barth received his medical education in Valletta (Malta), Rome and the University of Vienna. In 1774, he was appointed to the first chair in Ophthalmology in Europe by the Empress Maria Theresa. He established the Vienna School of Ophthalmology and wrote a book on cataract removal.

Also during this period, the official pharmacopoeias started to include some eye preparations. The 1618 *Pharmacopoeia Londinensis* (*London Pharmacopoeia*) included preparations purporting to correct the balance of the humours and strengthen the eyes to be taken by mouth. For example, Aloes Pills are stated by Culpeper in his 1649 *London Dispensatory* commentary on the *London Pharmacopoeia* to 'purgeth eyes of putrified humours'.

Other official ophthalmic preparations were: Oyntment of Tutty made from Tutty (zinc oxide), Lapis Calaminaris (calamine), Plantain water and oynment of roses. This was stated by Culpeper to 'dry up hot and salt humours'. Cephalic Plaister was made from rosin, black pitch, laudanum, turpentine, flowers of beans, doves' dung, myrrh, mastic, juniper gum and nutmegs. Again, according to Culpeper, this 'easeth the eyes of hot scalding vapours that annoy them'.

Nineteenth century

The nineteenth century marked the transition between the empirical tradition of earlier times and a more scientific approach to ophthalmic medicine. The discovery of the alkaloids started to provide improved treatments.

Atropine extracts from the Egyptian henbane were used by Cleopatra in the last century BCE to dilate her pupils, in the hope that she would appear more alluring – but with the disadvantage that her suitors would have been out of focus. In the Renaissance, women used the juice of the berries of deadly nightshade *Atropa belladonna* to enlarge the pupils of their eyes for cosmetic reasons. This practice resumed briefly in the late nineteenth and early twentieth century in Paris. The pupil dilating (mydriatic) effects of atropine were studied among others by the German chemist Friedlieb Ferdinand Runge (1795–1867). In 1831, the German pharmacist Heinrich F. G. Mein (1799–1864) succeeded in preparing atropine in pure crystalline form.

Physostigma venenosum, the Calabar bean, originated in the Cross-River state of what is now south-east Nigeria. The people there used them as 'ordeal beans' and gave them to persons accused of witchcraft or other crimes. When the person died it was considered a proof of guilt; if they vomited, they were considered innocent. The beans were first introduced to Britain in 1840. Thomas Fraser, an Edinburgh physician, investigated the effects of the bean for his MD thesis in 1862. He drew the drug to the attention of Douglas Argyll Robertson (1837–1909), a young physician who then investigated its use in ophthalmology.[10] Robertson found that it constricted the pupil in the eye and could be used to counteract the action of atropine in the eye. His 1863 paper was entitled 'The Calabar Bean as a New Ophthalmic Agent' and predicted that the drug would be used in the treatment of eye disorders. Jobst and Hesse isolated the active drug in the Calabar bean in 1864 and named it physostigmine. The first use of physostigmine as a treatment for glaucoma was by the German ophthalmologist Ludwig Laqueur in 1876, who himself suffered from glaucoma.

Gabriel Soares de Souza recorded in 1570 that the jaborandi plant was being used by the Indians in Brazil to treat mouth ulcers. In 1873, samples of *Pilocarpus pinnatifolius* were brought from Brazil to Paris by Symphronio Olympio Cezar Coutinho. He used the plant as a *sialogogue* – to stimulate flow of saliva in his patients, and to stimulate sweating. He published his findings and this aroused interest in the use of the herb. Sydney Ringer and Alfred Gould published a paper in the *Lancet* on the use of extract of jaborandi leaves on the eye in 1875, showing that it caused the pupil to contract. In the same year, Hardy and Gerrard isolated the alkaloid pilocarpine from the jaborandi plant and in 1877, the German ophthalmologist Adolf Weber introduced pilocarpine as a treatment for glaucoma.

In 1750, the French botanist and explorer Joseph de Jussieu sent a sample of the plant *Erythroxylon coca* to Europe. Albert Niemann

(1834–1861), working in Göttingen in 1860, was the first to isolate pure white crystals (which he named cocaine) from coca leaves; he was also the first to note that they had a numbing effect on the tongue. The Austrian ophthalmologist Carl Koller first applied cocaine to the eye in 1884 and found that it was a local anaesthetic. He announced his findings at a meeting of the Heidelberg Ophthalmological Society.[11]. A sample of the cocaine was brought straight from there to the Moorfields Eye Hospital in London. Robert Marcus Gunn was the house physician at the Moorfields and he carried out the first eye operation using the drug. The use of cocaine to anaesthetise the eye allowed measurements to be made of the pressure in the eye, because the early instruments had to press on the surface of the eye in order to measure its pressure.

The 1883 first edition of William Martindale's *Extra Pharmacopoeia of Unofficial Drugs* included a number of ophthalmic products.[12] It included four eye drops – Atropine Sulphate, Daturine Sulphate (hyoscyamine), Eserine (physostigmine), and Pilocarpine. Also included were three eye ointments – Atropine with Vaseline, IodoVaseline (a product containing the antiseptic compound iodoform), and Iodoform Ointment. Several solutions used as eye lotions or treatments were also mentioned – Boracic Acid Lotion, Atropine Solution, and Gelsemine Hydrochloride Solution (used to dilate the pupil for ophthalmic examinations). Gelsemine is the alkaloid from the roots of the Carolina jasmine plant.

One major problem with conventional eye drops is that volume of a drop is typically somewhere between 25 and 70 microlitres. But the product is rapidly removed from the eye by dilution with tears which usually run at about 1 microlitre per minute, and by blinking which removes 2 microlitres for each blink.[13] Only somewhere between 1 and 10 per cent of the dose permeates into the cornea and is absorbed into the eye. This means that eye drops often have to be given several times a day to get the required dose. A variety of ways have been used to try to extend the length of action of the product. One of the first attempts in the nineteenth century was the lamella, a minute gelatine/glycerol disc which was slipped under the lower eye lid and released its medicament over several days. The official 1885 *British Pharmacopoeia* included three small lamellae, made by pouring a film of gelatine and glycerol incorporating the drug then cutting tiny discs from the film.

The Atropine Lamella weighed about 1.3mg and contained 0.013mg of atropine sulphate. The Cocaine Lamella weighed about 1.3mg and contained 0.3mg cocaine. The Physostigmine Lamella again weighed 1.3mg and contained 0.065mg physostigmine. Lamellae were still used well into the twentieth century as they were included in the 1948 *British Pharmacopoeia*, but were discontinued in the 1958 edition.

Although Louis Pasteur's early discoveries in microbiology were published in the 1850s, it is noteworthy that there is no mention of the need for the lamellae to be sterile. It is not until the 1932 *British Pharmacopoeia* that any mention is made of the need for any of the equipment used in the manufacture of ophthalmic ointments to be sterile. And not until the 1948 *British Pharmacopoeia* was there a requirement that the eye ointments were to be made using aseptic techniques to avoid contamination with microorganisms during manufacture, and the need to use sterile tubes to package the eye ointments. All eye preparations now have to be sterile, and many eye drops are made in single use plastic dropper containers which minimises any risk of contamination with microorganisms by the patient.

See Picture 31 which shows some Levofloxacin antibiotic eye drops.

By the 1950s, a wider range of preparations was available for treatment of eye conditions, and included much more effective antibiotic preparations, such as those containing penicillin and sulfacetamide, to treat eye infections. The preparations included a range of eye lotions such as Adrenaline Compound Eye Lotion, Borax Compound Eye Lotion, Citric Acid Eye Lotion, Mercuric Oxycyanide Eye Lotion, Sodium Bicarbonate Eye Lotion, Sodium Chloride Eye Lotion and Zinc Sulphate Compound Eye Lotion. The range of eye ointments included ones containing boric acid, cocaine, hyoscine, penicillin and sulfacetamide. Eye drops included carbachol (used to constrict the pupil to treat glaucoma), mercuric chloride, and sulphacetamide. A range of ophthalmic tablets were apparently available weighing about 2.4mg which dissolved rapidly in the tear fluid.

In 1974, the Alza company marketed a device for controlled release of drug into the eye for treatment of glaucoma. This was the Ocusert.[14] The drug was pilocarpine alginate and it was enclosed in a reservoir where the rate of release of the drug was controlled through a membrane. The

Table 16.1: Current ophthalmic preparations.

Type of Drug	Examples	Drug Action	Condition Treated	Types of product used
Mydriatic	Tropicamide Cyclopentolate	Dilates pupil	Examination of eye	Eye drop, ointment
Miotic	Pilocarpine Carbachol	Constricts pupil	Glaucoma	Eye drops, ocular insert, gel
Beta-blocker	Timolol maleate Betaxolol	Reduction in eye pressure	Glaucoma	Eye drops, gel
Prostaglandin	Latanoprost Bimatoprost	Reduction in eye pressure	Glaucoma	Eye drops
Antihistamine	Antazoline Azelastine Olopatadine	Inhibition of inflammation	Allergic conjunctivitis	Eye drops
Anti-inflammatory	Betamethasone Dexamethasone	Inhibition of inflammation	Inflammation, allergic conjunctivitis	Eye drops, eye ointment, insert
Antibacterial	Chloramphenicol Levofloxacin Azithromycin	Bacteriostatic or bactericide	Eye infections	Eye drops, eye ointment
Antiviral	Aciclovir Gangiciclovir	Herpes simplex	Ophthalmic herpes viral infection	Eye drops, ointment
Diagnostic	Fluorescein sodium	Stain	Locating eye damage	Eye drops
Local anaesthetic	Oxybuprocaine hydrochloride	Blocks pain	Before surgery	Eye drops
Analgesic	Diclofenac sodium Flurbiprofen	Pain relief	After surgery	Eye drops
Artificial tears	Hypromellose Carmellose sodium	Eye lubrication	Dry eye	Eye drops, gel

device was 13.4mm long, 5.7mm wide and 0.3mm thick. Two strengths of the Ocusert were marketed: the Ocusert Pilo-20 and the Pilo-40. They were placed under the lower eyelid to release the pilocarpine at the rate of either 20 or 40 micrograms per hour over seven days.

Current types of ophthalmic products are summarised in Table 16.1.

Implants[15]

Macular oedema occurs when fluid and protein deposits collect on or under the macula at the back of the eye and cause it to thicken and swell. It is a possible complication of diabetes. One treatment for this is the Ozurdex implant (Allergan) containing the corticosteroid dexamethasone in a polymer matrix. The drug implant is injected with a special applicator into the vitreous humour (the liquid between the lens and the back of the eye). It gradually dissolves and releases the active ingredient over six months. Another treatment for diabetic macular oedema is the Iluvien implant (Alimera Sciences), which is again injected into the vitreous humour using a special applicator. The implant releases the corticosteroid drug fluocinolone acetonide over a period of thirty-six months – see Pictures 32 and 33.

Intravitreal injections

Lucentis (Novartis Pharmaceuticals) is an injection given at intervals of at least four weeks into the vitreous humour to treat diabetic macular oedema and the wet form of age-related macular degeneration (AMD).[16] AMD is a condition affecting the central part of the retina, the macula. It causes changes to the central vision, which can make everyday tasks difficult. The wet form of AMD is caused by the rapid growth of abnormal blood vessels under the macula. These new blood vessels leak blood and fluid that harm the central retina; the damage to the retina causes scarring and loss of vision. Lucentis contains the biotechnology drug ranibuzumab, an antibody made using recombinant DNA technology. This binds to the growth factor in the macula which is causing the new blood vessels to form and stops this growth factor working.

Photodynamic therapy

Photodynamic therapy is carried out by giving an intravenous injection of the drug verteporfin (Visudyne, Novartis), then activating the drug in the retina by illuminating the back of the eye after fifteen minutes with a red-light laser and a contact lens. This causes the release of free radicals from the verteporfin. Free radicals are unstable and they bond with other molecules. The reaction that follows between the free radicals and blood vessels causes locally increased levels of various chemicals, which in turn leads to constriction of the blood vessels in the retina, sealing of the blood vessels, and low oxygen levels in the blood vessels. This causes the harmful blood vessels to regress.

Chapter 17

Products via the Vagina and Rectum

Vaginal preparations

In Ancient Egypt the mortality between 3800 and 3000 BCE has been estimated.[1] Most individuals died before they reached the age of 15, so infant and child mortality was very high. The average life expectancy of those who survived was between 20 and 40 years old. In a later period between 2700 BCE and 300 CE the child mortality was lower but the average life expectancy was still only between 20 and 40 years. Even in a later Roman period, of those who survived childhood most could only expect to live until their thirties or forties. It is not surprising, therefore, that issues of fertility and reproduction loomed large in the practice of medicine, as families struggled to survive against the scourges of disease and famine during years of crop failure.

In women, particularly after delivery of a number of children, the muscles and other kinds of tissue that hold everything in place get stretched, and become weak, or torn. When that happens, some of the pelvic body parts can drop down and can even protrude from the vagina. This is called prolapse. Devices to try to hold everything in place are called pessaries. Medicated pessaries are also used to treat conditions of the vagina and uterus. The word is also used for a device used by women for contraception. This chapter will mention all three types of pessary.

Egyptian medicine

The Ebers papyrus from 1550 BCE included a number of gynaecological remedies.[2] One was for a displaced uterus using fumigation, where dried human excrement and incense was burnt and the woman bent over the fumes to let them penetrate into the vagina. To stop a pregnancy, acacia, colocynth and dates were ground in honey, and spread on a cloth which was introduced into the vagina. To start the process of childbirth in a pregnant woman, a pessary was made from juniper berries and pine resin and introduced into the vagina (recent animal studies have shown that juniper berry extract is an abortifacient). A remedy to cause a woman to be delivered of her baby was to apply peppermint to her bare posterior.

The *Hippocratic Corpus*

The *Hippocratic Corpus* included over 400 pessaries and vaginal applications.[3] The *Hippocratic Oath* specifically mentions pessaries. Part of it states:

> 'I will use treatment to help the sick according to my ability and judgment, but never with a view to injury and wrong-doing. Neither will I administer a poison to anybody when asked to do so, nor will I suggest such a course. Similarly, I will not give to a woman a pessary to cause abortion.' (W.H.S. Jones translation).[4]

The *Hippocratic Corpus* included a treatment for vaginal prolapse by placing a halved pomegranate soaked in wine into the vagina.

Uterine dropsy or hydrometra is an accumulation of fluid in the womb, caused by inflammation and general debility. During the first few months, the symptoms resemble those of pregnancy. The *Hippocratic Corpus* text *Nature of woman* recommended administering a purgative, then fumigating the womb with a cow–dung vapour bath. Then a pessary made from a cantharid beetle (Spanish or 'blister beetle') was inserted and after three days, a pessary made from bile. One day later, the woman douched herself with vinegar for three days. If the swollen stomach had emptied and menstruation occurred, she should have sex with her husband.

The *Corpus* included tests for fertility. One test was to place a clove of garlic, which had been cleaned and peeled, in the vagina as a pessary, then see if the next morning the odour of garlic could be smelt on the breath. If it could the woman would conceive. If it could not she would not conceive.

A key belief in Hippocratic medicine was of the importance of menstruation for the health of the female body; it was regarded as a necessary purgation. If there were issues with menstruation it was believed that women would accumulate waste matter. Thus, many of the treatments in Hippocratic and subsequently in Galenic medicine were to provoke the menses.

Dioscorides

Dioscorides book *De Materia Medica,* contained a huge number of references to the use of medicines involved in various ways in aspects of fertility and reproduction.[5] There were 78 references to abortifacients, 25 to aphrodisiacs, 18 to barrenness, 20 to childbirth, 7 to conception, 33 to female problems, 139 to menstruation, 3 to deterrents to sexual intercourse, 106 to the uterus and 28 to uterine suffocation (hysteria).

Examples of abortifacients were cardamom or bdellium (a gum resin extracted from *Commiphora wightii* and from *Commiphora africana* trees) burnt and used as a fumigation, and camel's thorn herb in a pessary. A variety of materials were claimed to be aphrodisiacs when drunk, including costus root (*Saussurea costus,* commonly known as costus, is a species of thistle) with honey, saffron, turnip seed, purslane and leeks with frankincense.

Pessaries made with spikenard (oil from *Nardostachys jatamansi,* a flowering plant of the valerian family) were used to stop uterine excretions and discharges. Costus root pessaries and saffron pessaries were also used for uterine ailments. A number of herbs such as spikenard, camel hay and tree moss were extracted with water to produce decoctions, which were then used in sitz-baths to treat uterine ailments. Internal douches of costus root or ointment of roses were also used for uterine complaints; fenugreek ointment was used for vaginal dryness. Marshmallow herb mixed with pork fat or with goose fat and turpentine was recommended for uterine inflammation.

In the Roman Republic and Empire, pessaries were also used to treat prolapse. An illustration is given in Picture 34 of a bronze ring pessary used to support the uterus.

Galen

Galen used many of the Hippocratic recipes. He mentions the condition of hysteria in women, which he felt was characterised by a variety of symptoms ranging from muscle contractions to lethargy, and asphyxia. He believed that the uterus could become withdrawn or inflamed, and endorsed the practice of fumigation with sweet-smelling herbs to attract the uterus back to its rightful position.

The School of Salerno and women's medicine

As mentioned in Chapter 5, the medieval school of medicine in Salerno was an important centre for the teaching of medicine and for translation of Arab texts into Latin. One text which originated in Salerno was *The Trotula*, which was a medieval compendium of women's medicine. It is now known that this is a combination of three different texts. The first and third texts *On the Condition of Women* and *On Women's Cosmetics* were anonymous. The second *On Treatments of Women* was attributed to a woman healer named Trota. Using the 2001 translation of *The Trotula* texts by Monica H. Green, we are able to see some of the conditions treated using pessaries.[6]

> Inducing menstruation: Bull's gall and natron (a sodium carbonate mineral) powder mixed with wild celery or hyssop, soaked into wool and pressed to make it hard to be able to insert into the vagina.
>
> Excessive menstrual flow: Plantain juice pessary
>
> Movement of the womb: Deer marrow or goose fat, red wax, butter, fenugreek and linseed made into a pessary
>
> Vaginal itching: Camphor, litharge (lead oxide), laurel berry and egg white made into a pessary.

Medicated pessaries remained a common form of treatment in the seventeenth and eighteenth centuries. The *Pharmacopoeia Londinensis, or the New London Dispensatory in Six Books* translated by William Salmon of 1716 contained three pessaries – Pessary for the Womb to prevent maternal fits and prolapse, an Opening Pessary for opening the womb and causing menstruation, and Mynsicht's astringent pessary which halted menstruation.[7] Adrian von Mynsicht (1603–1638) was a German alchemist and follower of Paracelsus. This same edition of the *New London Dispensatory* also contained three 'Injection' products introduced into the uterus using a syringe. These were an injection to stop menstruation, an injection to provoke menstruation and an injection to cleanse and heal the womb of all impurities, and to heal and dry ulcers.

Current medicated pessaries are mainly for treatment of vaginal thrush infections with *Candida albicans*. Up to three-quarters of women will have at least one attack of thrush in their lifetime. Most of the pessaries contain the antifungal drug clotrimazole.[8] A metal pessary mould from the twentieth century is shown in Picture 35.

Pessaries for managing pelvic organ prolapse

As mentioned, organs such as the uterus, bladder or bowel can protrude into the vagina because of weakness in the supporting tissues. A variety of devices were used over the centuries.[9] Philip Syng Physick (1768–1837) was trained in medicine in Philadelphia, London and Edinburgh, and returned to Philadelphia to practise. He has been dubbed the 'Father of American Surgery'. He invented the globe pessary when he saw an old billiard ball and realised that it was the right shape and size to stabilise the uterus. Hugh Lenox Hodge (1796–1873) was born in Philadelphia, trained in medicine and worked in Pennsylvania where he became the professor of obstetrics at the University of Pennsylvania. His invention of the Hodge pessary was apparently inspired by the steel hook on the ends of fire shovels and tongs.

Modern treatments include surgery and physiotherapy, with present-day pessaries made from latex or silicone rubber also available to help push the organs back to their proper position and relieve symptoms. There are a large variety of designs including the ring, dish, Gehrung, Hodge, cup, and oval. The Gelhorn, donut and cube designs are used for more advanced stages of prolapse.

Intrauterine contraceptive devices

The modern history of intrauterine contraceptive devices (IUCDs) begins in 1928, when Dr Ernest Grafenberg of Berlin reported on the use of handmade stars of silkworm gut which he had inserted into the uterus of some patients for contraception.[10] The stars were tied in the centre with silver wire. However, the device tended to be expelled by uterine contractions. Grafenberg then created a new device made by rolling silkworm gut into rings and binding with silver wire. Later he replaced the silkworm gut ring with a coil of silver alloy wire. This device became known as the Grafenberg ring. The Grafenberg ring was widely used in England and in the British dependencies, but not in the US. Grafenberg emigrated to the US in the 1930s but his device was considered ineffective and liable to cause infection. In the 1960s, there was a renewal of interest in IUCDs in the US and a number of different designs were evaluated. Also, positive evidence had emerged from Japan of extensive use of IUCDs using variants of the Grafenberg ring.

The new IUCD devices introduced in the 1960s included the Lippes loop made by Ortho, the Birnberg bow and others. These all had monofilament tails from the device into the vagina. The manufacturers felt that the tail enabled the device to be extracted more easily. They were controversial, however, as Grafenberg had always held that a tail increased the risk of infection from microbial invasion.

In the late 1960s and early 1970s, A.H. Robins Company marketed the Dalkon Shield IUCD. This had a multifilament tail. In the next four years there were many reports of septic abortion associated with the device. A septic abortion is an infection of the placenta and foetus in a very early pregnancy. There is risk of spreading to the uterus, causing pelvic infection or spreading more widely to cause sepsis and damage to other organs. It was reported that there was a near epidemic of infections in the pelvis associated with the Dalkon Shield due to the multifilament string upon which bacteria could travel into the uterus of users. More than 300,000 lawsuits were filed against the A.H. Robins Company in the US. The cost of the lawsuits and settlements, estimated at billions of dollars, led the company to file for Chapter 11 bankruptcy protection in 1985.

A further breakthrough in design of IUCDs was the discovery in 1969 by Zipper *et al* from the Worcester Foundation of the inhibitive effect of copper on sperm and this was used in a T-shaped device. The release of copper ions inhibits the mobility of the sperm and their viability so that they are unable to fertilise an egg.

There are currently two types of IUCD on the market – copper-releasing devices and hormone-releasing devices. The hormonal devices release the hormone drug levonorgestrel, which thickens the mucus in the cervix and prevents the sperm from reaching the egg. The drug is released in the uterine cavity and leads to a high concentration in the tissue but a low concentration in the blood. These devices are long-acting reversible contraceptives; the copper IUCDs can be used for up to ten years, the hormonal devices for up to five years.

Rectal preparations

Ancient Egypt

The Ebers papyrus from 1550 BCE contained a number of preparations to be used rectally:

E143: A remedy to cool the anus made from behen oil, colocynth juice, oil/fat, and honey.

E157: A remedy to cool the anus composed of mesentery from fat cattle [mesentery is the tissue which surrounds the organs of the gut, and suspends them from the abdominal wall] boiled with milk and honey, strained and then poured into the anus on one day.

E161: A remedy for haemorrhoids consisting of ox fat and acacia leaves bandaged on.

The *Hippocratic Corpus*

There are 200 recipes for enema preparations in the Hippocratic Corpus and 13 for suppositories. One of the treatises is the *Regime in Health*, and this emphasised the vital role of emetics and enemas. During winter, when most phlegm is produced and when the head and lungs are subject to diseases, emetics were recommended. As the body was full of bile, which caused a 'twisting of the bowels' (colic) during the summer, the use of enemas was preferred. The purpose of the enemas was to cool the body and draw down humours. Fat and moist patients were to receive enemas made from brine and sea water, while dry, lean and weak patients were to receive enemas made from milk, or water boiled with chickpeas.

An anal fistula is a small tunnel that develops between the end of the bowel and the skin near the anus (where faeces leave the body). Fistulas can also develop in the vagina. In *Fistulas*, the author recommended using a suppository made from deadly nightshade herb (*Atropa belladonna*), goose fat, and copper silicate. Fistulae are often infected so the copper salt would kill off bacteria.

Aulus Cornelius Celsus

In the second century CE Celsus, the author of *De Medicina*, recommended an enema made from pearl barley or rose oil with butter as a nutrient for those suffering from dysentery and unable to eat. Nutrient enemas continued to be used until the early twentieth century; they have now been superseded by enteral (tube) feeding directly into the stomach and by intravenous feeding with amino acids, glucose and lipids.

Dioscorides

Dioscorides' book *De Materia Medica* includes a variety of medicines for anal conditions.[11] Only one suppository was mentioned – saffron suppositories for afflictions of the anus. There were a large number of herbs which were smeared on the anal tissue to heal anal fissures and fistulas. These included pitch, dyer's buckthorn, chaste tree seeds, ash of calcined riverine crabs, teasel root, gillyflower flowers, the heads of mainis (fish) burned and ground up and sprinkled on. Fenugreek, sow thistle juice, boiled king's clover with grape syrup, rosemary frankincense, and lentil with melilot (sweet clover) and quince were all used to treat anal inflammation. Raw quince juice and violet leaves were used to treat prolapse of the anus. Another prolapse treatment was to use the electric ray fish which gave an electric shock. Fat from greasy wool (lanolin) and bull's bile were used to cure anal sores. Rosemary frankincense was used on a plaster to shrink haemorrhoids.

Arabic medicine

Ali ibn al-'Abbas al-Majusi (who died 982–994), Latinised as Haly Abbas, was a Persian physician from the Islamic Golden Age, who worked at the Al-Adudi Hospital in Baghdad. He is most famous for the *Kitab al-Maliki*, (the Complete Book of the Medical Art) or *Liber Regalis* (Royal Book) since it was dedicated to the Emir. Suppositories are mentioned in this book. Avicenna's *Canon of Medicine* does not list suppositories amongst the dosage forms.

Renaissance and Enlightenment medicine

A number of French authors mention the use of suppositories. The French surgeon Ambroise Paré (1509–1590) mentions the use of a variety of laxative suppositories, mild ones containing salt and honey, stronger ones containing scammony (*Convolvulus scammonia*, a bindweed native to the eastern Mediterranean), euphorbia or colocynth. They were made with soap or fat. A later writer, Jean de Renou (1568–1620), who was the physician to three French kings Henry II, III and IV, suggested in his book *Dispensatorium Medicum Continens Pharmaceuticarum, Lib V De Materia Medica, Lib III Pharmacopeam Itidem Sive Antidotarium Varium & Absolutissimum* that suppositories could be used as an alternative to the use of enemas. The French pharmacist Nicolas Lémery (1645–1715) included a chapter on suppositories in his *Pharmacopée Universelle* of 1715.

Modern suppositories

The early suppositories were made up of a variety of ingredients of animal, vegetable and mineral origin formed into an appropriate shape by hand to insert into the anus. During the Greco-Roman period, fabric or lint suppositories were also used where the material was soaked in a solution of medicaments. The weights of the suppositories were not standardised.

In the eighteenth century, a new era began with the discovery of cocoa butter, the vegetable fat extracted from the cocoa bean, the dried and fully fermented seed of *Theobroma cacao*.[12] In 1762, the French pharmacist and chemist Antoine Baumé (1728–1804) described in his book *Élémens de Pharmacie Theoretique et Pratique* (Elements of Theoretical and Practical Pharmacy) how cocoa butter could be melted and poured into a mould to make suppositories. In the US, the Philadelphia pharmacist Alfred B. Taylor in an 1852 article in the *American Journal of Pharmacy* mentioned the use of cocoa butter and quoted from François Dorvault's 1844 text *L'officine, ou, Répertoire Général de Pharmacie Pratique* (The Pharmacy, or General Directory of Practical Pharmacy); this contained recipes for suppositories containing belladonna, calomel (mercurous chloride) and quinine. These were made by forming paper cones in a bed of sand and pouring in the melted composition into the cone and allowing it to set. In America and Europe, inventors soon began designing different types of moulds for suppositories and pessaries. Griffenhagen has described much of the history of the suppository mould in an article in 1956.[13] There were two types, one for moulds used where the molten suppository mass was poured into the mould, and one which used a cold compression method.

The firm of Hall and Ruckel of New York City started selling a range of sizes of hollow suppositories in the UK in 1860 through S. Maw, Son and Thompson in London and other wholesale druggists. These were made from cocoa butter and had a hollow in them into which a pharmacist could insert his own medication. They included a cocoa butter stopper which was used to seal the suppository. However, they were not commercially successful as the amount of labour in filling them was as much as manufacturing the suppository from scratch.

Oil of Theobroma (cocoa butter) was included in the 1885 *British Pharmacopoeia*. There were eight suppositories in that edition: carbolic acid suppositories (used as an antiseptic), tannic acid suppositories, tannic acid suppositories with soap, mercurial suppositories, iodoform suppositories (antiseptic), and compound lead suppositories. Belladonna suppositories (used as an antispasmodic to relieve the pain of haemorrhoids or anal fistula) and glycerin suppositories (used as a laxative) were added in the 1898 *British Pharmacopoeia*. The 1948 *British Pharmacopoeia* added bismuth subgallate suppositories (for haemorrhoids), cocaine suppositories (local anaesthetic for relief of pain of haemorrhoids), suppositories of hamamelis (for haemorrhoids), and suppositories of hamamelis and zinc oxide. But by 1968 there were only two official suppositories in the *British Pharmacopoeia* – bisacodyl suppositories and glycerin suppositories, both of which were used as a laxative.

See Picture 38 for a typical suppository mould used in a pharmacy or hospital.

During the twentieth century, a large variety of suppository bases were developed: fatty bases such as hydrogenated fatty acids and compounds of glycerine with fatty acids, water-soluble and water-miscible bases such as polyethylene glycols, and other miscellaneous bases.

Suppositories have never been a popular way to take medicines in the UK or the US where it is preferred to take medicines by almost any other route. Suppositories are much more popular in France and Southern Europe. An Italian colleague once summed up their view for me as, 'The mouth is for the food and drink …' He preferred to take his medicines rectally and not spoil his palate for the better things of life. Despite this there are still a surprising number of commercial suppository products on the UK market. There are a variety of products for treating haemorrhoids; bisacodyl suppositories and glycerol suppositories as laxatives; aspirin and paracetamol as painkillers; indomethacin and diclofenac as painkillers and to treat inflammation; mesalazine and sulfasalazine for ulcerative colitis; and metronidazole for bacterial infections.

John Arderne's Treatises of Fistula in Ano, Haemorrhoids and Clysters

John Arderne (1307–1392) was educated as a surgeon in Montpellier and practised in France as a military surgeon on the English side during the One Hundred Years' War. He returned to England and practised in Wiltshire, Nottinghamshire and later, London. His book was written in 1376.[14] His description of the clyster (enema) syringe taken from an early fifteenth century translation of his book was as follows: 'Instrument for clystryez to be ministered. A pipe of wood – box, hazel or willow. To be length of six inches. Afterwards have a he a swine bladder, blown to much, for which thou shalt prepare to be kept.' The book includes a number of recipes for enemas. One remedy stated:

'Maluez common and green camomile and bruise them a little. Seeth them in water until it becomes green. Then take white bran as much as sufficeth and boil it a little, afterwards cool it and to be cooling add one handful of salt and clean honey or oil. Mix by hand or spatula. This will keep a fortnight.'

Arderne recommended using clysters to prevent illnesses such as constipation, by purging three or four times in winter, in summer once.

Enemas in the fifteenth to seventeenth centuries

Jean Fernel (1497–1558) was the physician to the French royal court. He is credited with the invention of the term 'physiology'. He wrote a number of books, including *Universa Medicina* which was in three parts: the *Physiologia*, the *Pathologia* and the *Therapeutice*. One chapter in *Therapeutice* was about purgation. The device he used to give enemas was a tube attached to a pig's bladder. He recommended the use of a salt solution with added honey and herbs.

The famous French surgeon Ambroise Paré (1510–1590) is credited with the invention of an apparatus for self-administration of enemas; the patient sat on the nozzle and pumped the liquid into his anus.

By the seventeenth century, clyster (enema) syringes were made of a variety of materials, usually of copper or porcelain, but also silver or mother of pearl for the wealthy and nobility for whom the use of enemas became a fashionable treatment. The French King Louis XIV (1636–1715) is reported to have received over 2,000 enemas during his life. The excessive use of enemas by some physicians made them a target of the satirists. The French actor and playwright Jean-Baptiste Poquelin, better known by his stage name of Molière, wrote a three-act comedy-ballet in 1673 entitled *Le Malade Imaginaire* (The Hypochondriac) where he described physicians using enemas for any and every condition. The cartoon in Picture 37 shows an apothecary preparing to administer an enema to a young lady patient, who has just escaped in fright. A French eighteenth-century enema syringe is shown in Picture 36.

Tobacco enemas

Tobacco had been discovered and used by the native people of the Americas for hundreds of years. Sir Walter Raleigh is often credited with bringing tobacco from Virginia to England in July 1586, but the truth is that the Spanish had already introduced tobacco to Europe in about 1528, and its use spread rapidly. The Spanish physician Nicolas Monardes had written a book on herbs and materials from the Americas and Caribbean, and this was translated into English by the merchant trader John Frampton in 1596 and called *Joyfull Newes out of the Newe Founde World*.[16] The book recommended the use of tobacco for the relief of toothache, falling fingernails, worms, halitosis, lockjaw and even cancer. Tobacco was included in some of the early pharmacopoeias.

Richard Mead (1673–1754), who was physician to George II, documented one of the earliest cases of the use of tobacco smoke to resuscitate victims of drowning in 1746, when a woman was treated by inserting the stem of a passing sailor's pipe into her rectum, covering the bowl with a piece of perforated paper and blowing hard.[17] The woman revived. The idea caught on and in the 1780s, the Royal Humane Society installed resuscitation kits including smoke enemas along the River Thames. The kit consisted of a nozzle, a fumigator and bellows to blow the smoke. Smoke enemas were apparently regarded as equally efficacious to artificial respiration.

Enemas of tobacco extract were also used to treat strangulated hernias and other intestinal obstructions. Enema Tabaci (tobacco) was included in the 1824 *London Pharmacopoeia*. It was made by soaking tobacco in boiling water for an hour, then straining before use. However, G.F. Collier in his translation of the text also includes an antidote to be used, as the tobacco contained nicotine which he said acted on the brain. Enema Tabaci was also included in the 1864 edition of the *British Pharmacopoeia* but it fell out of favour because of the effect of nicotine on the heart and was not included in the 1885 edition.

Enemas in the nineteenth and twentieth centuries

In the nineteenth century there were a number of different types of equipment used for giving enemas, including the bulb enema. Later the bag enema was developed, where the solution was placed in the bag to be hung above the patient and infused into the anus by gravity.

John Harvey Kellogg (1852–1943) was an American physician who became the medical director of the Battle Creek Sanitarium in Michigan. He advocated vegetarianism, nutrition and the benefits of a bland diet to reduce sexual stimulation. He is best known for the development of the cornflakes which bear his name, but he also invented a method of making peanut butter. He was a proponent of colonic irrigation to remove harmful bacteria which he accomplished by running several gallons of water through the patient's bowels.[18] This was followed by a pint of yoghurt to provide healthy bacteria for the gut, half to be eaten, the other half given as an enema.

Colonic cleansing is still used in alternative medicine by practitioners who believe that faecal matter in the intestine builds up and leads to illness, thus its removal detoxifies the body. In 1932, Dr W. Kerr Russell wrote a book entitled 'Colonic Irrigation'[19] and this was followed by many other books by other authors on the same topic. Today there are still a considerable number of colonic 'hydrotherapy' clinics and practitioners.

During the nineteenth century, enemas were chiefly used as purgatives. The 1864 *British Pharmacopoeia* included Enema Aloes, Enema of Asafoetida, Enema of Magnesium Sulphate (Epsom salts), Enema of Opium, Enema of Tobacco, and Enema of Turpentine. The Enema of Opium would have been used to relieve intestinal pain and colic. But by 1898 these had disappeared from official use. Enemas were still used in the twentieth century to evacuate the lower bowel in cases of severe constipation, and also in obstetrics to help stimulate contractions.

Current uses of enema products

A small number of enemas are still used today. These include a phosphate enema and a couple of micro-enema products (small volume enemas) used to treat constipation and to clear the bowel before surgery or before examinations of the bowel. Other enemas containing budesonide (a corticosteroid) or mesalazine are used to treat ulcerative colitis.

Other rectal dosage forms

A febrile convulsion is a fit or seizure caused by a sudden change in a small child's body temperature, and is usually associated with a fever. Febrile convulsions are alarming and very upsetting to witness for the parents. In the mid-1970s, a treatment using a rectal solution of diazepam was pioneered in Sweden by Stig Agurell and his colleagues from the Karolinska Sjukhuset, and then by Finn Knudsen in the Glostrup Hospital in Denmark.[20] This was shown to act within less than five minutes. A number of diazepam rectal solution products are now available packaged in polyethylene tubes which can be squeezed to inject the dose.

Other commercial rectal products which are available include a glyceryl trinitrate ointment for rectal fissures (tears in the anus caused by straining in passing hard stools when constipated), and steroid foam products for haemorrhoids.

Chapter 18

Medicines for Other Routes of Administration

Nasal products

The Greek *Hippocratic Corpus* from the fourth century BCE included treatments for nasal polyps (a benign tumour that grows in the lining of the nose or sinuses).[1] The text recommended that they should be cut out and cauterised (burnt with a heated instrument to seal the wound). The wounds were recommended to be dusted with black hellebore (*Helleborus niger*), cleaned with flower of copper then treated with honey. Flower of copper was composed of the purple globules which are thrown off when molten copper runs from the furnace, and which were then purified by the addition of clear water.

Pedanius Dioscorides' book *De Materia Medica* contained remedies for a number of nasal conditions.[2] He recommended camel's thorn or arsenic sulphide for sores in the nose. For discharges from the nose he used storax or sulphur and for nasal polyps, he recommended unguent of iris, or cypress chopped up in a fig, or dragon arum, or flower of copper. Ivy leaf juice was used to clear putrid humours of the nostrils.

Abū Bakr Muhammad ibn Zakariyyā al-Rāzī (854–925 CE), better known as Rhazes, was the first to describe seasonal irritation of the nose (hay fever) and its likely causes.[3] He also mentioned the different types of common cold.

At the end of the nineteenth century, more scientific treatments for nasal conditions started to become available. John Johnson Kyle's 1906 *Manual of Diseases of the Ear, Nose and Throat* listed some of the remedies for inflammations of the nose and chronic catarrh.[4] One product was protargol, a silver protein solution invented by Arthur Eichengrum in 1897 when he was working for Bayer in Germany. Another product was argyrol made from silver nitrate, gelatine and sodium hydroxide. Both products were astringent and killed bacteria. Kyle mentioned a range of strength of solutions of silver nitrate. He also mentioned the use of nasal suppositories and quotes a wide range of medicines that could be applied using suppositories – potassium chlorate, bismuth subnitrate, iodoform, mercuric chloride, boric acid, cocaine, and cocaine and morphine.

By the 1950s, the main preparations used for nasal conditions were nasal drops and nasal washes. Some medicines and antiseptic preparations mentioned by Kyle in 1908 were still in use such as nose drops of silver protein and mercuric salts and a borax nasal wash. For the treatment of colds and hay fever, nose drops of phenylephrine, ephedrine and naphazoline were used as decongestants.[5]

The 1980s and 1990s saw the earlier nasal administration devices evolve from pipettes, drops and plastic squeeze bottles to more sophisticated spray devices with improved dose accuracy and more efficient coverage of the nasal mucosa. The preparations currently available are nasal drops, liquid nasal sprays, nasal washes and nasal ointments and creams. During this period, the use of the nasal route of administration has increased for drugs that are difficult to give except by injection. Companies are also now researching using the nasal route for a range of vaccines. Influenza vaccination is now given to children from 2 to 17 years by a 0.1ml dose delivered to each nostril.

The nose provides part of the body's defence against inhaled bacteria, irritating chemicals and particles.[6] These stick to the thick mucus in the nose. The cells of the epithelium lining the nose have small hair-like protuberances (cilia) that carry the thick mucus backwards in the nose and down the throat. The cilia beat at about 1,000 strokes a minute and this means that about half of a drug administered via the nose is normally cleared in about fifteen minutes, will then go down the throat and be swallowed. Part of the product administered via the nose will therefore be absorbed from the nose and part from the gut after being swallowed. However, even if only a part is absorbed via the nose, it can still mean the drug is absorbed more rapidly than if given by mouth in a tablet or capsule. A good example of rapid absorption via the nose comes from the cocaine recreational drug users who get a 'high' within 3–5 minutes of sniffing the powdered drug. Prescription medicines which depend on rapid nasal absorption are the nasal sprays containing sumatriptan or zolmitriptan, both of which are used for the relief of migraine attacks.

Two painkillers for the relief of severe pain are also given via nasal inhalation: diamorphine hydrochloride (heroin) and fentanyl citrate. Another drug which relies on speedy absorption from the nasal route is naloxone, which is given as a nasal spray as an emergency antidote treatment for drug addicts who have overdosed on drugs such as heroin or morphine.

Another reason to use the nasal route to give a drug is when it is a medicine (for example, a peptide which is an amino acid compound), which would be broken down in the gut by the enzymes if it was taken by mouth, and which would otherwise have to be given by injection. One such medicine given by the nasal route is buserelin, which is used to treat prostate cancer.

The nasal spray delivery devices (nebulisers) are based on a mechanical pump. Pressure is applied on a chamber containing a liquid or suspension causing a spray to come out of a nozzle. Some of the products contain an antimicrobial preservative and some are preservative-free where the design of the device prevents contamination of the product. These devices are now used to package most of the nasal products on the market. The products include steroids used to treat hay fever, such as beclomethasone, budesonide, fluticasone, mometasone, and triamcinolone. Medicines such as azelastine and xylometazoline are used for nasal congestion due to colds or hay fever.

There are still some simple nose drop products on the market such as ephedrine nasal drops and xylometazoline drops. These are decongestants to relieve nasal congestion due to colds and catarrh. A nasal ointment is on the market containing mupirocin, and this is used to eliminate staphylococci from the nose. A menthol balm is used as a nasal decongestant.

Ear products

The Egyptian Ebers papyrus included a number of remedies for ear problems, including deafness:[7]

> E764: For reduced hearing: Red ochre, leaves of im–deciduous tree, finely ground in behen oil and introduced into the ear

E767: To treat a wound in the ear: Cut out destroyed tissue and then insert oil/fat and honey into the ear canal, then bandage over the ear.

E768: Remedy for a diseased ear: Behen oil, terebinth resin, and fluid dropped into the ear.

The *Hippocratic Corpus* included the first description of the membrane in the ear that comprises the eardrum and made the connection between the eardrum and hearing. The *Corpus* included a local application of honey diluted with water for discharge from the ears, and also pouring almond oil into the ear canal. In chronic cases a powder containing lead oxide and lead carbonate was used.

Asclepiades of Bithynia (124–40 BCE) established Greek medicine in Rome. He opposed the orthodox Hippocratic theory of medicine based on humours. He had a universal remedy for ear disease consisting of cinnamon, cassia, reed grass blossoms, castoreum, white and long pepper, amomum, myrobalan, incense, lavender, myrrh, saffron and sodium bicarbonate mixed with vinegar. For earache he recommended instilling oil in which an African snail had been boiled into the ear.

In his *De Medicina* written in the first century CE, Aulus Cornelius Celsus provided a survey of the existing therapy for ear complaints. For ear disease he recommended instillations of oil in which earthworms had been boiled, or juice of peach stones. For exudations from the ear he used juice from leeks mixed with honey, myrrh and crocus. To remove insects from the ear canal, he used sticky resin on cotton or an injection with an ear syringe to dislodge them.[8] This was one of the first mentions of the use of an ear syringe.

Galen, writing in the second century CE, recommended the use of fatty or oily substances such as oil of roses, or oil of nard, or goose fat for earache. In cases of worms in the ear, he used insufflations (powder blown into the ear) of white hellebore root or instillations of blackberry juice. For deafness he recommended a combination of diet, purgatives and applications to dissolve thick fluids.

The Persian physician Rhazes treated tinnitus (hearing noises in the head that aren't caused by an outside source) with opium mixed with oil of roses. He recommended instilling oil into the ear to remove accumulated ear wax, then putting water into the ear canal and removing the softened wax with cotton swabs. Worms in the ear were removed by instilling the juice of peach leaves and wormwood into the ear.

Avicenna (980–1036 CE) documented the anatomy of the ear: the external ear shaped to collect sound waves, the ear canal to protect the eardrum, and the thin membrane which responds to sound vibrations. Hearing is caused by the impact of sound waves on the eardrum.

The *Leechbook of Bald* was written in about 950 CE in Winchester. It included many Anglo-Saxon native remedies and some borrowed from much earlier Graeco-Roman cultures. There were many remedies for ear complaints, for sore ears, earache, for deafness, and for treating worms and earwigs in the ears.[9] Sore ears were treated with warm oil with various herbs infused in it, or henbane juice (which would have contained atropine, hyoscyamine and hyoscine). Animal bile was used to treat deafness.

Bernard de Gordon (1270–1330) was a French professor of medicine in Montpellier. His recommended method of removing water from the ears was to put a tube into the ear and get a person of low standing to suck on it. For removal of worms from the ear, he recommended laying the patient down and putting a cut ripe apple over the ear to entice the worm out of the ear.

Nicholas Culpeper's *London Dispensatory* of 1653 included several recipes for ear diseases. Black hellebore root dropped into the ears 'helps deafness coming of Melancholly'. Ground ivy juice helps noise in the ears (presumably tinnitus). Flower of Oyntment made from Rozin, Per-rozin, yellow wax, sheep suet, olibanum, myrrh and mastic was used for swelling of the ears.

In the tenth century, Rhazes recommended the use of oil to soften ear wax; ear drops of almond oil or olive oil are still used today for the same purpose. Other ear drops now in common use contain docusate sodium which softens the wax, and urea hydrogen peroxide drops, which release bubbles of gas to break up the wax.

Inflammation of the outer ear or ear canal is called 'otitis externa' or 'swimmer's ear'. Symptoms include ear pain or discharge. Inflammation is treated with steroid preparations such as betamethasone or prednisolone drops. If the ear is infected it is treated with antibiotic drops such as those containing neomycin sulfate or framycetin sulfate.

Earwigs were popularly supposed to crawl into the ears of sleepers and burrow into their brains. A number of authors have branded this as superstition, since there are no well-documented cases.[10] Nevertheless, as we have seen, a variety of physicians from Celsus to Bernard de Gordon have written about worms or insects getting into the ear. What is the truth? Kroukamp and Londt did a survey of ear-invading insects from 2001 to 2003 in the Tygerburg Hospital in South Africa and found that cockroaches and flies were the most frequent insects seen, and they were recovered by the use of forceps, suction or syringing.[11] Yaroko and Irfan did a survey in 2010 of insects found in patients' ears in the Universiti Sains Hospital in Malaysia.[12] They mainly found ticks and some beetles and cockroaches. If alive, the insect was killed with liquid paraffin and lignocaine local anaesthetic spray before being sucked out. Bhargava and Victor in 1999 reported on a case in Oman where a carabid beetle had entered the ear canal, chewed through the tympanic membrane and found its way into the middle ear, causing damage to the patient's hearing.[13] The offending insect had to be removed under a general anaesthetic.

Hair products

The Egyptian Ebers papyrus contains a number of recipes for products to treat greying of the hair and for baldness.[14]

E459: A treatment for greying: Blood of a black ox, added to oil/fat and then applied to the head.

E465: To cause hair to grow on a bald person: Lion fat, hippopotamus fat, crocodile fat, cat fat, serpent fat, ibex fat, all made into a mass and applied to the head.

One of the earliest treatments for dandruff is mentioned in Aulus Cornelius Celsus's book *De Medicina* written in the first century CE.[15] He felt the dandruff was caused by an excessive discharge of humour and treated it with labdanum (the resin from the *Cistus* shrub) with myrtle oil and wine, or myrobalans with wine. Myrobalans is the name given to the astringent fruits of several species of *Terminalia*, which are native to South Asia from India and Nepal east to south-west China, and south to Sri Lanka, Malaysia, and Vietnam.

The first hair colours were derived from plant sources and insects.[16] Henna is a brown/orange dye prepared from the plant *Lawsonia inermis*, also known as the henna tree. Natural blue indigo dye was obtained from plants in the genus *Indigofera*, native to the tropics, notably the Indian subcontinent. Chamomile highlights blonde or fair hair. These dyes were used to colour hair in ancient Egypt. Lemon juice, sulphur and honey were used to encourage bleaching of hair.

In his book *De Materia Medica*, Dioscorides described many materials which he claimed could be used to colour hair.[17]. These included cypress leaves with vinegar, henna leaves in quince juice, dyer's buckthorn, the shittah tree, holm oak bark boiled in water, sumac leaves, extract of myrtle, nettles, mulberry leaves boiled in water with leaves of the grapevine and black fig, ivy berries, sage, mullein flowers, burweed, elder roots and copper sulphate. These natural materials were all that was available until the nineteenth century.

In 1867, chemist E.H. Thiellay, with Leon Hugot, a hairdresser, showed that hydrogen peroxide could be used for lightening or bleaching hair.

William Perkin, a student at the Royal College of Chemistry (now Imperial College London), conducted a series of experiments in 1856, suggested by the college's director, the German chemist, Professor August Wilhelm von Hoffman. Hoffman was trying to make a synthetic quinine for the treatment of malaria, and asked Perkin to carry out this research. After one failed attempt, in which he oxidised a compound called aniline, Perkin washed out his flask with alcohol and noticed the reaction created a purple substance. A refined version of this substance, which Perkin called mauveine, became the first synthetic dye. Hoffman worked with Perkin's discovery and in turn made the molecule called para-phenylenediamine, which darkens on exposure to air.[18] In 1909, Eugène Paul Louis Schueller, a young French chemist, developed a hair dye formula using para-phenylene diamine which he called *Oréale*. He manufactured his own products, which he sold to Parisian hairdressers.

This was the beginning of the future cosmetics and haircare company L'Oréal.

Dioscorides in *De Materia Medica* described a wide range of herbal and other materials to restore hair to bald patches.[19] These included barley meal and pitch, burnt walnut husks mixed with wine and oil, sea horse ash mixed with pitch, bear's fat, radish with honey, onion and chicken fat, asphodel root ash, maidenhair, wild carrot juice, and iron rust. To strengthen hair and stop it falling out, he recommended the following treatments: myrrh mixed with gum labdanum, wine and myrtle ointment, ground cabbage leaves, rock rose mixed with wine, myrrh and oil of myrtle, or aloes and wine. Gum labdanum is a sticky brown resin obtained from *Cistus* (rockrose) shrubs; it was collected by combing the beards and thighs of goats and sheep that had grazed on the shrubs. Olive oil or meal of fenugreek were used to treat scurf (dandruff).

During the nineteenth century and until the middle of the twentieth century, the prescription books from individual pharmacies showed that they also manufactured their own hair products – tonics and similar items. These contained ingredients such as rum and tincture of cantharides (the blister beetle) which would have irritated and stimulated the scalp. Hospital pharmacies also made their own in-house hair tonic products for patients. The 1941 Indexed Registry for University College Hospital Dispensary included two formulae for hair lotions.[20]

The pharmaceutical historian Peter Homan has reviewed the development of cures for baldness in the ancient world through to the twentieth century.[21] During the nineteenth century, proprietary products such as Harlene Hair Tonic produced by The Edwards Company of High Holborn in London were sold with the claim that 'Harlene produces luxuriant hair'. The 1873 edition of *Squire's Companion to the British Pharmacopoeia 1873* written by Peter Squires (chemist to Queen Victoria) included a formula for a hair lotion which contained cantharidin, the active drug from the cantharides blister beetle. This was still mentioned in the 1958 edition of *The Extra Pharmacopoeia, Martindale* as Squire's Hair Liniment.

The development of the drug minoxidil to treat alopecia (baldness) has been mentioned in Chapter 9 of this book.

Nail products

The Egyptian Ebers papyrus includes some remedies for nail disorders:[22]

E619: Remedy for a toenail: Honey and ochre ground with oil/fat and then applied and bandaged.

E622: For the treatment of a nail if it drops to the floor: Prepare natron, terebinth resin, oil/fat and ochre and spread on the toe.

Aulus Cornelius Celsus in his first century CE treatise *De Medicina* was the first to deal in any detail with skin, hair and nail problems as a group.

Most skin infections are due to a group of fungi called the dermatophytes. Dermatophytes are the main cause of athlete's foot and the fungal infections of the toenail and fingernail.[23] The German physician Georg Meissner (1829–1905), whilst still a student, was the first person to describe fungi in the nails of patients.[24] In 1854, the German physician and pathologist Rudolf Virchow gave the name *onychomycosis* to the fungal disease in nails. The fungus *Trichophyton rubrum* is the major cause of these conditions. It originated in West Africa, South-east Asia, Australia and Indonesia and spread to Europe and the US in the late nineteenth and early twentieth centuries.

The use of socks with modern shoes and boots, and changing rooms has led to many more cases of onychomycosis. The *Trichophyton* fungus mainly penetrates the nail and nail bed around the edges of the nail.

The first to apply a treatment for onychomycosis was Neumann in 1870, who used a solution of sodium hydroxide, mercuric chloride and terebinth oil (oil made from the turpentine tree). In 1880, the American dermatologist Edward Wigglesworth realised that an issue with this infection was the need to penetrate through the nail. He recommended scraping the nail with glass, then wetting it frequently with a solution of mercuric chloride. The British dermatologist Arthur Whitfield (1868–1947) devised Whitfield's ointment, which consisted of benzoic acid (a weak antifungal compound) and salicylic acid in a base of soft paraffin and coconut oil.[25] In 1907, this ointment was shown to have some effect on onychomycosis, and it was used for several decades.

After the Second World War, a number of antifungal products such as griseofulvin and ketoconazole were developed, which could be taken by mouth to treat fungal skin infections. A range of oral medicines have now been developed including terbinafine and itraconazole (approved in 1995).

Two newer medicines for fungal nail infections are amorolfine (discovered in 1978) and tioconazole (approved in 1982), and these are now available as nail lacquers which are painted onto the infected nail for between six and twelve months.[26]

Dental products

One of the Mesopotamian cuneiform tablets (VAT 8256) contains a collection of prescriptions for dental products. It includes what is probably the first mention of the tooth worm, felt for hundreds of years to be the cause of toothache. An herbal preparation which was used against the toothworm was the root of the false carob. Galbanum resin was used for loose teeth.[27]

An Egyptian dental cream from 3000 to 5000 BCE contained powdered ashes from oxen hooves, egg shells, pumice and myrrh. It was used to remove debris from the teeth. Twigs were used as toothpicks to remove food and debris.

The Ebers papyrus contains a number of recipes for remedies for tooth complaints:[28]

E740: A remedy for filling teeth: Scrapings of millstone, ochre, honey, made into a mass.

E741: Treatment for toothache: Notched sycamore figs, beans, honey, malachite, ochre, ground and powdered together and applied to the tooth.

Aulus Cornelius Celsus (25 BCE–50 CE) included a chapter on toothache in Book VI of his medical encyclopaedia *De Medicina*. A paste of poppy juice was applied inside and outside the tooth to relieve pain. If the tooth had to be removed, Celsus suggested that a peppercorn without its coating be inserted into the cavity of the tooth to split the tooth so it falls out. Also shredded alum could be put into the tooth to loosen it. For treatment of dental decay, Celsus recommended scraping the tooth and smearing it with crushed rose petals to which ox gall and myrrh had been added.

Dioscorides in his *De Materia Medica* included a large number of remedies for toothache, loose teeth and for cleaning teeth.[19] Olive oil, mastic, the juice of pickled olives, an extract of pomegranate flowers, vinegar with squill and alum with vinegar were all used to tighten loose teeth. Pine boiled in vinegar, cedar in vinegar, pressed olives boiled to a thick consistency, sumac gum, hart's horn boiled in vinegar, capers when chewed, ranunculus, sulphurwort, and spurge all treated toothache. One more dramatic remedy was to use a stingray to sting in the mouth causing the affected tooth to shatter and be ejected. Murex (sea snails) calcined (heated to a high temperature), calcined land snails, cuttlefish bone, aristolochia and ground pumice stone were all used to clean teeth. The bone and pumice stone would have provided abrasives.

Galen writing in the second century CE quoted a prescription from Diocles of Carystos (375–295 BCE), the Greek physician. This was for toothache and consisted of gum resin, opium, pepper, wax, lousewort, and Cnidic mezereum (a *Daphne* species, also known as the spurge laurel). These were all mixed and painted on the tooth.

Up until the nineteenth century there was no anaesthesia, so toothache was a misfortune that had to be endured and the only treatments were to use remedies which may or may not have been very effective. The Anglo-Saxon *Leechbook III* stated that toothache could be treated by chewing pepper, or cooking henbane roots in vinegar or wine, putting them next to the sore tooth and chewing. Since it was believed that tooth decay was caused by toothworms, some remedies were used to get rid of the worms. The *Leechbook III* recommended getting rid of toothworms by taking oak meal, henbane seed and wax, mixing them together and making them into a wax candle, which was burnt and the smoke allowed into the mouth to drive the worms out. The worms could then be collected on a sheet under the patient.

Abū Bakr Muhammad ibn Zakariyyā al-Rāzī (Rhazes) (854–925 CE) included a formula for a toothpowder in his works. This consisted of birthwort, ocean crab and mussels' ashes, honey, soda, borax, juniper, pumice, emery, mugwort and burnt wild thyme. For teething pain in infants he recommended massaging the gums with rabbit brain, chicken fat with grape juice and rose oil. For toothache he used colocynth pulp, opoponax, resin, myrrh and borax.

Hildegard of Bingen (1098–1179 CE) was a German Benedictine abbess, writer, composer, philosopher, and Christian mystic. Her writings on natural history include herbal remedies for diseases. For toothache, deadly nightshade warmed in water was applied to the jaw, and extracts of wormwood and vervain cooked in wine given to be drunk. She recommended curing the toothworm with the smoke of aloes and myrrh.

In 1528, Johannes Stockerus, the municipal physician in Ulm in Germany recommended the use of an amalgam of vitriol and mercury as a filling material for cavities in teeth.

Toothbrushes made from hog bristles were found in China from the era of the Tang Dynasty (619–907 CE). They began to be imported into Europe by travellers. There is a reference in the 1690 autobiography of the Oxford antiquary Anthony Wood to using a toothbrush which he had bought from a J. Barret.

Culpeper's *London Dispensatory* of 1653 contains reference to the burnt ashes of vine sticks being used 'to scour the teeth and make them as white as snow'. The 'Froath of the Sea' was also used to make teeth white – this sea foam would have contained natural surfactants. Bistort bruised and boiled in white wine and used as a mouthwash was stated to help inflammation and soreness of the mouth and fasten loose teeth.[30]. Bistort is a species of flowering plant in the dock family *Polygonaceae* native to Europe and north and west Asia.

In 1780, William Addis started to manufacture toothbrushes. He had been jailed for causing a riot in 1770, and whilst in prison had used a bone from a meal to design a toothbrush using bristles he obtained from one of his guards. After his death, his son took over running of the business and it continued as a family business until 1996.[31]

During the eighteenth century, toothpowders came into common use. They contained abrasives such as brick dust, orris, cuttlefish and earthenware together with sodium bicarbonate. The powders were coloured with cochineal, and often had an essential oil added for flavour.

At the end of the century, sodium borate was added which caused a foaming effect.

A dentist named Peabody was the first person to add a soap to toothpowder in 1824, when he used sodium palmitate. In the 1850s, John Harris added chalk (calcium carbonate). An American dentist Dr Washington Sheffield and his son founded the Sheffield Dentifrice Company in 1880 and also started selling a mouthwash. Two years later they started selling a tooth cream in a collapsible tube [32]. The formula of the cream included chalk, orris, soap, cuttlefish, carmine, myrrh, cinchona, syrup, glycerine, mint, fennel and wintergreen essence. Colgate and Company also started selling toothpaste in the late nineteenth century.

In 1892, Sir James Crichton-Browne, who was a leading British psychiatrist, neurologist and medical psychologist, speculated on the reasons for the large proportion of children whose teeth were affected by dental decay. His essay in the *Lancet* was entitled '*An Address on Tooth Culture*'.[34] One reason was that he felt that the diet of children had changed and that they no longer received sufficient fluoride in their diet to maintain the health of their teeth.

In the late nineteenth century, a number of dentists started using cocaine solution as a local anaesthetic to dull the pain of dental procedures and in 1903, the German surgeon Heinrich Braun recommended the addition of adrenaline to cause narrowing of the blood vessels so that the effect of anaesthetic drugs were kept to a small area. A new local anaesthetic medicine, procaine, was developed in 1905 by Alfred Einhorn and Richard Willstätter. The product was marketed by the firm of Hoechst under the trade name 'Novocaine'. Heinrich Braun introduced procaine into clinical medicine. It was used in conjunction with adrenaline for dental operations.

In 1914, British Patent GB 3034 was filed for 'improvements in or relating to dentifrices' containing sodium fluoride, although the first fluoridated toothpastes were not sold until the 1950s. After the Second World War, the soap in the toothpaste was replaced by the synthetic surfactant sodium laurilsulfate. The formulation of toothpastes gradually improved to improve stain removal, combat tooth decay, to add antiplaque agents such as triclosan, to desensitise teeth, add dyes for visual appeal and flavours for breath-freshening. Today's toothpastes can contain up to twenty ingredients.

Animal bristles in toothbrushes were replaced just before the Second World War by synthetic materials, usually nylon. The first electric toothbrush, the Broxodent, was invented in Switzerland in 1954.

Notes

Preface
1. Wellcome Library, MS 5661 *1880 Prescription Book*, R. Woollatt and Boyd Chemists.
2. Wellcome Library, MS 5664 *1901/2 Prescription Book*, R. Woollatt and Boyd Chemists.
3. Wellcome Library, GC/100/1 *1899/1900 Prescription Dispensing Book*, Armitage Dispensing Chemists.
4. Wellcome Library, GC/100/27 *1938/1939 Prescription Dispensing Book*, Armitage Dispensing Chemists.
5. Royal London Hospital Archives, RLHLH/PH/1/2 *1899–1902 Drug Purchase Ledger*.
6. Royal London Hospital Archives, RLHLH/PA/1/3 *1910–1914 Drug Register*.
7. Royal London Hospital Archives, RLHBH/PH/2/1 *1944–1945 Brompton Hospital Formulae for Tablets*.
8. Herbal Medicines Market Size and Forecast, *Hexa Research September 2017 Market Research Report*.
9. Posadzki, P. et al., Prevalence of herbal medicine use by UK patients/consumers: a systematic review of surveys, *Focus on Alternative and Complementary Therapies*, 18: 19–26 (2013).

Chapter 1: Early Medicines: From Prehistory to Mesopotamian and Egyptian Medicine
1. Samorini, G., *Animals and Psychedelics. The Natural World and the Instinct to Alter Consciousness*, English translation, Park Street Press, Rochester, Vermont (2002).
2. Pope, H.G., *Tabernanthe iboga*: an African Narcotic Plant of Social Importance, *Economic Botany*, 23(2), 174–184 (1968).
3. Hart, B.L., Behavioural defences in animals against pathogens and parasites: parallels with the pillars of medicines in humans, *Phil. Trans. R. Soc.*, 366, 3406–3417 (2011).
4. Huffman, M.A and Caton, J.M., Self-induced Increase of Gut Motility and the Control of Parasitic Infections in Wild Chimpanzees, *International Journal of Primatology*, 22(3): 329–345 (2001).
5. Huffman, M.A., Chapter 2 in *Monkeys, Apes and Humans*, Springer Japan (2013).
6. Wrangham, R.W. & Nishida, T., *Aspilia* spp. Leaves: A puzzle in the feeding behaviour or wild chimpanzees, *Primates* 24(2): 276–282 (1983).
7. Barelli, C. and Huffman, M.A., Leaf swallowing and parasite expulsion in Khao Yai white-handed gibbons, the first report in an Asian ape species, *Am. J. Primatol.* 79: 1–7 (2016).
8. Mee, A. et al., Observations of Parrots at a Geophagy Site in Bolivia, *Biota Neotropica* 5(2): 1–4 (2005).
9. Gilardi, J.D. et al., Biochemical Functions of Geophagy in Parrots: Detoxification of Dietary Toxins and Cytoprotective Effects, *Journal of Chemical Ecology*, 25(4): 897–922 (1999).
10. Dediu, D. and Levinson, S.C., On the antiquity of language: the reinterpretation of Neanderthal linguistic capabilities and its consequences, *Frontiers in psychology* 4: 1–17 (2013).

11. De Rios, M.D, *Hallucinogens. Cross-Cultural Perspectives*, Prism Press (1990).
12. Hardy, K, and Kubiak-Martens, L., *Wild harvest: Plants in the hominin and pre-agrarian worlds*, Oxford Books (2016).
13. Sistiaga, A. et al., The Neanderthal Meal: A New Perspective Using Faecal Biomarkers, PLOS ONE 9(6): e101045 (2014).
14. Hardy, K. et al., Neanderthal medics? Evidence for food, cooking and medicinal plants trapped in dental calculus, *Naturwissenschaften* 99: 617–626 (2012).
15. Solecki, R., Shanidar IV, a Neanderthal Burial in Northern Iraq, *Science* 190(4217): 880–881 (1975).
16. Martkoplishvili, I. and Kvavadze, E., Some popular medicinal plants and diseases of the Upper Palaeolithic in Western Georgia, *Journal of Ethnopharmacology* 166: 42–52 (2015).
17. Dillehay, T.D. et al., Early Holocene coca chewing in Northern Peru, *Antiquity* 84(326): 939–953 (2010).
18. De Rios, M.D, *Hallucinogens. Cross-Cultural Perspectives*, Prism Press (1990).
19. Merlin, M.D., Archaeological Evidence for the Tradition of Psychoactive Plant Use in the Old World, *Economic Botany* 57(3): 295–323 (2003).
20. Xie, M. et al., Interdisciplinary Investigation on Ancient Ephedra Twigs from Gumugou Cemetery in Xinjiang Region, Northwest China, *Microscopy Research and Technique* 76; 663–672 (2013).
21. Fowler, B., *Iceman, Uncovering the Life and Times of a Prehistoric Man found in an Alpine Glacier*, Macmillan (2000).
22. Glob, P.V., *The Mound People. Danish Bronze-Age Man Preserved*, Faber and Faber (1974).
23. McGovern, P.E., *Uncorking the Past. The Quest for Wine, Beer and other Alcoholic Beverages*, University of California Press (2009).
24. Kramer, S.N., *From the Tablets of Sumer*, Falcon's Wing Press (1956).
25. Campbell-Thompson, R., *Assyrian Medical Texts*, Oxford University Press (1923).
26. Geller, M.G., *Ancient Babylonian Medicine. Theory and Practice*, Wiley-Blackwell (2010).
27. Nunn, J.F., *Ancient Egyptian Medicine*, British Museum Press (1996).
28. Ghalioungui, P., *The Ebers Papyrus. A New English Translation*, Academy of Scientific Research and Technology, Cairo (1987).
29. Al-Snafi, A.E., Chemical constituents and pharmacological effects of Citrullus colocynthis – A review, *IOSR Journal of Pharmacy* 6(3); 57–67 (2013).
30. Roy, R.K. et al., Effect of Citrullus colocynthis on Hair Growth in Albino Rats, *Pharmaceutical Biology* 45(10): 739–744 (2007).
31. Haimov-Kochman, R. et al,, Reproduction concepts and practices in ancient Egypt mirrored by modern medicine, *European Journal of Obstetrics and Gynaecology and Reproductive Biology* 123: 3–8 (2005).
32. Nunn, J.F., *Ancient Egyptian Medicine*, British Museum Press (1996).

Chapter 2: Hippocrates and Greek Medicine

1. Arnott, R., Healing and medicine in the Aegean Bronze Age, *Journal of the Royal Society of Medicine* 89: 265–270 (1996).
2. Warren, C.P.W., Some aspects of medicine in the Greek Bronze Age, *Medical History* 14(4): 364–377 (1970).
3. Merlin, M.D., Archaeological Evidence for the Tradition of Psychoactive Plant Use in the Old World, *Economic Botany* 57(3): 295–323 (2003).
4. Jouanna, J., *Hippocrates* translated by M.B. DeBevoise, John Hopkins University Press (1999).

5. Scarborough, J. ed., *Folklore and Folk Medicine, Recognition of Drugs in Classical Antiquity*, American Institute of the History of Pharmacy (1987).
6. Totelin, L., *Hippocratic Recipes. Oral and Written Transmission of Pharmacological Knowledge in Fifth- and Fourth-Century Greece*, Brill, Leiden (2009).
7. Touwaide, A. & Appetiti, E., Food and medicines in the Mediterranean tradition. A systematic analysis of the earliest extant body of textual evidence, *Journal of Ethnopharmacology* 167: 11–29 (2015).
8. Jones, W.H.S, *Hippocrates. With an English translation*, William Heinemann Ltd (1931).
9. Thanos, C., *Chapter 1 on Aristotle and Theophrastus on plant-animal interactions in Plant-Animal Interactions in Mediterranean-Type Ecosystems edited Arianoutsou, M and Groves, R.H*, Kluwer Academic Publishers (1994).
10. Gow, A.S.F. and Scholfield. A.F., *Nicander, the Poems and Poetical Fragments*, Cambridge University Press (1953).

Chapter 3: Galen and Roman Medicine

1. Celsus, *De Medicina. With English translation by W.G. Spencer*, William Heinemann Ltd Loeb Classical Library (1935).
2. ibid.
3. Scribonius, Largus, *Compositiones Médicales. Text established, translated and commented on by J. Jouanna-Bouchet*, Les Belles Lettres, Paris (2016).
4. Jourdan, P., *Notes de Critique Verbale sur Scribonius Largus*, Librairie C. Klincksieck, Paris (1919).
5. Riddle, J.M., *Dioscorides on Pharmacy and Medicine*, University of Texas Press, Austin (1985).
6. Pedanius Dioscorides of Anazarbus, *De Materia Medica. Translated by L.Y. Beck*, Alterumwissenschaftliche Texte und Studien Band 38, Olms-Weidmann (2017).
7. Mattern, S.P., *The Prince of Medicine. Galen in the Roman Empire*, Oxford University Press (2013).
8. Galeni, Claudii, *Opera Omnia. Editionem curavit Kühn, C. G.* Reprinted Leipzig, Georg Olms (1964/5).
9. Grant, M., *Galen on Food and Diet*, Routledge (2002).
10. Hankinson, R.J. ed., *The Cambridge Companion to Galen*, Cambridge University Press (2008).
11. Debru, A. ed., Galen on Pharmacology: Philosophy, History and Medicine, *Proceedings of the Vth International Galen Colloquium, Lille, 16–18 March 1995*, Brill, Leiden (1997).
12. Davies, R.W., Some Roman Medicine, *Medical History* 14(1): 106–107 (1970).
13. Summerton, N., *Medicine and Healthcare in Roman Britain*, Shire Archaeology Book (2007).

Chapter 4: Avicenna and the Arabian Period

1. Browning, R. and Nutton, V., *"Oribasius", from The Oxford Classical Dictionary Hornblower. S and Spawforth A, ed.*, Oxford University Press (2003).
2. Bouros-vallianatos, P., Clinical Experience in Late Antiquity: Alexander of Tralles and the Therapy of Epilepsy, *Med. Hist.* 58(3): 337–353 (2014).
3. Forrest, R.D., Early history of wound treatment, *Journal of the Royal Society of Medicine* 75: 198–205 (1982).
4. Francis Adams, *Seven books of Paulus Aegineta. Translated from the Greek by Francis Adams*, The Sydenham Society (1844).

5. Modanlou, H., A Tribute to Zakariya Razi (865–925 AD), An Iranian Pioneer Scholar, *Arch Iranian Med* 11(6): 673–677 (2008).
6. Lakhatakia, R., A Trio of Exemplars of Medieval Islamic Medicine. Al-Razi, Avicenna and Ibn Al-Nafis, *Sultan Qaboos University Med J.* 14(4): 455–459 (2014).
7. Mcginnis, J., *Avicenna*, Oxford University Press (2010).
8. Goodman, L.E., *Avicenna*, Routledge (1992).
9. Gruner, O.C., *A Treatise on The Canon of Medicine of Avicenna Incorporating a Translation of The First Book*, Augustus M. Kelley, New York (1970).
10. Heydari, M et al., Medicinal Aspects of Opium As Described in Avicenna's Canon of Medicine, *Acat med-hist Adriat* 11(1): 101–112 (2013).

Chapter 5: Medicines in the Medieval World

1. Kyle, E., *The English Correspondence of St Boniface. Translated and Edited with an Introductory Sketch of the Saint's Life*, Chatto and Windus, London (1911).
2. Cameron, M.L., *Anglo-Saxon Medicine*, Cambridge University Press (1993).
3. Pettit, E., *Anglo-Saxon Remedies, Charms, Prayers from the British Library MS Harley 585. The Lacnunga*, Edward Mellen Press, Lampeter (2001).
4. Arsdall, A. Van, *Medieval herbal remedies: The Old English Herbarium and Anglo-Saxon medicine*, Routledge (2002).
5. Kristeller, O.P., The School of Salerno. Its development and its contribution to the history of learning, *Bulletin of the History of Medicine (Baltimore)*, 17: 138–194 (1945).
6. Singer, C and Sigerist, H.E., *The Origins of the Medical School of Salerno, the First University, An Attempted Reconstruction*, Verlag Seldwyla, Zurich (1924).
7. Conrad, L.I. et al., *The Western Medical Tradition 800 BC to AD 1800*, Cambridge University Press (1995).
8. Hammond, E., Physicians in Medieval English Religious Houses, *Bulletin of the History of Medicine* Vol XXXII(2): 105–120 (1958).
9. Barry, G. and Carruthers, L.A., *A History of Britain's Hospitals*, The Book Guild (2005).
10. Getz, F., *Gilbert the Englishman*, Oxford Dictionary of National Biography (2016).
11. McVaugh, M., An early discussion of medicinal degrees at Montpellier by Henry of Winchester, *Bulletin of the History of Medicine* 49(1): 57–71 (1975).
12. Demaitre, L.E., *Doctor Bernard de Gordon: Professor and Practitioner*, Pontifical Institute of Medieval Studies. Toronto (1980).
13. Trease, G., *Pharmacy in History*, 45–46. Baillière, Tindall and Cox (1964).
14. Chaucer, G., *The Canterbury Tales. A Rendering for Modern Readers by F.E. Hill*, George Allen and Unwin (1936).
15. Capener, M., Chaucer and John of Gaddesden, *Ann Roy Coll Surg* 50: 283–300 (1972).
16. Trease, G., *Pharmacy in History*, Baillière, Tindall and Cox (1964).

Chapter 6: Paracelsus, the Alchemists and their Legacy

1. Haq, S.N., *Names, Natures and Things: The Alchemist Jabir ibn Hayyan and his Kitab al-Ahjar (Book of Stones)*, Springer Science and Business Media (1995).
2. Debus, A.G., *Chemistry and Medical Debate, Van Helmont to Boerhave*, Science History Publications, USA (2001).
3. Ball, P., *The Devil's Doctor. Paracelsus and the World of Renaissance Magic and Science*, William Heinemann, London (2006).
4. Shackleford, J., *A Philosophic Path for Paracelsian Medicine. The Ideas, Intellectual Context, and Influence of Petrus Severinus*, Museum Tusculanum Press, University of Copenhagen (2004).

5. Rosenfeld, L., The Last Alchemist – The First Biochemist: J.B. van Helmont (1577–1644), *Clinical Chemistry* 31(10): 1755–1780 (1985).
6. Walton, M.T., *The Chemical Philosophy and Kabbalah in Bridging Traditions. Alchemy, Chemistry and Paracelsian Practices in the Modern Era. Edited Parshall, K et al.* Early Modern Studies 15, Truman State University Press, Missouri (2015).
7. Trevor-Roper, H., *Europe's Physician. The Various Life of Sir Theodore de Mayerne*, Yale University Press (2006).
8. Cushing, H., *A Bio-Bibliography of Andreas Vesalius*, Yale University (1943).
9. Wright, Thomas, *Circulation: William Harvey's Revolutionary Idea*, London: Chatto (2012).
10. Drygas, A., Was Valerius Cordus the Discoverer of Ether? *Archiwum Historii Filozofi Medcyny* 60(4): 427–444 (1997).
11. Cartwright, A.C., *The British Pharmacopoeia, 1864 to 2014*, Ashgate (2015).
12. Colledge of Physicians, Certain Necessary Directions as well as For the Cure of the Plague, *Printed by John Bill and Christopher Barker, Printers to the Kings most Excellent Majesty* (1665).
13. Malcolmson, J.G., *A Practical Essay on the History and Treatment of Beriberi*, Vepery Mission Press, Madras (1835).
14. Morton, H.V., *A Traveller in Italy*, Methuen and Co Ltd (1964).
15. Wall, C., *A History of the Worshipful Society of Apothecaries of London. Revised, annotated and edited by Underwood, E.A.*, Oxford (1963).
16. Wallis, P. and Jenner, M.R., *Medicines and the Market in England and its Colonies, c. 1450–c. 1850*, Palgrave Macmillan (2007).
17. Anon., *The Oriental Navigator or Directions for Sailing To and Fro from the East Indies. To which is added The India Officers and Traders Guide in purchasing Drugs and Spices of Asia and the East Indies*, James Humphreys, Philadelphia (1801).
18. Mortimer, I., *The Dying and the Doctors. The Medical Revolutions in Seventeenth-Century England*, Boydell Press (2009).
19. Mackintosh, A., The Patent Medicines Industry in Late Georgian England: A Respectable Alternative to both Regular Medicine and Irregular Practice, *Social history of medicine* 30(1): 22 (2016).
20. Holloway, V., *The Mighty Healer. Thomas Holloway's Victorian Patent Medicine Empire*, Pen & Sword (2016).

Chapter 7: Medicines from Natural Products

1. Holmes, O.W., Currents and Counter-Currents in Medical Science, Address to Massachusetts Medical Society (30 May 1860). In *Medical Essays 1842–1882*, 202–3 (1891).
2. Calder, R., *The Life Savers*, Pan Books Ltd, London (1961).
3. Travilian, T.E. ed., *Pliny the Elder, the Natural History Book VII*, Bloomsbury Academic (2015).
4. Pedanius Dioscorides of Anazarbus, *De Materia Medica. Third revised edition. Translated by Beck, L. Y.*, Olms-Weidmann (2017).
5. Arber, A., *Herbals – Their Origin and Evolution. A Chapter in the History of Botany. Third Edition*, Cambridge University Press (1990).
6. Anderson, F., *An illustrated history of the Herbals*, Columbia University Press (1977).
7. Parkinson, A., *Nature's Alchemist, John Parkinson, Herbalist to Charles I*, Frances Lincoln Ltd. (2007).

8. Parkinson, J., *Paradisi in Sole Paradisus Terrestris. Faithfully Reprinted From The Edition of 1629*, Methuen and Co. (1904).

9. Parkinson, J., *Theatrum Botanicum*, Tho Cotes (1640).

10. Woolley, B., *Nicholas Culpeper and the fight for medical freedom*, Harper Perennial (2004).

11. Grieve, M., *A Modern Herbal. First published 1931, edited and introduced by Leyel, C.F.* Peregrine Books (1976).

12. Chast, F., *Histoire contemporaine des médicaments*, Editions La Découverte (1995).

13. Stone, W., An Account of the Success of the Bark of the Willow in the Cure of Agues. Letter to Rt Hon. George Early of Macclesfield from Rev. Edmund Stone, *Philosophical Transactions* 53(1763): 195–200 (1763).

14. Nicolaides, A., Assessing Medical Practice and Surgical Technology in the Egyptian Pharaonic Era, *Medical Technology SA.* 27(1): 20–25 (2013).

15. Doetsch, R.N., Studies on Biogenesis by Sir William Roberts, *Medical History* 7: 232–240 (1963).

16. Zhang, L. & Demain, A.L., *Natural Products: Drug Discovery and Therapeutic Medicine*, Totowa, N.J.: Humana Press (2005).

17. Worboys, M., *Fleming, Sir Alexander (1885–1955)*, Oxford Dictionary of National Biography, Oxford University Press (2011).

18. Wainright, M. & Swan, H.T., C.G. Paine and the Earliest Surviving Clinical Records of Penicillin Therapy, *Medical History* 30; 42–56 (1986).

19. Pringle, P., *Experiment Eleven: Deceit and Betrayal in the Discovery of the Cure for Tuberculosis*, Bloomsbury Publishing (2012).

20. Keith, G.W., Benjamin Minge Duggar: 1872–1956. *Mycologia* 49(3): 434–438 (1957).

21. Doyle, L., Myxoedema: some early reports and contributions by British authors, *J Royal Soc Medicine* 84: 103–106 (1991).

22. Mellanby, E., An Experimental Investigation on Rickets, *Nutrition Reviews* 34(11): 338–340 (2009).

23. Dobson, M., Experiments and observation of the Urine in diabetes, *Med Obs Inq* 5: 298–316 (1766).

24. Lee, M.R., William Withering (1741–1799): A Birmingham Lunatic, *Proc Royal Coll Physicians Edinburg.* 31: 77–83 (2001).

25. Proskurnina, N.F. and Areshkina, L.J., On the alkaloids from Galanthus Woronowi *Z. obst. Chem.* 22: 1899–1902 (1947).

26. Mucke, H.A.M, The case of galantamine: repurposing and late blooming of a cholinergic drug, *Future Science OA.* Published Online:3 Sep 2015 https://doi.org/10.4155/fso.15.73 (2015).

27. Newman, D.J. & Cragg, G., Natural Products As Sources of New Drugs over the 30 Years from 1981 to 2010, *Journal of Natural Products* 75: 311–335 (2012).

28. *WHO Traditional Medicine Strategy 2014–2023*, World Health Organization, Geneva (2013).

29. Anon., CBI Trade Statistics: Natural Ingredients for Health Products in Europe, *CBI Market Intelligence, The Netherlands* (2015).

30. Anon., CBI Trade Statistics. Natural Ingredients for Health Products in France, *CBI Market Intelligence, The Netherlands* (2015).

31. Anon., CBI Product Factsheet: Natural Ingredients for Health Products in the United Kingdom, *CBI Market Intelligence, The Netherlands* (2015).

32. Arrête Royal du 29 Août 1997 relatif à la fabrication et au commerce de denrées alimentaires composées ou contenant de plantes ou préparations de plantes. (M.B. 21 XI.1997)

https://www.health.belgium.be/sites/default/files/uploads/fields/fpshealth_theme_file/consolidated_version_rd_29_august_1997_v10-02-2017_fr.pdf (Accessed 2 April 2019).

33. Ernst, E., The Risk-Benefit Profile of Commonly Used Herbal Therapies: Gingko, St John's Wort, Ginseng, Echinacea, Saw Palmetto, and Kava, *American College of Physicians Annals of Internal Medicine* 156(1): 42–50 (2002).

34. Bent, S. et al., Valerian for Sleep: A Systematic Review and Meta-Analysis, *The American Journal of Medicine* 119: 105–1012 (2006).

Chapter 8: The First Synthetic Medicines

1. Bause, G.S. & Sim, P.P., Valerius Cordus Synthesizes Sulfuric Ether – the Wood Library-Museum's "New" Tome from 1561, *American Society of Anesthesiologists Monitor* 73: 20–23 (2009).

2. Ball, P., *The Devil's Doctor. Paracelsus and the World of Renaissance Magic and Science*, William Heinemann (2006).

3. Butler, T.C., The Introduction of Chloral Hydrate into Medical Practice, *Bulletin of the History of Medicine* 44(2): 168–172 (1970).

4. Brune, K. & Hinz, B., The Discovery and Development of Antiinflammatory Drugs, *Arthritis and Rheumatism* 50(8): 2391–2399 (2004).

5. Ugurlucan, M. et al., Aspirin: From a Historical Perspective, *Recent Patents on Cardiovascular Drug Discovery* 7: 71–76 (2012).

6. Anon., Bicentenary of Nitrous Oxide. *British Medical Journal* 2(5810): 367–368 (1972).

7. Stratmann, L., *Chloroform – The Quest for Oblivion*, Sutton Publishing (2003).

8. Marsh, N. & Marsh, A., A Short History of Nitroglycerine and Nitric Oxide in Pharmacology and Physiology, *Clinical and Experimental Pharmacology* 27: 313–319 (2000).

9. Bosch, F. & Rosich, L., The Contributions of Paul Ehrlich to Pharmacology: A Tribute on the Occasion of the Centenary of His Nobel Prize. *Pharmacology* 82(3): 171–179 (2008).

10. Raviña, E., Fathers of chemotherapy, pp 48–50 in The *Evolution of Drug Discovery*, Wiley-VCH Verlag GmbH and Co (2011).

11. Gilbert, M., *Winston S. Churchill, Volume VII*, London, Heinemann (1986).

12. Rang, H.P., The receptor concept: pharmacology's big idea, *British Journal of Pharmacology* 147: S9–S16 (2006).

13. Quirke, V., Putting Theory into Practice: James Black, Receptor Theory and the Development of the Beta-Blockers at ICI, 1958–1978, *Medical History* 50: 69–92 (2006).

Chapter 9: Modern Medicine Developments

1. Walpole, H., *Letter of 28 January 1754 written to Horace Mann* (1754).

2. Ban, T., The role of serendipity in drug discovery. *Dialogues in clinical neuroscience* 8(1): 335–344 (2006).

3. Ghofrani, H.A. et al., Sildenafil: from angina to erectile dysfunction to pulmonary hypertension and beyond, *Nature Living* 5: 689–693 (2006).

4. Li, J.J., *Blockbuster Drugs – The Rise and Decline of the Pharmaceutical Industry*, Oxford University Press (2014).

5. Maehle, A-H., A binding question: the evolution of the receptor concept, *Endeavour* 33(4): 135–140 (2009).

6. Smith, C.G. & O'Donnell, J.T. ed., *The Process of New Drug Discovery and Development. Second Edition*, Informa Healthcare (2006).

7. Higuchi, S. et al., Alcohol and aldehyde dehydrogenase polymorphisms and the risk for alcoholism, *Am J Psychiatry* 252(8): 1219–1221 (1995).

8. Fredrick, E.E., Glucose-6-Phosphate Dehydrogenase Deficiency in Congenital Hemolytic Disease, *Journal of the National Medical Association* 54(5): 576–583 (1962).
9. Becquemont, L. et al., Practical recommendations for pharmacogenomics-based prescription: 2010 ESF-UB Conference on Pharmacogenetics and Pharmacogenomics, *Pharmacogenomics* 12(1): 113–124 (2011).
10. Zhou, S. et al., Thalidomide – A Notorious Sedative to a Wonder Anticancer Drug, *Curr Med Chem* 20(33): 4102–4108 (2013).

Chapter 10: Biotechnology, Biopharmaceuticals and Biosimilars

1. Hammarsten, J.F. et al., Who discovered smallpox vaccination? Edward Jenner or Benjamin Jesty? *Trans Am Clin Climatol Assoc* 90: 44–55 (1979).
2. Riedel, S., Edward Jenner and the History of Smallpox and Vaccination, *Baylor University Medical Center Proceedings* 18(1): 21–25 (2005).
3. Nutton, V., The seeds of disease: An explanation of contagion and infections from the Greeks to the Renaissance, *Medical History* 27: 1–34 (1983).
4. Plotkin, S. ed., *History of vaccine development*, Springer New York (2011).
5. Blevins, S.M. & Bronze, M.S., Robert Koch and the 'golden age' of bacteriology, *International Journal of Infectious Diseases* 14: e744–e751 (2010).
6. Kantha, S.S., A Centennial Review; the 1890 Tetanus Antitoxin Paper of von Behring and Kitasato and the Related Developments, *Keio J Med* 40(1): 35–39 (1990).
7. Marks, L.V., *The Lock and Key of Medicine. Monoclonal Antibodies and the Transformation of Healthcare*, Yale University Press (2015).
8. Hughes, S.S., Making dollars out of DNA. The first major patent in biotechnology and the commercialization of molecular biology, 1974–1980, *Isis* 92(3): 541–575 (2001).
9. Bhopale, G.M. & Nanda, R.K., Recombinant DNA expression products for human therapeutic use, *Current Science* 89(4): 614–622 (2005).
10. Robinson, J., Preparing for the big biologic switch, *Pharmaceutical Journal* 301(7916): 88–91 (2018).

Chapter 12: Medicines Taken by Mouth

1. Campbell J., Campbell, J. & David, R., An Insight into the Practice of Pharmacy in Ancient Egypt, *Pharmaceutical Historian* 35(4): 62–68 (2005).
2. Campbell, J., An assessment of the pharmaceutical and therapeutic merit of remedies within the Kahun, Edwin Smith, Ebers and Chester Beatty ancient Egyptian medical papyri, *PhD thesis University of Manchester* (2007).
3. Schlosser, S., Distillation – from Bronze Age till today, *Proceedings of the Thirty-eighth International Conference of Slovak Society of Chemical Engineering* 1–12 (2011).
4. *Pharmacopoeia Augustana, 1927 Facsimile edition with introductory essays by Theodore Husemann* published by the State Historical Society of Wisconsin.
5. Culpeper, N., *Pharmacopoeia Londinensis or the London Dispensatory*, Printed for Peter Cole (1653).
6. *Apothecary's Account Book, Odiham, 1774–1782*, MS 3974 Wellcome Library.
7. *Apothecary Prescription Book for the 1770s, Batt family*, MS 5201 Wellcome Library.
8. Cooley, A.J., *A Cyclopaedia of Practical Receipts and Collateral Information in the Arts, Manufactures, Professions and Trades, Page 334*, John Churchill (1856).
9. *Pharmaceutical Journal* (1870–71), 1(3): 149.
10. *Record of Prescriptions from Lewis's Chemists, West Street, Ware, 1854–1855*, DE/X1008/1/2, Hertfordshire Archives.

11. *Record of Prescriptions from Lewis's Chemists, West Street, Ware 1896 to 1900*, DE/ X1008/1/3, Hertfordshire Archives.

12. Armitage Dispensing Chemist, *Prescription Dispensing Book 1899–1904*, GC/100/1, Wellcome Library.

13. Brown, P.S., Medicines Advertised in Eighteenth-Century Bath Newspapers, *Medical History* 20: 152–168 (1976).

14. Armitage Dispensing Chemist, Blackheath, *Prescriptions Register 1938–1940*, GC/100/27 Wellcome Library.

15. Cook, I.J. & Kahrilas, P.J., AGA Technical Review on Management of Oropharyngeal Dysphagia, *Gastroenterology* 116: 455–478 (1999).

16. Smith, S.M., Schroeder, K. & Fahey, T., Over-the-counter (OTC) medications for acute cough in children and adults in community settings, *Cochran Systematic Review* (2014).

17. Olabisi, O. et al., Honey for acute cough in children, *Cochran Systematic Review* (2018).

18. Pariente, L., Note sur un procédé nouveau pour l'administration de certaines substances médicanmenteuses, Guilliermond M A in *Naissance et Evolution de Quinze Formes Pharmaceutiques, Editions Louis Pariente, Paris, p. 36* (1996).

19. Brierly, R. & Higby, G.J., The history of dosage forms, in *Encyclopaedia of Pharmaceutical Technology, Eds Swarbrick J, Boylan J C*: 1993, 7: 299–339 (1993).

20. Corley, T. A. B., *Beecham's from pills to pharmaceuticals*, Lancaster, Crucible Books (2011).

21. Jackson, W. A., Brockedon's press, *Pharm Hist*, 1987, 17: 2–3 (1987).

22. Anon, Brockedon's patent process, *Pharm J*, 1844, 3: 554 (1844).

23. Kebler, L. F., The tablet industry – its evolution and present status – the composition of tablets and methods of analysis, *J Amer Pharm Assoc*, 3: 820–848 (1914).

24. van Itallie, P. H., Pioneers of tablet making, *J Amer Pharm Assoc, Practical Pharmacy Edition* 20: 724–725 (1959).

25. Anon., The science and art of dispensing, *Pharm J* 87: 464–465 (1911).

26. Anon., A new tablet machine, *Pharm J*. 70: 512 (1903).

27. Foote, P. A., The Evolution of the Tablet Machine, Bulletin of the University of Wisconsin 1: 5–66 (1928).

28. Fairhome, R. F., Pharmaceutical notes, *Pharm J*. 27: 103–103 (1881).

29. Rogerson, M. and Son, British Enterprise at a Discount, *Chemist and Druggist*, 23: 510 (1881).

30. Newbery F. and Son, American compressed remedies, *Chemist and Druggist*, 23: 555 (1881).

31. Jones, T. M., Tablets, Tabloids … and tabloids, *Pharm J*. 230: 301–307 (1983).

32. 'Galen', Tabloids and the new British Pharmacopoeia, *Pharm J*. 54: 232 (1895).

33. Burroughs Wellcome & Co, Tabloids and Tablets, *Chemist and Druggist* 40: 785 (1892).

34. 'Apprentice', Compressed tablets, *Pharm J*. 51: 204 (1891).

35. Anon, The passing of the tablet fad, *Pharm J*. 54: 583–584 (1895).

36. Editorial, The tendency of tablet medication, *Pharm J*. 57: 535 (1896).

37. Parry E. J. & Estcourt P. A., Compressed drugs. Accuracy of dosage in tablets, *Pharm J*. 53: 592–593 (1894).

38. McFerran, J. A., On the compression of compressed tablets, *Pharm J*. 52: 972–974 (1893).

39. Editorial, Factory made medicines, *Pharm J*. 52: 1035 (1893).

40. Wall, W. A., Compressed tablet machine, *Pharm J*. 54: 432 (1895).

41. Foster, F., Compressed tablet machine *Pharm J*. 54: 452 (1895).

42. Gibbs, R. D., A new tablet compressing machine, *Pharm J*. 58: 548 (1897).

43. Anon, Tablets and Tabellae, *Chemist and Druggist* 37: 492, 531, 563, 603, 655 and 695 (1890).

44. Jones, B. *The history of the medicinal capsule, in Pharmaceutical Capsules, second edition Podczeck F, Jones B. E.*, London, Pharmaceutical Press 1–22 (2004).

Chapter 13: Medicines Given by Injection
1. Bestetti, R.B. et al., Development of Anatomophysiologic Knowledge Regarding the Cardiovascular System: From Egyptians to Harvey, *Arq Bras Cardio* 103(6): 538–545 (2014).
2. Amr, S.S. & Tbakhi, T., Ibn Al-Nafis: Discoverer of the Pulmonary Circulation, *Ann Saudi Med* 27(5): 385–387 (2007).
3. Trueta, J., Michael Servetus and the Discovery of the Lesser Circulation, *The Yale journal of biology and medicine* 21: 1–15 (1948).
4. Harvey, W., *Exercitatio anatomica de motu cordis et sanguinis in animalibus. Translated and edited by Keynes, G.* Palo Alto, California (1998).
5. Gibson, W.C., The Bio-medical Pursuits of Christopher Wren, *Medical History* 14: 331–341 (1970).
6. Reinbacher, W.R.,. *Leben, Arbeit und Umwelt des Arztes: Johann Daniel Major (1634–1693), Eine Biographie Aus Dem 17. Jahrhundert, Mit Neuen Erkenntnissen*, M. Kroeber (1998).
7. Gladstone, E., The Lure of Medical History. Johann Sigismund Elsholtz (1623–1688), I Introduction, *California and Western Medicine XXXVIII* (6), 432–434 (1933).
8. Gladstone, E., The Lure of Medical History. Johann Sigismund Elsholtz. II, *California and Western Medicine XXXIX* (1): 45–47 (1933).
9. Woodcroft, B. ed. and translator, *The Pneumatics of Hero of Alexandria*, Taylor, Walton and Maberly (1851).
10. Price, J., Dominique Anel and the Small Lachrymal Syringe, *Medical History* 13(4) : 340–354 (1969).
11. Champlan, D., *Un Novateur. Charles-Gabriel Pravaz*, Marcel Vigné, Paris (1931).
12. Blake, J.B., Mr Ferguson's Hypodermic Syringe, *Journal of the History of Medicine and Allied Sciences* 15(4): 337–341 (1960).
13. Hunter, C., *On the Speedy Relief of Pain and Other Nervous Affections By Means of The Hypodermic Method*, John Churchill & Sons (1865).
14. Schwidetzky, O., The History of Needles and Syringes, *Anesthesia and Analgesia* 23: 34–39 (1944).
15. Sacha, G. et al., Pre-filled syringes: a review of the history, manufacturing and challenges, *Pharmaceutical Development and Technology* 20(1): 1–11 (2015).
16. Kivitz, A. & Segurado, O.G., Humira Pen: a novel autoinjection device for subcutaneous injection of fully human monoclonal antibody adalimumab, *Expert Review Medical Devices* 4(2): 109–116 (2007).
17. Dauphin, A. et al., Les solutés de perfusion ; histoire d'une forme pharmaceutique majeure née à l'hôpital, *Revue d'Histoire de la Pharmacie* 338 : 219–238 (2003).
18. Latta, T., Malignant cholera, *Lancet* 1832 ; 1831–2, 2 : 274–277 (1832).
19. Asaleh, F.M. et al., Insulin pumps; from inception to the present and toward the future, *Journal of Clinical Pharmacy and Therapeutics* 35(2): 127–138 (2010).
20. Skyler, J.S., Continuous Subcutaneous Insulin Infusion–An Historical Perspective *Diabetes Technology & Therapeutics* 12(Supplement 1): S5–S9 (2010).
21. Graham, F. & Clark, D., The Syringe Driver and the Subcutaneous Route in Palliative Care: The Inventor, the History and the Implications, *Journal of Pain and Symptom Management* 29(1): 32–40 (2005).

22. Ravi, A.D. et al., Needle-free injection technology: A complete insight, *Int J Pharm Investig* 5(4): 192–199 (2015).
23. Potts, M. & Paxman, J.M., Depo-Provera – ethical issues in its testing and distribution, *Journal of medical ethics* 1: 9–20 (1984).
24. Valenstein, M. et al., Adherence assessments and the use of depot antipsychotics in patients with schizophrenia, *J Clin Psychiatry* 62(7): 545–551 (2001).

Chapter 14: Medicines Delivered On or Through the Skin

1. Geller, M.J. *Ancient Babylonian Medicine. Theory and Practice*, Wiley-Blackwell (2010).
2. Ghalioungui, P., *The Ebers Papyrus. A New English Translation, Commentaries and Glossaries*, Academy of Scientific Research and Technology, Cairo (1987).
3. Hawkins, J. *Investigating Antibacterial Plant-Derived Compounds from Natural Honey*, PhD Thesis School of Pharmacy and Pharmaceutical Sciences, Cardiff (2015).
4. Dioscorides, P., *De Materia Medica. Translated by Beck, L. Y. Third Revised Edition*, Olms-Weidmann. (2017).
5. Harrison, A.P. et al., Transdermal Opioid Patches for Pain Treatment in Ancient Egypt, *Pain Practice* 12(8): 620–625 (2012).
6. Cameron, M.L., *Chapter 12: Rational Medicine* in *Anglo-Saxon Medicine*, Cambridge University Press (1993).
7. Shim, K.M. et al., Effects of Aucubin on the Healing of Wounds, *In vivo* 21: 1037–1042 (2007).
8. White, P.A.S. et al., Antioxidant Activity and Mechanisms of Action of Natural Compounds Isolated from Lichens: A Systematic Review, *Molecules* 19: 14496–14527 (2014).
9. Rai, A., The Antiinflammatory and Antiarthritic Properties of Ethanol Extract of Hedera Helix, *Indian Journal of Pharmaceutical Sciences* 75(1): 99–102 (2013).
10. Culpeper, N., *Pharmacopoeia Londinensis, or The London Dispensatory Further Adorned by the Studies and Collections of the Fellows*, Printed for Peter Cole (1653).
11. Cartwright, A.C., *The British Pharmacopoeia, 1864 to 2014*, Ashgate (2015).
12. Griffenhagen, G., The lost art of plaster spreading, *Amer Journal Professional Pharmacist* 23(2): 139–143 (1957).
13. Kilmer, F.B., Manufacture of Medicinal Plasters, *Amer. Journal Pharmacy* 82(9): 416–428 (1910).
14. Pastore, M.N. et al., Transdermal patches: history, development and pharmacology, *British Journal of Pharmacology* 172(9): 2179–2209 (2015).
15. Walters, A. ed., *Chapter 4: Skin Transport in Dermatological and Transdermal Formulations*, Marcel Dekker Inc. (2002).
16. Paul Audouit of Havre, France, Improvement in Medicated Plasters, *US Patent Office Letters Patent No. 146,503* (1873).
17. Fiore, M.C. et al., The Effectiveness of the Nicotine Patch for Smoking Cessation, *JAMA* 271(24): 1940–1947 (1994).
18. Bariya, S.H., Micro-needles: an emerging transdermal drug delivery system, *Journal of Pharmacy and Pharmacology* 64(1): 11–29 (2012).

Chapter 15: Medicines Delivered to the Lungs

1. Shehata, M.A., History of Inhalation Therapy, *International Journal of Inhalation Health* 9: 1–12 (2008).
2. Herodotus, *Histories, Volume IV. New English Version edited with notes by George Rawlinson*, D. Appleton and Co, New York (1859/1860).

3. Dioscorides, P., *De Materia Medica, Translated by Beck, L. Y. Third, revised edition*, Olms-Weidmann (2017).

4. Stern, P., *Medical advice to the consumptive and asthmatic people of England: wherein the present method of treating disorders of the lungs is shewn to be futile and fundamentally wrong, and a new method of cure proposed*, Printed for J. Almon (1767).

5. Jackson, M., "Divine Stramonium"; The Rise and Fall of Smoking for Asthma, *Medical History* 54: 171–194 (2010).

6. Elliott, H.L. & Reid, J.L., The Clinical Pharmacology of a Herbal Asthma Cigarette, *Br J Clin Pharmacol* 10: 487–490 (1980).

7. Bisgard, H. et al. ed., *Drug Delivery to the Lung*, Marcel Dekker (2002).

8. Adams, J., On an Improved Apparatus for Spray Inhalations, *Glasgow Medical Journal* 182–197 (1868).

9. Doig, R.L. Epinephrin: Especially in Asthma, *California State Journal of Medicine* III(2): 54–55 (1905).

10. Nikander, K. & Sanders, M., The early evolution of nebulizers, *Medicamundi* 54(3): 47–53 (2010).

11. Stein, S.W. & Thiel, C.G., The History of Therapeutic Aerosols: A Chronological Review, *Journal of Aerosol Medicine and Pulmonary Drug Delivery* 30(1): 20–41 (2017).

12. Stein, S.W., Advances in Metered Dose Inhaler Technology: Hardware Development, *AAPS PharmSciTech* 15(2): 326–338 (2014).

13. Self-propelling compositions for inhalation therapy containing a salt of isoproterenol or epinephrine. *US Patent 2868691 A* (1956).

14. Anderson, P.J., History of Aerosol Therapy: Liquid Nebulization to MDI to DPIs, *Respiratory Care* 50(9): 1139–1150 (2005).

15. De Boer, A.H. et al., Dry powder inhalation: past, present and future, *Expert Opinion on Drug Delivery* 14(4): 499–512 (2017).

Chapter 16: Medicines for the Eye

1. Herodotus, *The Histories. New Translation by Waterfield, R*, Oxford University Press (1998).

2. Andersen, S.R, History of Ophthalmology. The eye and its diseases in Ancient Egypt, *Acta Ophthalmologica Scandinavica* 75: 338–344 (1997).

3. Dioscorides P., *De Materia Medica. Translated by Beck, LY. Third, revised edition*, Olms-Weidmann (2017).

4. Nielsen, H., *Ancient Ophthalmological Agents*, Odense University Press (1974).

5. Pérez-Cambrodi, R.J. et al., Collyria Seals in the Roman Empire, *Acta med-hist Adriat* 11(1): 89–100 (2013).

6. Harrison, F. et al, A 1,000-Year Old Antimicrobial Remedy with Antistaphylococcal Activity, *Mbio* 6(4): e01129–15 (2015).

7. Nejabat, M. et al., Avicenna and Cataracts: A New Analysis of Contributions to Diagnosis and Treatment from the Canon, *Iran Red Crescent Med J* 14(5): 265–270 (2012).

8. Smith, E.S., Drug Therapy in Trachoma and its sequelae as presented by Ibn al-Nafis, *Pharmacy in History* 14(3): 95–110 (1972).

9. Packer, M. and Brandt, J.D., Ophthalmology's Botanical Heritage, *Survey of Ophthalmology* 36(5): 357–365 (1992).

10. Snyder, C., *Our Ophthalmic Heritage*, Little, Brown and Company, Boston (1967).

11. Collins, E.T., *The History and Traditions of the Moorfields Eye Hospital. One Hundred Years of Ophthalmic Discovery and Development*, H.K. Lewis and Co. (1929).

12. Martindale, W., *The Extra Pharmacopoeia*, H.K. Lewis (1883).

13. Gibson, M., *Ophthalmic Dosage Forms. Second Edition. Volume 199 of Drugs and the Pharmaceutical Sciences.* Informa (2009).
14. Kumari, A. et al., Ocular inserts – Advancement in therapy of eye diseases, *Journal of Advanced Pharmaceutical Technology & Research* 1(3): 291–295 (2010).
15. Bertens, C.J.F. et al., Topical drug delivery devices: A review, *Experimental Eye Research* 168: 149–160 (2018).
16. Mitchell, P. et al., Ranibizumab (Lucentis) in neovascular age-related macular degeneration: evidence from clinical trials, *British Journal of Ophthalmology* 94(1): 2–13 (2010).

Chapter 17: Medicines *via* the Vagina and Rectum

1. Sterling, S., Mortality Profiles as Indicators of Slowed Reproduction Rates. Evidence from Ancient Egypt, *Journal of Anthropological Archaeology* 16: 319–343 (1999).
2. Ghalioungui, P., *The Ebers Papyrus. A New English Translation, Commentaries and Glossaries*, Academy of Scientific Research and Technology, Cairo (1987).
3. Totelin, L.M.V., *Hippocratic Recipes. Oral and Written Transmission of Pharmacological Knowledge in Fifth- and Fourth-Century Greece*, Brill, Leiden (2009).
4. Hippocrates *English translation by W.H.S. Jones*, William Heinemann, London (1923–1931).
5. Dioscorides, P., *De Materia Medica. Translated by Beck, L. Third, revised edition*, Olms-Weidmann (2017).
6. Green, M.H., *The Trotula: a medieval compendium of women's medicine. Edited and translated by Green, M.H.* University of Pennsylvania Press (2001).
7. Sansom, W., *Pharmacopoeia Londinensis, or the new London Dispensatory in six books. Translated into English by William Sansom*, Printed by J. Dawks (1716).
8. Watson, M.C. et al., Oral versus intra-vaginal imidazole and triazole anti-fungal agents for the treatment of uncomplicated vulvovaginal candidiasis (thrush): a systematic review, *British Journal of Obstetrics and Gynaecology* 109: 85–95 (2002).
9. Moses, M., *Lost in the Museum. Buried Treasures and the Stories they tell. Chapter 4: Pessaries*, Altamira Press (2008).
10. Margulies, L., History of intrauterine devices, *Bull N.Y. Academy Medicine* 51(5): 662–667 (1974).
11. Dioscorides, P., *De Materia Medica. Translated by Beck, L. Third, revised edition*, Olms-Weidmann (2017).
12. Allen, L.V. ed., *Chapter 2: History and development of the suppository, Dennis Worthen in Suppositories*, Pharmaceutical Press (2008).
13. Griffenhagen, G., Tools of the Apothecary. 4. Suppository Molds, *J. Amer. Pharm. Assoc Pract Pharm Ed* 17(6): 402–403 (1956).
14. Arderne, J., *Treatises of Fistula in Ano, Haemorrhoids and Clysters. An Early Fifteenth Century Manuscript Translation. Edited by D'Arcy Power*, Kegan, Paul, Trench, Trübner and Co Ltd (1910).
15. Doyle, D., Per rectum: a history of enemata, *J Royal College of Physicians of Edinburgh* 35: 367–370 (2005).
16. Monardes, N., *Joyfull newes out of the new-founde worlde. Wherein are declared, the rare and singular vertues of divers herbs, trees, plants, oyles and stones, with their applications, as well as to the use of phisicke. Translated by Frampton, J.*, Printed by E. Allde (1596).
17. Lawrence, G., Tobacco smoke enemas. *Lancet* 359(9315): 1442 (2002).
18. Kellogg, J.H., *Rational Hydrotherapy, a treatise on the physiological and therapeutic effects of hydriatic procedures*, International Tract Society (1900).

19. Russell, W.K., *Colonic irrigation*, E & S Livingstone (1932).
20. Knudsen, F.U., Rectal administration of diazepam in solution in the acute treatment of convulsions in children, *Archives of Disease in Childhood* 54: 855–857 (1979).

Chapter 18: Medicines for Other Routes of Administration
1. Tsoucalas, G. and Sgantzos, M., Hippocrates (ca 460–370 BC) on nasal cancer, *JBUOM* 21(4): 1031–1034 (2016).
2. Pedanius Dioscorides of Anazarbus, *De Materia Medica. Translated by Lily Y. Beck, Third, revised edition*, Olms-Weidmann (2017).
3. Shehata, M. *Ear, Nose and Throat Medical Practice in Muslim Heritage.* Available from http://muslimheritage.com/article/ear-nose-and-throat-medical-practice-muslim-heritage [accessed 26 March 2019].
4. John Johnson Kyle, *Manual of Diseases of the Ear, Nose and Throat. Second Edition*, Sidney Appleton, pp 169–174 (1908).
5. *The Extra Pharmacopoeia Martindale, Volume I, Twenty-fourth Edition*, London, The Pharmaceutical Press (1958).
6. Illum, L., Nasal drug delivery: new developments and strategies, *Drug Discovery Today* 7(23): 1184–1189 (2002).
7. Ghalioungui, P., *The Ebers Papyrus. A New English Translation, Commentaries and Glossaries*, Academy of Scientific Research and Technology, Cairo (1987).
8. Rousseau, N. and Mudry, A., Auricular Clyster, Otenchytes, and Pyoulcos: Precursors of the Ear Syringe, *Oncology and Neurology* 39: 506–512 (2018).
9. Cameron, M.L., *Anglo-Saxon Medicine*, Cambridge University Press (1993).
10. Berenbaum, M., Lend me your earwigs, *American Entomologist* 53(4): 196–197 (2007).
11. Kroukamp, G. and Londt, G.H., Ear-invading arthropods: A South African survey, *SAMJ* 96(4): 290–291 (2006).
12. Yaroko, A.A. and Irfan, M., An annual audit of the ear foreign bodies in Hospital Universiti Sains Malaysia, *Malays Fam Physician* 7(1): 2–5 (2012).
13. Bhargava, D. and Victor, R., Carabid beetle invasion of the ear in Oman, *Wilderness and Environmental Medicine* 10: 157–160) (1999).
14. Ghalioungui, P., *The Ebers Papyrus. A New English Translation, Commentaries and Glossaries*, Academy of Scientific Research and Technology, Cairo (1987).
15. *A Corn. Celsus of Medicine in Eight Books. Translated with Notes Critical and Explanatory by James Grieve*, Edinburgh University Press (1814).
16. Chaudhri, S.K. and Jain, N.K., History of cosmetics, *Asian Journal of Pharmaceutics* July-September 164–167 (2009).
17. Pedanius Dioscorides of Anazarbus, *De Materia Medica. Translated by Lily Y. Beck. Third, revised edition*, Olms-Weidmann (2017).
18. Clausen, H. et al., *Hair Preparations. Ullmann's Encyclopaedia of Industrial Chemistry*, Wiley-VCH Verlag GmbH & Co (2011).
19. Pedanius Dioscorides of Anazarbus, *De Materia Medica. Translated by Lily Y. Beck, Third, revised edition*, Olms-Weidmann (2017).
20. *Royal London Hospital Archive RLHBH/PH/2/2* Indexed Registry for University College Hospital Dispensary (1941).
21. Homan, P.G., Baldness: A brief history of treatments from antiquity to the present, *Pharmaceutical Historian* 49(1): 24–31 (2019).
22. Ghalioungui, P., *The Ebers Papyrus. A New English Translation, Commentaries and Glossaries*, Academy of Scientific Research and Technology, Cairo (1987).

23. Murdan, S., Nail disorders in older people, and aspects of their pharmaceutical treatment, *International Journal of Pharmaceutics* 512(2): 405–411 (2016).

24. Sigurgeirson, B., The History of Onychomycosis. *In Onychomycosis Diagnosis and Effective Management. Edited by Rigopoulos, D et al.* Wiley-Blackwell (2018).

25. Williams, D.L., The Whitfield Tradition of Therapy, *British Medical Journal* Aug 20 2(4937): 453–455 (1955).

26. Yau, M. et al., How to treat fungal nail effectively, *Pharm. J.* 20 November (2018).

27. Hoffmann-Axthelm translated by Koehler, H.M., *History of Dentistry*, Quintessence Publishing Co. Inc. (1981).

28. Ghalioungui, P., *The Ebers Papyrus. A New English Translation, Commentaries and Glossaries*, Academy of Scientific Research and Technology, Cairo (1987).

29. Pedanius Dioscorides of Anazarbus, *De Materia Medica. Translated by Lily Y. Beck. Third revised edition*, Olms-Weidmann (2017).

30. Culpeper, N., *Pharmacopoeia Londinensis, or the London Dispensatorium*, Peter Cole (1653).

31. Jardim, J. J. et al., The history and global market of oral home-care products, *Braz. Oral Res.* 23(1): 17–22 (2009).

32. Lippert, F., *An Introduction to Toothpaste – its Purpose, History and Ingredients. Monographs in Oral Science* S. Karger AG 23: 1–14 (2013).

33. Crichton-Browne, J., An Address on Tooth Culture. *Lancet* 2: 6–10 (1892).

Index